Advance Praise for

"An ambitious goal, accomplished. This thoughtfully organized, highly educational case study manual successfully teaches while entertaining ... a rare achievement.

Bouncebacks begins each chapter with a real patient case as it actually presented. The reader is given all information that is obtained. Then we are left to consider if and how we might have approached the patient differently... anticipating an outcome (*Bouncebacks*) that will necessitate additional care.

We are next engaged by the always delightfully entertaining and insightful Greg Henry. He, without foreknowledge, predicts what might go wrong, while scoring the patient management and case risk. Dr. Henry occasionally exhorts us with Shakespeare, while at other times, just 'down-home' good sense.

The course of each patient's illness is provided, sometimes with a relatively benign outcome, other times with a devastating result. Always, we the readers are able to say, 'Yes, this could have been considered and dealt with more effectively.'

Just when our appetite to know more is whetted, we are sated with the case discussion. The final section of each case contains a consistently organized discussion of each diagnosis. Accomplished guest reviewers treat us with the presentation, management, the teaching points and a germane list of references.

Let us learn from the mistakes of others. *Bouncebacks* can be used effectively by all students of emergency medicine, beginners and veterans alike. At my hospital, we have begun using it, a case at a time, for regular educational in-services to members of our ED team, as well as discussions for our department meetings. This is a book that will be dog-eared."

Robert Strauss Jr., MD, FACEP
Associate Chairman of the department of emergency medicine
Saint Francis Hospital, Poughkeepsie, N.Y.
ACEP Award for Outstanding Contribution in Education, 1999
Co-author, *Emergency Department Management: Principles and Applications*

"Case based teaching can be very effective—particularly when the cases are ones where something went wrong! The cases in this book range from the obvious to the subtle to the extraordinarily unusual just like they do in real life. Many of them bring up important topics that we all need to think about. While the teaching value of the topic discussions, written by multiple authors, is not surprisingly a bit varied, a very welcome (and delightful) constant is the thoughtful, informed and literate commentaries (on all the cases) by the inimitable Greg Henry."

Jerry Hoffman, MD, FACEP
Professor of Medicine and Emergency Medicine, UCLA
Associate Editor, *Emergency Medical Abstracts*
ACEP award for outstanding contribution in education, 1996
AAEM Peter Rosen award, 2003

"Learn from the mistakes of others in this lively and gripping set of emergency medicine cases gone awry. Greg Henry's legendary razor-sharp insight is in top form."

Steven M. Green, MD, FACEP
Professor of Emergency Medicine & Pediatrics
Loma Linda University Medical Center & Children's Hospital

"In my view, there are three main factors to assure excellence in emergency medicine—qualified physicians working in fair practice environments and committed to lifelong education.The authors have done a remarkable job assisting us with the later by organizing a wealth of didactic information in a manner that makes logical sense to practicing emergency physicians. They elegantly demonstrate how to really close-the-loop on proper management and supportive documentation so that patient safety is optimized. Congratulations on a job well done!"

Tom Scaletta, MD FAAEM
Assistant Professor, Department of Emergency Medicine, Rush Medical College
President, American Academy of Emergency Medicine (AAEM)
Author, *Emergent Management of Trauma* and *Bioterrorism On Hand*
Editor of *Rules of the Road for Emergency Medicine Residents and Graduates*

"Innovative approach to a common hi-risk encounter in the ED, with pithy perceptive comments from the incomparable Dr. Henry, and analysis with recommendations from seasoned respected emergency physicians—this book is a valuable tool to improve patient care and reduce litigation for all emergency care providers."

Robert A. Bitterman, MD JD FACEP
Vice-Chairman, Board of Governors, Emergency Physician Insurance Co., Auburn, CA
President, Bitterman Healthlaw Consulting Group, Inc., Charlotte, NC.
Member, ACEP Medical-Legal Committee
Chairman, ACEP EMTALA Task Force
Editorial boards, *Managed Care Emergency Department* and the *Emergency Department Legal Letter*
Author, *EMTALA: Providing Emergency Care Under Federal Law*

"*Bouncebacks! Emergency Department Cases: ED Returns*—an exception to the rule that medical books are boring. This book is an entertaining and informative page-turner—easy reading that informs. The cases are interesting cases that most of us can relate to from our own practices. The commentaries by Dr. Henry are entertaining and informative, as usual! The experts' reviews are well-written and informative. A great read!"

Catherine A. Marco, MD, FACEP
Clinical Professor, Department of Surgery, Medical University of Ohio, Toledo, Ohio
Attending Physician, St. Vincent Mercy Medical Center
President elect, Ohio chapter American College of Emergency Physicians (ACEP)
Board of Directors, Society for Academic Emergency Medicine (SAEM)
Associate editor, *Academic Emergency Medicine* (journal)

"*Bouncebacks!* reaffirms the fact that a medical text need not be dull to deeply inform the reader. Its format allows us the pleasure of reaching our own conclusions before learning the outcome. The learning ante is raised even higher because we also get to measure our thinking against that of Dr. Greg Henry, who makes witty and brilliant comments on each case before knowing the ultimate outcome himself. Each situation is then capped by an in-depth, topic-based discussion written by emergency physicians clearly chosen as much for their writing skills as their academic reputations and expertise. I love this book and copies will be given to each member of my group. Bravo to *Boucebacks!* Let other specialties envy and emulate."

Frank J. Edwards, MD, FACEP
Assistant Professor of Medical Humanities, University of Rochester, NY
Author, *M&M files: Morbidity and Mortality Rounds in Emergency Medicine*
President, Delphi Emergency Physicians, LLC

"Dr. Weinstock and Dr. Longstreth hit a homerun! Read these cases! Greg Henry is right on point as only he can be. The cases presented scream with pathology. Reaffirms 'salute the red flags.' Let's learn from our colleagues and keep the lawyers at bay..."

Alan R. Grillo MD
Medical Director Emergency Department Spectrum Health Reed City Campus
Reed City, Michigan

"*Bouncebacks* is an exceptional book and is a must read for all emergency care providers. Greg Henry's comments are priceless and really help in remembering the pearls of each case. The case discussions are very thorough and up-to-date, yet concise and easy to read. I would love to see more cases and look forward to the next edition!"

Ghazala Q. Sharieff, MD, FACEP, FAAEM, FAAP
Associate Clinical Professor, Children's Hospital and Health Center/University of California, San Diego
Director of Pediatric Emergency Medicine, Palomar-Pomerado Hospital/California Emergency Physicians, San Diego, CA.
American Academy Emergency Medicine (AAEM) Young Educator of the Year, 2003
Member, ACEP Pediatric Emergency Medicine Committee
Editorial Board, *Journal of Emergency Medicine*

"*Bouncebacks* is a collection of interesting cases and even more interesting discussion. What is unique about this is that the cases range from the obvious to ones in which it would be highly unlikely that any emergency physician would make the diagnosis on first presentation. As anyone who reviews these cases, does quality assurance or participates in morbidity mortality conferences knows, it's frequently the basics of emergency medicine that need adherence. The authors and commentators clearly present actions that are important in the workup, documentation, and follow-up of patients. Even more interesting is the sometimes subtle and sometimes not so subtle differences among the discussants. It highlights the disagreements that honest expert witnesses can have looking at the same set of facts. The reader will appreciate the clarity of the writing here and the diverse of ways in which common complaints can sometimes evolve into complex problems. This book is appropriate reading for all emergency physicians from residents to experienced clinicians."

Charles Emerman, MD
Chairman, Department of Emergency Medicine, The Cleveland Clinic
Professor and Chairman, Department of Emergency Medicine, Case Western Reserve University
ACEP award for outstanding contribution in research, 1998

"Overall it's a fun and easy read, with many cases that are fairly certain to make their way into residency M&M's and real life practice. ... We will be looking at this in our Education committee for possible opportunities to incorporate into our EMR1 curriculum."

Carey Chisholm, MD, FACEP
Director, IU-Methodist Emergency Medicine Residency Program
Clinical Professor of Emergency Medicine
Associate editor, Academic Emergency Medicine editorial board
Immediate Past president, Society for Academic Emergency Medicine (SAEM)

"The unique format and real-life presentations in Bouncebacks! Emergency Department Cases: ED Returns make it a pleasure to read, and outstandingly educational. Readers learn best when they can identify with a specific case or set of facts, and picture themselves 'on the line.' The format of including discussion along the way, and after the fact keeps your interest, and the more academic discussion that follows has the perfect setting- the actual case at hand. The academic discussions are concise and up to date. A great read for all Emergency and primary care physicians!"

Neal Little, MD, FACEP
Clinical instructor, University of Michigan Medical School
Co-author, "Neurologic Emergencies: A Symptom-Oriented Approach, 2nd ed."
Co-presenter, Medical practice risk assessment: Continuing medical education for Emergency Physicians

"*Bouncebacks! Emergency Department Cases: ED Returns* by Drs. Weinstock and Longstreth is a text unique to Emergency Medicine that reviews ED cases. A verbatim case presentation is followed by an exciting and comprehensive analysis of the medical aspects of the case emphasizing practical teaching points. The case is also associated with a brief medicolegal assessment of what went wrong or could have gone wrong with the case. The cases are very representative and relevant to all practicing emergency physicians and the unique format makes for easy and enjoyable reading. Compared to standard texts this is a breath of fresh air that is recommended to emergency physicians at both the resident and attending levels."

Adam J. Singer, MD, FACEP
Professor and Vice Chairman for Research, Department of Emergency Medicine, Stony Brook University and Medical Center
Associate Editor, Journal of Academic Emergency Medicine
Member, Scientific Review Committee, ACEP
Program Committee, SAEM
Author, *Emergency Medicine Pearls and Lacerations and Acute Wounds: An Evidence-Based Guide*

"I just completed reading the book. Outstanding idea, structure, easy to read, and most valuable discussion for every chapter on very important topics and challenging or common diagnosis. I also got to see outstanding management strategies described by many specialty leaders, colleagues and friends.

I had a hard time putting the book down, once I started reading the first 2-3 cases. Within 4 hours, I had already gone through 20 of the 30 cases. I simply enjoyed reading it and experiencing what was being reported as if these were my cases in the ED.

Thank you Mike and Ryan for a great book and product. This will be of great use to so many of our emergency physicians in the trenches of our ED."

Antoine Kazzi, MD, FAAEM
Associate Professor of Clinical Medicine, University of California, Irvine
Chief of Service & Medical Director, Emergency Medicine, The American University of Beirut, Lebanon
Immediate Past President, American Academy of Emergency Medicine (AAEM)
Chief editor, *AAEM's Rules of the road for Medical Students*

(For more comments please see last page)

Bouncebacks!

Emergency Department Cases: ED Returns

Michael B. Weinstock, MD
Ryan Longstreth, MD, FACEP

Case by Case Commentary by:

Gregory L. Henry, MD, FACEP

Illustrations by:

Hudson Meredith

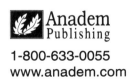
Anadem
Publishing

1-800-633-0055
www.anadem.com

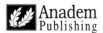
Anadem
Publishing

3620 North High Street
Columbus, OH   43214
Tel: 1 (800) 633-0055
www.anadem.com

Bouncebacks!
Emergency Department Cases: ED Returns

Michael B. Weinstock
Ryan Longstreth
Commentary by Gregory L. Henry

Illustrations by Hudson Meredith

Bouncebacks! is based upon information from sources believed to be reliable. In developing this book the publisher, authors, contributors, reviewers, and editors have made substantial efforts to make sure that the regimens, drugs, and treatments are correct and are in accordance with currently accepted standards. Readers are cautioned to use their own judgment in making clinical decisions and, when appropriate, consult and compare information from other resources since ongoing research and clinical experience yield new information and since there is the possibility of human error in developing such a comprehensive resource as this. Attention should be paid to checking the product information supplied by drug manufacturers when prescribing or administering drugs, particularly if the prescriber is not familiar with the drug or does not regularly use it.

Readers should be aware that there are legitimate differences of opinion among physicians on both clinical and ethical/moral issues in treating patients. With this in mind, readers are urged to use individual judgment in making treatment decisions, recognizing the best interests of the patient and his/her own knowledge and understanding of these issues. The material in Bouncebacks! is not intended to substitute for the advice of a qualified attorney or other professional. You should consult a qualified professional for advice about your specific situation. Readers are cautioned to use their own judgment in making decisions on the issues covered in this book because there are on-going changes in these matters. The publisher, authors, reviewers, contributors, and editors disclaim any liability, loss or damage as a result, directly or indirectly, from using or applying any of the contents of Bouncebacks!

Second printing 2007

PRINTED IN THE UNITED STATES OF AMERICA

ISBN 1-890018-61-9

Initially inspired by the morbidity and mortality conferences at Mt. Carmel-St. Ann's Emergency Department, this book has been several years in the making; we hope to capture the excitement and suspense of those conferences in the format of this book. We think that you will be captivated, perhaps a bit frightened, and at times enlightened. This book is unique as these are all real patients—the ED record you are about to read is the actual documentation recorded on the chart by the physician and staff. The chart includes typos, strange abbreviations and, at times, glaring omissions. This is the time for *you* to be the "Monday morning quarterback"… or the defense attorney—whichever role seems most comfortable!

We have compiled 30 cases of patients who presented to the ED, most of whom were subsequently sent home, and then "bounced back" to receive a different diagnosis. A few arrested shortly after returning to the ED, some were again discharged (one patient had 6 ED visits), and most were admitted. The patients all presented with common problems such as headache, fever, abdominal pain, back pain, and chest pain, complaints which could have occurred in any ED, urgent care or primary care physician's office. In fact, almost half of our patients *did* see their primary care physician before their final ED visit!

Our primary goal is to improve patient safety. Although these patients were not entirely mismanaged, often important "red flags" are not recognized. Additional goals include continuing education in documentation, risk management, and discussion on evaluation and management of common ED complaints and diagnoses.

Each chapter begins with documentation of the initial patient visit. Then Gregory Henry, the past president of the American College of Emergency Physicians (ACEP) and CEO of Medical Practice Risk Assessment, Inc. (Ann Arbor, MI), comments on the physician's evaluation and documentation from both a medical and risk management perspective. He makes his comments while "blinded" to the eventual ED diagnosis. His comments are insightful, humorous, and memorable. Next, we present the final ED visit, diagnosis, and hospital/surgical course. Finally, national experts provide a referenced discussion of the appropriate ED approach to the presenting complaint and final diagnosis of each patient, referring to the case presented.

Each case has an accompanying illustration, intended to capture the "teaching points," without giving away the final diagnosis. Most have a time displayed (clock on the wall/wristwatch), which corresponds to the sentinel event which occurred in the case.

We close with a tongue-in-cheek discussion of medical malpractice issues, entitled; "So you want to be sued for malpractice; the top 10 ways to *maximize* your risk," written by several leading defense attorneys.

We hope you enjoy reading as much as we have enjoyed writing. So let the action begin—"Remember that patient you saw last night…"

Michael Weinstock, MD   mweinstock@ihainc.org
Ryan Longstreth, MD, FACEP   rlongstreth@ihainc.org
May 1, 2006

Michael B. Weinstock, MD

Michael and Beth Weinstock and their three children, Olivia (7), Eli (5) and Theo (1), live in Columbus, Ohio. Michael is an ED Attending and the Director of Medical Education in the Emergency Department at Mt. Carmel St. Ann's. He also works part time in the HIV/AIDS clinic at Ohio State University as a Clinical Assistant Professor in the Division of Infectious Diseases. He has authored *The Resident's Guide to Ambulatory Care*, a 500 page handbook of management strategies for common ambulatory conditions which is now in its 5th edition. He has practiced volunteer medicine in Papua New Guinea, Nepal, and the West Indies and is an avid traveler, skier, and blues guitar and harmonica player.

Ryan Longstreth, MD, FACEP

Ryan and his wife Amy live in Galena, Ohio with their two young children, Max and Drew. Ryan completed his EM residency at William Beaumont Hospital in Royal Oak, Michigan and now works as an ED attending at Mt. Carmel St. Ann's Hospital in Westerville, Ohio. He is the Assistant Director of the ED and the Director of the Observation Unit. In his spare time, he enjoys spending time with his family, golf, baseball, and red wine.

Gregory L. Henry, MD, FACEP

Gregory L. Henry is a Clinical Professor in the Department of Emergency Medicine at University of Michigan Medical Center. He was the President of the American College of Emergency Physicians (ACEP) from 1995–1996 and is currently the President and CEO of Medical Practice Risk Assessment, Inc. and President of Savannah Assurance Limited, LTD. He is on the editorial boards of *Emergency Medicine Practice*, *Emergency Department Management*, and *Foresight* and recently of the *Emergency Department Legal Letter*. He is the recipient of numerous awards including the "Over the top" lecturer award and the "Outstanding speaker of the Year" award from ACEP. He is the author of *Neurologic Emergencies: A Symptom-Oriented Approach, 2nd ed*. He currently staffs the Emergency Department at St. Joseph Mercy Hospital in Ann Arbor, Michigan, and Saline Hospital in Saline, Michigan.

FOREWORD

Homer's *Odyssey* is based on the Greek concept of "Xenia;" the guest-host relationship that dominated the ancient world—it was expected that people of breeding would offer food, shelter, and conversation to all travel weary individuals. Xenia is poorly understood today—except in our emergency departments.

No matter how reprehensible the person or implausible the story, everyone is a welcome guest at the local emergency department. If your momma doesn't love you and the police don't want you, the welcome mat is always out at the ED!! The emergency physician functions while suffering insults from intoxicated patients, while trying to solve (unsolvable) social problems, and within the framework of a plethora of paper work and healthcare regulations. Picking apart a perplexing case is rarely a problem when patients present one at a time, as during grand rounds, but this is infrequent in real life.

This book is an attempt to raise the emergency physician's index of suspicion on cases which turned into both medical and medico-legal nightmares. In a busy emergency department, events occur rapidly; the patient's personality and ability to coherently tell a story often determine the quality of their health care.

 The smart doctor is not one who learns from his own mistakes, but from the mistakes of others. Here's hoping that this book is read by a lot of smart doctors.

Gregory L. Henry, MD, FACEP
CEO, Medical Practice Risk Assessment, Inc., Ann Arbor, Michigan (www.mp-ra.com)
Clinical Professor, Department of Emergency Medicine
  University of Michigan Medical School, Ann Arbor, Michigan
Past President, American College of Emergency Physicians (ACEP)

TABLE OF CONTENTS & CONTRIBUTORS

Michael B. Weinstock, MD
Clinical Assistant Professor, Division of Emergency Medicine
  The Ohio State University, College of Medicine, Columbus, Ohio
Attending ED physician, Director of Medical Education
  Mt. Carmel St. Ann's Emergency Department, Westerville, Ohio

Ryan Longstreth, MD, FACEP
Attending ED Physician
  Mt. Carmel St. Ann's Emergency Department, Westerville, Ohio
Assistant ED Director, St. Ann's Emergency Department

Case by Case Commentary
Gregory L. Henry, MD, FACEP
CEO, Medical Practice Risk Assessment, Inc., Ann Arbor, Michigan
Clinical Professor, Department of Emergency Medicine
  University of Michigan Medical School, Ann Arbor, Michigan
Past President, American College of Emergency Physicians (ACEP)

Wesley P. Eilbert, MD, FACEP
Clinical Associate Professor and Resident Research Director
  Department of Emergency Medicine, University of Illinois College of Medicine
Director of Undergraduate Education, Department of Emergency Medicine
  Mercy Hospital and Medical Center, Chicago, Illinois

Scott W. Melanson, MD, FACEP
Associate Program Director, Emergency Medicine Residency
Chair, Disaster Committee, St. Luke's Hospital, Bethlehem, Pennsylvania
Clinical Associate Professor, Temple University, Philadelphia, Pennsylvania

M. Jacob Ott, MD
Ohio Chapter, American College of Emergency Physicians
  Ultrasound Instructor
Attending ED physician & ED Ultrasound Director
  Mt. Carmel St. Ann's Emergency Department, Westerville, Ohio

Andy Jagoda, MD, FACEP
Professor and Vice Chair
  Department of Emergency Medicine
  Mount Sinai School of Medicine, New York, New York
Chair, ACEP Clinical Policies Committee
Chair, ACEP Clinical Policy Subcommittee on Acute Headache
Editor-in-Chief, Emergency Medicine Practice

John Bruns, Jr., MD
Assistant Professor
  Department of Emergency Medicine
  Mount Sinai School of Medicine, New York, New York

Ann Dietrich, MD, FAAP, FACEP
Attending, ED physician, Columbus Children's Hospital
Associate Professor, The Ohio State University College of Medicine, Columbus, Ohio
Editor-in-chief, Pediatric Emergency Medicine Reports
Editor-in-chief, Trauma Reports
ACEP, Pediatric Emergency Medicine Committee

Stephen A. Colucciello, MD, FACEP
Associate Chair, Department of Emergency Medicine
  Carolinas Medical Center, Charlotte, North Carolina
Adjunct Professor, Department of Emergency Medicine
  University of North Carolina at Chapel Hill, Chapel Hill, North Carolina
Former Member, ACEP Clinical Policies Committee
Former Member, ACEP Clinical Policies Subcommittee on Abdominal Pain
Chair (1998-2000), ACEP Clinical Policies Subcommittee on Syncope

Amal Mattu, MD, FAAEM, FACEP
Associate Professor and Residency Director
  Emergency Medicine Residency Program
  University of Maryland School of Medicine, Baltimore, Maryland
Author, *ECG's for the Emergency Physician*
Consulting Editor, Emergency Medicine Clinics of North America
Section Editor for Best Practices in Emergency Medicine, Journal of Emergency Medicine
American Academy of Emergency Medicine (AAEM) Young Educator of the Year, 2002

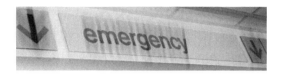

A TWO STEP APPROACH TO AVOID "BOUNCEBACKS"

Commentary:
Michael B. Weinstock, MD

Clinical Assistant Professor, Division of Emergency Medicine
  The Ohio State University, College of Medicine
  Columbus, Ohio
Attending ED physician, Director of Medical Education
  Mt. Carmel St. Ann's Emergency Department
  Westerville, Ohio

Ryan Longstreth, MD, FACEP

Attending ED Physician
  Mt. Carmel St. Ann's Emergency Department, Westerville, Ohio
Assistant ED Director, St. Ann's Emergency Department

BOUNCE BACK STUDIES

Each year there are approximately 115 million visits to emergency departments in the United States. Approximately 3% of these patients will "bounce back" within 72 hours (3.3 million occurrences per year)[1-4] and 0.6% will "bounce back" and require admission (660,000 occurrences per year).[1,5] Of the patients who return, 18–30% return due to a possible medical error made during the initial visit (600,000 to 1 million occurrences per year).[2,7,8] Not all bouncebacks are related to medical errors; for example, we may ask a patient with an abscess to return for packing removal, a patient with ureterolithiasis may return for intractable pain, or a patient may return for unrelated problems.

DEATH WITHIN 7–8 DAYS OF ED DISCHARGE—TWO STUDIES

In 1994, Kefer, et al., performed a retrospective chart review of 2,665 medical examiner (ME) cases in Milwaukee County and found 42 deceased patients who had been evaluated and released from an ED within 8 days of their death. They found that 21% (9) of these deaths were unexpected and directly related to the initial ED evaluation. The patients' ages ranged from 9 months to 91 years, and the most common cause of death was ruptured aortic abdominal aneurysm (3 of the 9 patients). Other chief complaints and causes of death included a 26 year old initially diagnosed with pneumonia who died from a pulmonary embolus, a 76 year old initially diagnosed with nasal contusion who died from a traumatic brain injury, and a 45 year old initially diagnosed with cough and chest pain who died from pneumonia.[6] It should be noted that the total number of deaths is likely underestimated since the data does not include bounceback admissions which eventually resulted in death, deaths presenting to a different hospital or different ME, and deaths without a definitive link to initial ED visit. Finally, this data does not include patients with poor outcomes—only those who died.

In May 2007, Sklar, et al., performed a retrospective cohort of ED patients who were discharged to home from the University of New Mexico Health Sciences Center, an urban tertiary-care facility. The geographic location makes this study unique since the Health Sciences Center is New Mexico's only medical school and only Level I trauma center, making it more likely that all unanticipated deaths were captured. The main outcome was death within 7 days of ED discharge. A 10 year data review identified 117 patients, equating to a death rate of 30/100,000 patients discharged from the ED. Subjects were aged 10 years and older, representing 387,334 ED visits. Of the 117 patients, 50% (58 total patients) died of complications related to the initial visit. Sixty percent of these 58 patients died due to a possible medical error (35 of the total 117 patients).[7] Extrapolated, this equates to over 10,000 potentially avoidable deaths per year in the US in patients discharged from our emergency departments.

A closer look at the 117 patients found that:

- 17 (15%) of the deaths were expected (i.e., terminal cancer, etc.)
- 58 (50%) died from a condition related to the initial visit and the death was unexpected
- 35 of the total (60% of the 58 unexpected deaths) were due to a possible medical error
- Frequent initial complaints included CNS symptoms (seizure, HA, dizziness), abdominal pain, chest pain, shortness of breath, or weakness

Common characteristics of the possible medical error cases include:

1. Atypical presentation of unusual problem.
2. Chronic disease with decompensation (e.g., CHF).
3. Abnormal vital signs. Note: tachycardia occurred in 25 out of 35 (71%) of "possible error" cases.
4. Mental disability, psychiatric problem, or substance abuse make it less likely patient will return for worsening problems.

BRINGING IT HOME (TO YOUR HOME!)

Three percent of patients will bounce back within 3 days, 0.6% will bounce back and be admitted, 30/100,000 will die within 7 days of ED discharge, and 9/100,000 will die within 7 days of ED discharge secondary to a possible medical error. In 2005 (115 million ED visits), we can estimate that 34,500 patients died within 7 days of their initial ED visit, including 10,350 unexpected deaths related to the initial ED visit in which a possible medical error occurred.

If you work 30 hours per week and see 3 patients per hour, you will see about 4,500 patients per year. 135 of these patients will bounce back each year, which is nearly one patient per shift; 24 to 40 of the 135 patients will bounce back because of a possible medical error. If your career spans 30 years, you will see a total of 135,000 patients. *During the course of your career, you will send home 17 patients who will die within 7 days of ED discharge, due to a possible medical error.*

HOW CAN WE USE THIS INFORMATION TO IMPROVE PATIENT SAFETY?

In his 2004 study, *Risk factors for 72-hour admission to the ED*, Martin-Gill states that "by identifying high risk patients prospectively, physicians will be better able to make informed decisions when considering the depth of evaluation, timing of d/c decisions, and extent of follow up care."[5] In his 2007 study, *Unanticipated Death After Discharge Home From the Emergency Department*, Sklar states that "These data may inform efforts to decrease medical errors and identify high-risk patients, such as developing better methods for assessing the significance of abnormal vital signs."

Just as many parents will take a "second look" both ways before taking their children across a busy street, we propose a similar "extra check" when discharging patients with a potential for a poor outcome. Our approach is a simple, quick, no-cost method to potentially avoid ED errors and deaths; we call it "The Two Step Approach." The two step approach involves a minimal amount of time (about 1–2 minutes per "high risk" patient, equal to perhaps 5–10 minutes per shift).

THE TWO STEP APPROACH:

The two step approach is straightforward: 1) Identify "high risk" patients who are being discharged from the ED, and 2) Review their ED evaluation before they leave.

The approach seems so simple as to be obvious, but the charts of litigious patients with poor outcomes are rife with inconsistencies, abnormal vital signs, and inadequate/poor documentation. The two step approach encourages a "second look" at patients who have an increased risk of bouncing back or dying within 7 days of initial ED evaluation.

A high risk patient is one with a potentially life- or limb-threatening illness who leaves the ED without a definitive diagnosis. Pre-discharge review involves ensuring their evaluation, as reflected in the documentation, was consistent, logical, and thorough.

Step 1: Identify high risk patients

- High risk complaint without definitive diagnosis on discharge (e.g., abdominal pain, chest pain, headache and fever, etc.)
- Abnormal vital signs
- Condition making it less likely patient will return for worsening symptoms (mental/psychiatric/substance abuse)
- Chronic disease with decompensation
- Difficulty obtaining accurate data (language, dementia, inebriation, etc.)
- Advanced age
- Upset patients
- Unmet patient expectations
- Bouncebacks (a patient return, usually within 72 hours)
- Summary: A patient you will worry about after you are finished with your shift

Step 2: Review your evaluation prior to ED discharge

- Address all documented complaints in H&P
- Confirm history is accurate
- Consider potentially serious diagnoses
- Explore abnormal findings
- Write a progress note explaining the medical decision-making process (if unclear from the H&P)
- Assure that aftercare instructions are specific and follow-up is timely and available
- Confirm that patient understands and is comfortable with the plan
- Summary: Complete a medically and legally defensible evaluation, which is reflected in the documentation on the chart

As you read the cases in this book, many of these errors will be obvious, others more subtle. "Red flags" can easily be overlooked in a well appearing patient who presents to a busy ED. We hope that this "Two Step" approach will better enable us to identify patients at high risk for a poor outcome, and to "look both ways" twice, before sending them home.

REFERENCES

1. Gordon JA, An LC, Hayward RA, et al. Initial emergency department diagnosis and return visits: risk versus perception. Ann Emerg Med 1998;32: 569-73.
2. Pierce JM, Kellermann AL, Oster C. "Bounces": An analysis of short-term return visits to a public hospital emergency department. Ann Emerg Med 1990;19:752-7.
3. Wilkins PS, Beckett MW. Audit of unexpected return visits to an accident and emergency department. Arch Emerg Med 1992;9:352-6.

4. O'Dwyer F, Bodiwala GG. Unscheduled return visits by patients to the accident and emergency department. Arch Emerg Med 1991;8:196-200.
5. Martin-Gill C, Reiser RC. Risk factors for 72-hour admission to the ED. Am J Emerg Med 2004; 22:448-53.
6. Kefer MP, Hargarten SW, Jentzen J. Death after discharge from the emergency department. Ann Emerg Med 1994;24:1102-7.
7. Sklar DP, Loeliger E, Edmunds K, et al. Unanticipated death after discharge home from the emergency department. Ann Emerg Med 2007;49:735-45.
8. Nunez S, Hexdall A, Aguirre-Jaime A. Unscheduled returns to the emergency department: an outcome of medical errors? Qual Saf Health Care 2006;15:102-8.

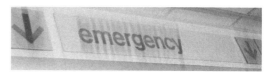

CASE 1

18 YEAR OLD MALE WITH LEFT HAND PAIN

Commentary:
Gregory L. Henry, MD, FACEP

CEO, Medical Practice Risk Assessment, Inc., Ann Arbor, Michigan
Clinical Professor, Department of Emergency Medicine
   University of Michigan Medical School, Ann Arbor, Michigan
Past President, American College of Emergency Physicians (ACEP)

Discussion:
Wesley P. Eilbert, MD, FACEP

Clinical Associate Professor and Resident Research Director
   Department of Emergency Medicine
   University of Illinois College of Medicine
Director of Undergraduate Education, Department of Emergency Medicine
   Mercy Hospital and Medical Center, Chicago, Illinois

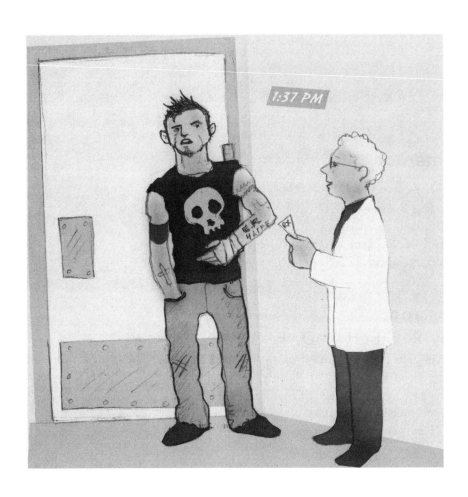

18 YEAR OLD MALE WITH LEFT HAND PAIN

—Initial Visit*—

*Authors' Note: The history, exam and notes are the actual documentation of the physicians and providers, including abbreviations (and spelling errors)

CHIEF COMPLAINT (at 11:02): Left hand pain

```
VITAL SIGNS
 Time      Temp(F)      Pulse       Resp        Syst        Diast
11:12       96.6         66          16         110          68
```

HISTORY OF PRESENT ILLNESS (at 11:20): 18 year old left-handed male without a significant PMH presents with complaints that he was messing around with some friends the night before and they were close to a brick wall and a brick was loose and came down and landed on the dorsum of his left hand over the third MCP joint. The injury occurred 15 hours prior to the ED presentation. He complains of edema and redness and a laceration. Also c/o limited movement of the finger with pain with flexion and extension. No c/o fever, chills, night sweats. No allergies. Tetanus unknown.

PAST MEDICAL HISTORY/TRIAGE:
Medications: None
Allergies: None
PMH: None
PSH: None

EXAM (at 11:23):
General: Alert and oriented, no acute distress
Ext: 1 cm laceration over the third MCP joint on the dorsum and edema and erythema and swelling between the second and fourth metacarpal clear to the base of the metacarpals; even passive ROM of the third MCP causes pain with both flexion and extension
Skin: No red streaks
Neurovasc: Cap refill brisk. Sensation WNL

ORDERS/RESULTS (at 11:58): XR negative for fracture

PROGRESS NOTES (at 12:45): Anesthetized with 0.5% Marcaine, prep, drape, thorough irrigation with sterile saline and explored. The extensor tendon was intact, but the tendon sheath was frayed. Cleaned again with 10% betadine solution. Two loose 4-0 ethilon sutures were placed to the skin. Ancef 1 g IM and dT. Wound dressed with polysporin, adaptic and a volar OCL splint.

DIAGNOSIS: Left hand laceration, fifteen hours old, with cellulitis

DISPOSITION: The patient was discharged to Home ambulatory at 13:37. Prescription for Keflex. Referral to a plastic surgeon to follow up in a couple of days and return to the ED with worsening symptoms or if unable to get in to see Plastic Surgeon.

Phone call to ED the next day: Patient called the next day (1 day after initial ED presentation) with complaints of swelling of the hand and fingers and pain. Has been taking Advil because he cannot afford Rx. Advised to return to the ED to be checked.

Gregory L. Henry comments:

"Not even apes, who walk on their knuckles, use them to protect themselves when they fall"

Patients lie a lot. Even without seeing the end of this case, I know the end of this case. No 18 year-old has anything happen to his knuckles, unrelated to a fight. The great story; "I tripped and fell," is always a lie. Not even apes, who walk on their knuckles, use them to protect themselves when they fall. A significant injury over the MCP joint is caused by a human mouth until proven otherwise. People do not want to admit how various things happen, and this is true not only of emergency patients.

The evaluation of this patient is not unreasonable. It should be noted that whenever a patient has pain with passive motion of the digit, tenosynovitis, must be suspected. Advanced tenosynovitis almost always results, even with effective therapy, in scarring of the tendon sheath and some limitation or aggravation with motion. Pain with passive range of motion should be a clue that this is not just a simple laceration.

The documentation of this case is reasonable, but the documented mechanism of injury is questionable.

The diagnosis in the case is concerning. Cellulitis involves inflammation of skin and soft tissues. Tenosynovitis, a more specific diagnosis, involves the tendon and tendon sheaths. This was clearly documented in the physical exam and should have been reflected in the diagnosis. It is also somewhat troubling that the follow up program was longer than expected; if someone has an active infection in a hand, follow-up should be within the first 24 hours.

The therapy with IV Ancef and then Keflex, although not unreasonable in most cases of cellulites, was not appropriate for a potential human bite wound.

- Thoroughness of Documentation: 8 out of 10.
- Thoroughness of Patient Evaluation: 9 out of 10.
- Risk of Serious Illness Being Missed: High risk.
- Risk Management Legal Rating: High risk.

18 YEAR OLD MALE WITH LEFT HAND PAIN

—Second Visit: 5 Days Later—

CHIEF COMPLAINT (at 01:03): Severe left hand pain

VITAL SIGNS					
Time	Temp(F)	Pulse	Resp	Syst	Diast
01:08	100.3	104	20	132	78

HISTORY OF PRESENT ILLNESS (at 01:44): He said that the pain suddenly increased when his girlfriend kicked it by mistake and he felt like the wound opened up and he had some drainage from the site. The pain extends from the wound down into his hand. No complaints of fever, nausea, vomiting or red streaks going up the hand. He is taking his girlfriend's Percocet (which she had from an old ankle injury), but it is not providing adequate relief. He did not fill his prescription for Keflex.

PAST MEDICAL HISTORY/TRIAGE:
  Allergies: None
  PMH: None
  PSH: None

EXAM (at 01:48):
  General: Seems very uncomfortable, holding his left hand above his head, face in a grimace from pain
  Hand: 1.5 cm laceration over the dorsal aspect of the MCP of the middle finger with 2 stitches loosely in place. Small amount of purulent drainage from the wound. Extreme pain with motion at the MCP joint and also pain when the MCP joint is immobilized and the PIP joint is moved. Pain with palpation along the tendon which overlies the metacarpal bone of the middle finger on the dorsal and plantar aspect. Minimal erythema of the skin around the wound.
  Skin: No red streaks.

PROGRESS NOTES (at 02:30): Unasyn 3g IVPB, Demerol 25mg IV and Phenergan 12.5mg IV. Wound culture was obtained. Volar OCL placed up to DIP joint. Consulted plastic surgeon and patient will be admitted to his service. He recommended Betadine and water soaks every 8 hours and the patient kept NPO for surgery in the morning.

RESULTS:

Test	Value	Units	Ref. Range
WBC	11.1	K/μL	4.6-10.2
HGB	13.2	G/DL	13.5-17.5
PLT	253	K/μL	142-424

DIAGNOSIS: Acute left hand cellulitis with probable tendon sheath infection versus MCP septic arthritis. He was transferred to the floor at 04:10.

HOSPITAL COURSE:

Progress note (per hand surgeon): Taken to the OR and wound opened and incision extended. A large laceration in the extensor mechanism was found which exposed the joint. There was pus within the joint. It was irrigated and a small drain was left in the wound. Skin was closed and a bulky dressing applied. Culture results (below) suggest etiology of injury was a human bite wound. Infectious disease was consulted and they recommended 2-4 weeks of IV antibiotic therapy. The patient was discharged in good condition.

Culture results: Eikenella species, Streptococcus viridans

FINAL DIAGNOSIS: Hand laceration secondary to human bite wound

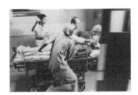

DISCUSSION OF CLENCHED FIST INJURIES, ANIMAL BITE WOUNDS, AND ADHERENCE TO THERAPY

Wesley P. Eilbert, MD, FACEP

I. GENERAL APPROACH TO CLENCHED FIST INJURIES

Lacerations over the dorsal surface of the third, fourth and fifth MCP joints of the dominant hand must be considered clenched fist injuries (CFIs) until proven otherwise. The patient in this case exemplifies the typical CFI patient; these patients are overwhelmingly male, between 12 and 34 years old, and usually seek medical attention only after enough time has elapsed for symptoms of infection to emerge.[1,2] These injuries are more common in the summer months and on weekends.[3] Patients with CFIs often have a history of recent drug or alcohol use, are notoriously noncompliant, and frequently offer an alternative explanation for the cause of their injury.[1,2,4] The type of hand injury sustained by this patient is also typical of CFIs – a small (<1cm) laceration over the dorsal aspect of the third, fourth or fifth MCP joint of the dominant hand.[5] CFIs have also been described over the dorsal aspect of the proximal interphalangeal joints.[6]

It would be difficult, if not impossible, to reliably determine what percentage of patients in the emergency department lie about their injuries, though we all know this occurs. Our patient told the physician on his first visit that a brick had fallen on his hand; when he returned his culture revealed eikenella (oral flora), indicating that the true nature of the injury was a "fight bite." Identifying those types of injuries and patient characteristics that are frequently associated with patient dishonesty is the first step in eliciting "the real story." Any injuries which may have resulted from child or domestic abuse, alternative sexual practices, illegal drug use or interpersonal violence, as well as injuries with potential legal ramifications, should alert the emergency physician to consider a different mechanism of injury than that described by the patient.

While everyone has a personal style of obtaining an accurate history from an otherwise reluctant patient, here are some time-tested techniques to keep in mind when treating this type of patient:

1. Make patient aware of the potentially bad outcomes if the correct cause of the injury isn't known. This "scare tactic approach" will work occasionally.

2. Make the patient's family or friends aware of the potentially bad outcomes if the true cause of the injury isn't known. In my experience, this "guilt-inducing technique" has a higher yield than the "scare tactic approach."

3. Assure the patient of the confidential nature of their treatment. This may not be true in all circumstances however, depending on local laws (e.g., injuries involving a firearm, child abuse, etc.).

As is often necessary in highly suspicious cases, it would have been wise to treat this patient on the first visit as a CFI, regardless of the patient's story.

The unique anatomy of the hand, with its relatively thin protective covering of skin on its dorsal surface, makes it vulnerable to fractures, osteomyelitis, tendon sheath injury, as well as joint space injury and infection. Not surprisingly, CFIs have consistently high rates of deep structure damage. Damage to underlying bones occurs in 17%–58% of CFIs, 52%–62% violate a joint capsule (typically the MCP joint), and 15%–20% have associated tendon injury.[7]

II. PHYSICAL EXAMINATION AND X-RAYS OF THE HAND

The initial exam of potential CFI should take place after appropriate anesthesia in a bloodless field. A tourniquet or inflated blood pressure cuff can be used for this purpose. Extending the margins of the laceration is often necessary to allow for adequate visualization of the underlying structures. The underlying joint capsule extensor tendon should be inspected. The examiner must take into account the flexed position of the interphalageal and MCP joints at the time of injury. An injured segment of tendon will retract proximally in the unclenched, open hand and will be missed if the wound is examined only in this position. The tendon's strength through its range of motion should be tested. Weakness of extension when compared with the same digit on the uninjured hand may indicate partial disruption. It should be noted, however, that patients may possess normal strength with up to 90% disruption of the tendon.[8] While nonspecific, pain during movement may also be an indicator of partial tendon disruption. Physical examination on the initial visit revealed that "even passive ROM of the third MCP causes pain with both flexion and extension," unusual for a simple laceration. Strength testing was not documented. If performed, it may have been a clue that this was not simply a laceration.

Radiographs should be obtained, looking not only for fractures, but also foreign bodies (i.e., tooth fragments) and intraarticular air, indicating joint penetration. Any known or potential damage to important underlying structures (e.g., tendons, arteries, nerves, bones or joints) warrants consultation with a hand specialist in the ED.

Since many CFIs, like this case, present only after the initial symptoms of infection appear, a high index of suspicion for these complications must be maintained. A warm, swollen joint under a CFI which is painful with passive or active range of motion is typical of septic arthritis. An elevated erythrocyte sedimentation rate (>30mm/hr), while not specific, is highly sensitive (>95%) for septic arthritis and is useful as a screening test.[9]

 ESR

III. MANAGEMENT OF BITE WOUNDS TO THE HAND

Wound care of CFIs should proceed as with any animal bite to the hand. Cleaning, debridement, and irrigation are the most important factors in preventing wound infection and optimizing outcome. The area around the wound should be cleaned with an antibacterial agent such as 1% povidone-iodine solution. Povidone-iodine surgical scrub and 10% solution should not be used since both are toxic to native tissue.[7] Scrubbing of the wound itself is controversial, though probably reasonable with grossly contaminated wounds if done gently. Debridement of devitalized tissue should be performed as with any traumatic wound.

Irrigation is the most effective means of decontaminating bite wounds and has been shown to decrease their rate of infection fivefold.[10] Which solution to use for irrigation is a matter of some debate, with normal saline, diluted povidone-iodine and tap water all having been proven efficacious. Ideally, the irrigant should be delivered through a 19 gauge needle or angiocath attached to a 20cc syringe with a moderate amount of hand pressure. A volume of 100-300cc is sufficient for most CFIs.

It is generally accepted that CFIs should not be closed primarily.[2,5,7,11-18] In this case, even it if was assumed the patient's laceration was not a CFI, suturing an infected wound is never a good idea. Ideally, CFIs should be left open with a bulky dressing, and the hand splinted in a position of function for 2–3 days. The patient should be instructed to keep the hand elevated to decrease edema; a sling may be used for this purpose. Given their high propensity for infection, all CFIs should be reevaluated in 24–48 hours. If cosmesis is an issue, CFIs can be closed in a delayed primary fashion after 4 days if no evidence of infection is present.

Clenched fist injuries have alarmingly high rates of osteomyelitis (16%), septic arthritis (12%) and tenosynovitis (22%).[7] For this reason, virtually all authorities recommend prophylactic antibiotics as part of their treatment.[2,5,6,7,11,12,14,17-20] However, only one study to date has proven conclusively the value of prophylactic antibiotics for human bites to the hand.[21] Prophylactic antibiotics should ideally be given within 3 hours of the initial injury. This means, practically stated, it's wise to give the first dose in the E.D. Oral antibiotics have been found to be equivalent to intravenous antibiotics when used for this purpose.[21] Infections from CFIs are usually polymicrobial with an average of 4 species present on culture, and approximately half are mixed aerobic/anaerobic infections. Streptococcus and Staphylococcus species are the most common infecting organisms, present 82% and 57% of the time, respectively. Eikenella corrodens, as cultured in our patient, is a fastidious bacteria which is resistant to multiple antibiotics, and present approximately one-third of the time.[22] Penicillin will cover most of these organisms well, except for the Staphylococcus species, which typically produce beta-lactamase. For this reason, an anti-staphylococcal penicillin or non-beta-lactam must be given. Amoxicillin/clavulanate is the prophylactic monotherapy of choice for CFIs.[7,22,23] Penicillin plus dicloxacillin is a cheaper alternative, though the q.i.d. dosing can contribute to patient noncompliance. For penicillin-allergic patients, clindamycin combined with ciprofloxacin or

clinda + cipro / PCN + Diclox
or Tri/Sulfa

trimethoprim-sulfamethoxazole is a reasonable alternative.[7,23]   Prophylactic antibiotics should be continued for 3 to 5 days.[7]

IV. DISCUSSION OF THE CASE

There is no question that this patient required admission on his second ED visit. His physical findings, consistent with a septic joint or tenosynovitis, make the need for admission obvious. It would have probably been wise on this second visit to repeat an x-ray, looking for evidence of osteomyelitis or gas in the soft tissues. Even without evidence of tenosynovitis or a septic joint, some authorities recommend operative exploration of any clinically infected CFI presenting after 24 hours.[1,25]

V. TREATMENT OF SEPTIC ARTHRITIS

Unasyn

Treatment of septic arthritis begins with prompt administration of I.V. antibiotics. Ampicillin/sulbactam was an excellent choice in this case. Other antibiotic options for the inpatient treatment of CFIs include: ticarcillin/clavulanate, piperacillin/tazobactam, cefoxitin, and clindamycin plus ciprofloxacin for those allergic to penicillin.[7,22,23] Drainage of the infected joint by a hand specialist, either by formal arthrotomy or serial joint aspirations, should be performed as soon as possible.

VI. APPROACH TO ANIMAL BITE WOUNDS TO THE HAND

This discussion would not be complete without some mention of occlusional bites to the hand. Occlusional bites are those caused by occlusion of the perpetrator's teeth onto the victim's skin. Dogs and cats cause the vast majority of occlusional hand bites. Dogs have powerful jaws capable of exerting pressures over 200 pounds per square inch, resulting in an increased risk of crush injury to the underlying structures. Cats have sharp, slender teeth which easily penetrate skin and underlying tissues, causing a deep puncture wound with a relatively benign external appearance. Evaluation and treatment of occlusional hand bites should proceed in a similar fashion as described for CFIs. It is important to look for damage to deep structures, which includes obtaining x-rays and extending the margins of puncture wounds near joints to inspect for possible joint capsule violation. Like CFIs, occlusional hand bites should not be closed primarily and should receive prophylactic antibiotics.[7] Antibiotic options for occlusional human bites to the hand are similar to those for CFIs. Like human bites, amoxicillin/clavulanate is the monotherapy of choice for dog and cat bites. Other alternatives include penicillin plus cephalexin, and clindamycin combined with either ciprofloxacin or trimethaprim-sulfamethoxazole for penicillin-allergic patients.[7,23,26]

VII. ADHERENCE ISSUES IN THE EMERGENCY DEPARTMENT

Like the young man in this case, many of the patients seen in the emergency department do not obtain the medications we've prescribed. In fact, a 1996 study found that 12% of patients discharged from the ED were noncompliant with prescribed medication.[24] This study also noted these noncompliant patients were significantly more likely to be uninsured and have an annual income of less than $25,000. Oftentimes it is up to the emergency physician to find a creative way to get these patients the medications they need. Some suggestions to keep in mind:

1. Know the cheaper alternatives. As discussed above, a combination of penicillin and dicloxacillin would be significantly cheaper than amoxicillin/clavulanate when used prophylactically for CFIs.

2. Prescribe medications that have generic equivalents.
3. With a patient whose insurance plan will cover treatment in the hospital but not prescriptions, give the first dose of medication in the ED before the patient leaves. While I doubt the young man presented in this case had any type of insurance coverage, giving him the dose of IM cefazolin prior to his discharge was definitely a good idea. (Even though IM ampicillin/sulbactam would have been a better choice.)
4. Ask a social worker for help. No one in the hospital will know more about what services or alternatives are available to cover health care costs than the people in the social services department.

TEACHING POINTS ABOUT CASE 1:

- If the injury the patient has doesn't match the history given, assume the patient is lying and treat as such. Lacerations over the dorsal surface of the third, fourth and fifth MCP joints of the dominant hand must be considered clenched fist injuries (CFIs) until proven otherwise.
- CFIs are high morbidity injuries that require significantly different treatment than standard hand lacerations.
- The preferred antibiotic for human bite wounds is amoxicillin/clavulanate, not cephalexin.
- Lack of funding is a common cause of patient noncompliance with prescribed therapy. Using equivalent, more affordable therapies and the expertise of the social services department can go a long way in combating this problem. A brilliant diagnosis is overshadowed when a patient does not fill the prescription.

REFERENCES

1. Basadre JO, Parry SW. Indications for surgical debridement in 125 human bites to the hand. Arch Surg 1991; 126:65-7.
2. Bunzli WF, Wright DH, Hoang AT, et al. Current management of human bites. Pharmacotherapy 1998; 18:227-34.
3. Marr JS, Beck AM, Lugo JA Jr. An epidemiologic study of the human bite. Public Health Rep 1979; 94:514-21.
4. Phair IC, Quinton DN. Clenched fist human bite injuries. J Hand Surg [Br]1989; 14:86-7.
5. Perron AD, Miller MD, Brady WJ. Orthopedic pitfalls in the ED: fight bite. Am J Emerg Med 2002; 20;114-7.
6. Patzakis MJ, Wilkins J, Bassett RL. Surgical findings in clenched-fist injuries. Clin Orthop 1987; (220):237-40.
7. Eilbert WP. Dog, cat, and human bites: providing safe and cost-effective treatment in the ED. Emerg Med Prac 2003; 5:1-20.
8. Hart RG, Uehara DT, Wagner MJ, eds. Emergency and primary care of the hand. Dallas, TX, 2001.
9. Li SF, Henderson J, Dickman E, et al. Laboratory tests in adults with monarticular arthritis: can they rule out a specific joint? Acad Emerg Med 2004; 11:276-80.
10. Callaham ML. Treatment of common dog bites; infection risk factors. J Plast Reconstr Aesthet Surg 1978; 7:83-7.
11. Itzhak B, Human and animal bite infections. J Fam Prac 1989; 28:713-718.
12. Callaham ML. Controversies in antibiotic choices for bite wounds. Ann Emerg Med 1988; 17:1321-30.

13. Chadaev AP, Jukhtin VI, Butkevich AT, et al. Treatment of infected clenched-fist human bite wounds in the area of metacarpophalangeal joints. J Hand Surg [Am] 1996; 21:299-303.
14. Harrison BP, Hilliard MW. Emergency department evaluation and treatment of hand injuries. Emerg Med Clin North Am 1999; 17:793-822.
15. Mayo DD, Mayo KP, Matta A. Emergency department management of dog, cat and human bite wounds. Crit Dec Emerg Med 2001; 16:1-6.
16. Taplitz RA. Managing bite wounds. Currently recommended antibiotics for treatment and prophylaxis. Postgrad Med 2004; 116:49-52, 55-56, 59.
17. Griego RD, Rosen T, Orengo IF, et al. Dog, cat and human bites: a review. J Am Acad Dermatol 1995; 33:1019-29.
18. Brook I. Microbiology and management of human and animal bite wound infections. Prim Care 2003; 30:25-39.
19. Tsai E, Failla JM. Hand infections in the trauma patient. Hand Clin 1999; 15(2): 373-86.
20. Mennen U, Howells CJ. Human fight-bite injuries of the hand. J Hand Surg [Br] 1991; 16B:431-5.
21. Zubowicz VN, Gravier M. Management of early human bites of the hand: a prospective randomized study. Plast Reconstr Surg 1991; 88:111-4.
22. Talan DA, Abrahamian FM, Moran GJ, et al. Clinical presentation and bacteriologic analysis of infected human bites in patients presenting to emergency departments. Clin Infect Dis 2003; 37:1481-9.
23. Gilbert DN, Moellering RC Jr, Eliopoulos GM, et al. eds. The Sanford guide to antimicrobial therapy, 34th ed. Hyde Park, VT: 2004.
24. Thomas EJ, Burstin HR, O'Neil AC, et al. Patient noncompliance with medical advice after the emergency department visit. Ann Emerg Med 1996; 27:49-55.
25. Dreyfuss MD. Singer M. Human bites of the hand: a study of one hundred six patients. J Hand Surg 1985; 10A:884-9.
26. Talan DA, Citron DM, Abrahamian FM, et al. Bacteriologic analysis of infected dog and cat bites. Emergency Medicine Animal Bite Infection Study Group. N Engl J Med 1999; 340:85-92.

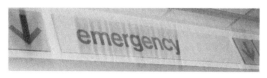

CASE2

33 YEAR OLD MALE WITH
ABDOMINAL PAIN

Commentary:
Gregory L. Henry, MD, FACEP

CEO, Medical Practice Risk Assessment, Inc., Ann Arbor, Michigan
Clinical Professor, Department of Emergency Medicine
   University of Michigan Medical School, Ann Arbor, Michigan
Past President, American College of Emergency Physicians (ACEP)

Discussion:
Scott W. Melanson, MD, FACEP

Associate Program Director, Emergency Medicine Residency
Chair, Disaster Committee, St. Luke's Hospital, Bethlehem, Pennsylvania
Clinical Associate Professor, Temple University, Philadelphia, Pennsylvania

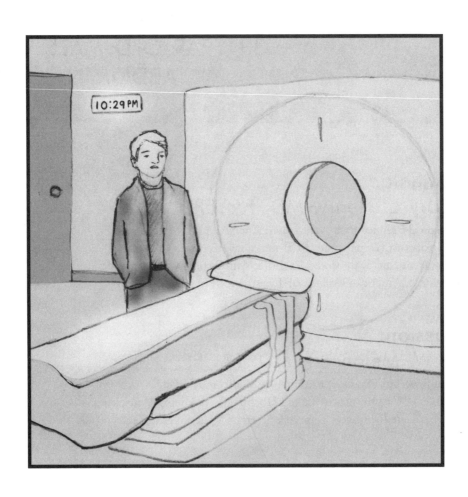

33 YEAR OLD MALE WITH ABDOMINAL PAIN

—Initial Visit*—

*Authors' Note: The history, exam and notes are the actual documentation of the physicians and providers, including abbreviations (and spelling errors)

CHIEF COMPLAINT (at 20:50): Abdominal pain

```
VITAL SIGNS
Time      Temp    Pulse   Resp    Syst    Diast   Pain
21:16     98.0    72      18      128     60      10
23:33             76      16      104     64      2
```

HISTORY OF PRESENT ILLNESS (at 21:06): He is a 33 year old male who states that at 7pm, after having normal BM, he developed gradual onset of RLQ and lower abdominal pain. He describes it as a bloating, spasm pain. After BM, pt noted urinary stream cut off and was no longer able to urinate. Gradually pain got worse, intermittent RLQ pain radiated into the right groin and testicles. Pain is 8/10 with spasms, mild nausea with pain. No dysuria, hematuria, testicular swelling, flank pain, chest pain, or fever/chills. Pt has no history of kidney stones but grandfather had many kidney stones.

PAST MEDICAL HISTORY/TRIAGE:
Medications: Claritin D
Allergies: No known allergies.
PMH: None
PSH: None

EXAM (at 21:15):
General: Well-appearing; well-nourished; A&O X 3, in no apparent distress
Head: Normocephalic; atraumatic.
Eyes: PERRL
Nose: The nose is normal in appearance without rhinorrhea
Resp: Normal chest excursion with respiration; breath sounds clear and equal bilaterally; no wheezes, rhonchi, or rales
Card: Regular rhythm, without murmurs, rub or gallop
Abd: Non-distended; Tender RLQ but no rebound. Mild right flank/side pain. No rigidity, rebound or guarding
Skin: Normal for age and race; warm and dry; no apparent lesions
GU Exam: External genitalia normal, no urethral discharge, testes descended bilaterally. No lesions noted on penis or scrotum. Epididymus normal bilaterally.

ORDERS (at 21:25): Dilaudid 1 mg IVP, Toradol 30 mg IVP, Phenergan 12.5 mg IVP, .9NS-500cc bolus then 125cc/hr.

RESULTS (at 22:09):
Urine dip: WNL except: Bilirubin - 1 mg/dL

Noncontrast helical CT of the abdomen/pelvis (at 22:29) - Unremarkable helical CT of the abdomen and pelvis.

PROGRESS NOTE (at 23:23): Pt felt much better but still had pain into the lower abd. bilaterally with sitting up.

DIAGNOSIS - Abdominal pain, unspecified site, Suspect bladder spasms.

DISPOSITION (at 23:41) - The patient was discharged to Home ambulatory. Follow-up with primary care physician in 2 days. Prescription for Vicodin 5mg. Aftercare instructions for abdominal pain and kidney stone/renal colic.

Gregory L. Henry comments:

"The male genitalia as a source of discomfort is quickly excluded on physical examination—we are then left with a limited number of abdominal structures as a source of right lower quadrant pain. "

Any human with pain below the umbilicus can have appendicitis. CT scanning, while not as accurate as originally thought, is appropriate.

The history describes bloating and spasm, not uncommon complaints in adults with appendicitis. The complaint of urinary difficulty is essentially a smoke screen; the bottom line is that we have a 33-year-old male with right lower quadrant pain. In a male, the structures located in the right lower quadrant are few and far between—males are not females! The male genitalia as a source of discomfort is quickly excluded on physical examination—we are then left with a limited number of abdominal structures as a source of right lower quadrant pain.

The evaluation of this patient was typical and the abdominal examination seems to be in order. Right lower quadrant tenderness, without rebound or guarding, was noted, although these findings are always dependent upon the examiner's skill. No comment was made of an obturator sign, which may be helpful in a case that is equivocal. The external genitalia were properly examined, and no evidence of hernia or genital abnormality could be found. This, along with clean urine, makes a genitourinary infection unlikely.

I agree that medication for pain relief is appropriate; there is no evidence that a diagnosis is influenced one way or the other after the use of analgesics. With a family history of kidney stones, a helical CT was appropriately performed, which ruled out kidney stone or aortic aneurysm as the problem. The patient was then discharged home to follow up with the primary doctor in 2 days.

obturator sign

The biggest problem in this case is not the evaluation, but the discharge program. A patient with a negative workup, and persistent right lower quadrant pain needs to be told that appendicitis is still a reasonable possibility; timeframe for follow-up should be 6 to 8 hours. If the patient is not completely pain free by this time, have the patient return to the ED for re-evaluation, or set up a re-evaluation with the patient's private physician. Most abdominal processes declare themselves within 12 hours.

The initial workup was not overly aggressive from a laboratory standpoint and this is a good thing. No specific blood test would answer any questions about this patient. Slight elevations in the white blood count can be seen with virtually any process and do not help decision making. The risk management problem here is not the history, physical, or laboratory studies—it is the discharge program.

- Thoroughness of Documentation: 8 out of 10.

- Thoroughness of Patient Evaluation: 8 out of 10.

- Risk of Serious Illness Being Missed: High risk.

- Risk Management Legal Rating: High risk secondary to the inadequate discharge program.

33 YEAR OLD MALE WITH ABDOMINAL PAIN

—Second Visit: Less than 24 Hours Later—

CHIEF COMPLAINT (at 17:18): Abdominal pain

VITALS SIGNS						
Time	Temp	Pulse	Resp	Syst	Diast	Pain
17:29	98.3	115	24	144	92	10
18:54		120	16	100	50	9
20:30		112	16	140	80	5

HISTORY OF PRESENT ILLNESS (at 18:17): The patient is a 33-year-old male who developed right-sided abdominal pain yesterday. He states he was fine yesterday during the day and went to work. When he came home, he had a bowel movement. He subsequently described the pain in his right lower quadrant, which he states felt like a gaseous pain and then it developed to a sharp-burning pain that was intermittently sharp. The patient had some slight nausea at that time and had 1 episode of emesis. He presented to this ER last evening. The patient had a urinalysis which was reportedly unremarkable, received IV pain medication, and helical CT scan to rule out kidney stone and told this was unremarkable. The patient was sent home. He states that he woke up at 4 o'clock this morning with continued pain in the right lower quadrant of his abdomen. He denies any radiation of the pain. He continues to feel nauseous and threw up once today. He has had nothing to eat today. About 2 p.m., the patient began feeling febrile. The patient denies any radiation of the pain into his testicles or into his flank. Denies chest pain, shortness of breath, calf muscle pain, leg/foot edema, diarrhea, bloody stools, dysuria, urinary frequency, hematuria, no urinary incontinence, rhinorrhea, cough, no loss of consciousness, or paresthesias.

PAST MEDICAL HISTORY/TRIAGE:
Medications: Claritin D
Allergies: No known allergies.
PMH: None
PSH: None

PHYSICAL EXAMINATION (at 18:25):
General: A white male who appears quite ill.
Vital: Afebrile. Vital signs are stable as documented on the chart.
Lungs: Clear to auscultation without wheeze.
Cardiovascular: Regular rate and rhythm.
Back: There is no CVA tenderness.
Abdomen: Positive bowel sounds, soft, and tender to palpation in the right lower quadrant with referred pain in the left lower quadrant and over to the right lower quadrant. There is mild guarding. No rebound.
Genitourinary: Testicular examination shows no masses. Epididymis is nonenlarged, and there is no hernia palpable.

ORDERS (at 18:28):
Demerol 50 mg IVP, Phenergan 12.5 mg IVP, Cefotan 1 g IVPB
IV: .9NS-500cc bolus then to 125cc/hour

RESULTS (at 19:04):

Test	Flag	Value	Units	Ref. range
WBC	H	16.0	K/uL	4.6-10.2
HGB		14.5	G/DL	13.5-17.5
PLT		235	K/uL	142-424
NA		136	MMOL/L	135-144
K		3.7	MMOL/L	3.5-5.1
CL		94	MMOL/L	98-107
AGAP		12.4	MMOL/L	6.0-18.0
CO2		28	MMOL/L	22-29
GLU		129		70-119
BUN		11	MG/DL	7-18
CREAT		1.1	MG/DL	0.6-1.3

Urinalysis - WNL

DIAGNOSIS (at 20:17):
Acute appendicitis without mention of peritonitis

DISPOSITION (at 20:21):
Admitted to surgical service

HOSPITAL COURSE:

********** Operative Report **********
Preoperative diagnosis: Appendicitis.
Postoperative diagnosis: Locally ruptured appendix.
Procedure: On opening the peritoneum, we immediately get return of yellow purulent fluid, which we aspirated up and then also cultured. We immediately encounter the appendix, which is lateral retrocecal in location. Grossly, it is obvious that there is appendicitis. In fact, there are a couple of areas of necrosis and one small pinpoint perforation near the mid-to-distal portion of the appendix from which there is a small amount of purulent fluid draining.

Surgeon progress note:

The patient was admitted to the hospital with right lower quadrant pain. He was felt to have ruptured appendicitis. He underwent an appendectomy, and at the time of surgery, he was found to have a ruptured appendix. He was treated with intravenous fluids and antibiotics. Postoperatively, he became quite distended and had developed a postoperative ileus. This required placement of an NG tube. The NG tube helped decompress the intestinal tract slowly over the time. Eventually, we were able to wean him off the intravenous pain medicine and gradually advanced his diet when his intestinal tract returned to some degree of function. Ultimately, he was able to be advanced on a diet to the point of tolerating food and no longer developing any distention. He then had some return of intestinal function that was adequate to allow him to be discharged 5 days after admission.

FINAL DIAGNOSIS: Ruptured appendicitis and postoperative ileus.

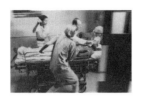

DIAGNOSIS AND MANAGEMENT OF ABDOMINAL PAIN

Scott W. Melanson, MD, FACEP

I. INTRODUCTION

Every day emergency physicians are faced with decisions concerning patients with abdominal pain; who needs laboratory testing, imaging, or emergent referral? Over the last decade imaging studies, particularly CT scanning, have improved our ability to diagnose abdominal pain - CT has been particularly helpful in evaluating patients with possible appendicitis. In order to best utilize imaging tests, the emergency physician (EP) must understand how these studies are performed and understand their limitations.

II. OVERVIEW OF CASE AND DIFFERENTIAL DIAGNOSIS

This 33 year old patient presented with complaints of right lower quadrant (RLQ) abdominal pain. Possible causes of RLQ pain in a male include appendicitis, diverticulitis (more commonly presents with left sided symptoms), pyelonephritis, bowel obstruction, ureteral calculi, cancer, AAA, testicular torsion, and the ever-famous "nonspecific abdominal pain." Urinary tract infection and AAA are very unlikely given the normal urine dip and his young age, respectively. The normal testicular exam removed torsion from the differential diagnosis. The diagnosis of nonspecific abdominal pain can be made only after more serious causes have been eliminated. Lack of prior abdominal surgery makes bowel obstruction less likely, but it is still a remote possibility. The patient's stool history and the quality and presence of bowel sounds is not recorded, but might have been helpful. The remaining diagnoses under consideration include ureteral calculi, appendicitis, nonspecific abdominal pain, bowel obstruction, cancer, and diverticulitis; the last 3 diagnoses are least likely.

III. LABORATORY TESTING

Laboratory testing is seldom diagnostic in patients with abdominal pain. Lipase and/or amylase are quite good, but not perfect, for the diagnosis of pancreatitis. Urine dip can be helpful in diagnosing urinary tract infection and renal colic but can be misleading; an inflamed appendix overlying the ureter can result in pyuria or hematuria. Similarly, hematuria has been seen with AAA; the most common misdiagnosis made in patients with AAA is renal colic. Conversely, patients with ureteral calculi can present without hematuria.

IV. GI IMAGING—CT, PLAIN FILMS, ULTRASOUND

The ability of CT to evaluate abdominal pain has dramatically increased with the advent of helical, or spiral scanning, compared to the older method of taking discrete, individual radiographic slices. Helical CT scans have a rotating tube that has multiple x-ray detectors mounted directly across from the source of the x-rays. When the patient moves through the CT scanner, the rotating tube spins around the patient, creating a helical pattern of x-ray beams. Now, the entire abdomen and pelvis can be scanned in less than 30 seconds. This rapid scanning allows all the images to be obtained during a single breath-hold. The images are reconstructed in 3 dimensions, without concern for unequal breaths causing misregistration, which occurred with conventional CT scanning. Helical scanning collects much more data than conventional scanning and allows for image slice widths of less than 5 mm. This degree of resolution is necessary for detection of tiny objects such as appendicoliths and uroliths.

In the case presented, the EP appropriately decided that further testing was required, and ordered a noncontrast CT scan of the abdomen and pelvis. EPs must decide what question they would like answered before ordering this test, so that the appropriate imaging protocol can be followed. For example, when looking for ureteral calculi, the CT scan should be done without GI or IV contrast since the scan is looking for a radiographically white stone along the course of the ureter. When IV contrast is administered, it will be excreted by the kidney into the ureter, obscuring the stone. Hydronephrosis, if present, will still be evident when IV contrast is used, but hydronephrosis is not always present with symptomatic ureteral calculi.

The optimal protocol for CT scanning for appendicitis has been a matter of debate in the literature in recent years. The standard approach in most hospitals currently is to use IV and oral contrast. The literature suggests that other approaches may be viable, and EPs need to be aware of these issues to best treat the broad range of patients they encounter. For example, IV contrast can cause renal compromise, especially in patients with preexisting renal insufficiency. Oral contrast often requires more than 45 minutes to cause opacification of the appendix; this delay may be acceptable in a 33 year old man with abdominal pain, but is not acceptable when AAA is a possibility.

Other imaging options for patients suspected of having appendicitis include plain radiographs and ultrasound. There are several nonspecific plain film findings in appendicitis such as a focal RLQ ileus (the sentinel loop) or a RLQ soft tissue mass, but the only finding that is specific for appendicitis is an appendicolith. While CT scan can demonstrate an appendicolith in 40–50% of patients with appendicitis, <10% will be evident of plain films; therefore, they are not recommended for the evaluation of suspected appendicitis. The only clear indications for plain abdominal films are for suspected pneumoperitoneum, bowel obstruction, and radiopaque foreign bodies in the GI tract.

Ultrasound has been used for over 20 years to assist in the diagnosis of appendicitis and more than 3 dozen studies have been published in the medical literature looking at its accuracy. It is a technically challenging exam that involves graded compression of the RLQ in search of the appendix. Good analgesia is required to be successful. There are 3 sonographic findings which suggest appendicitis: a noncompressible appendix that has a diameter > 6 mm, the presence of a complex mass in the RLQ, and the presence of an appendicolith. The literature suggests an extremely wide variation exists in the ability of various hospitals to perform ultrasonography accurately for appendicitis. Studies have found that ultrasound can have a sensitivity as low as 36%[18] or as high as 99%.[19] Similarly, specificities range from 68%[19] to 97%.[20] Ultrasonography for appendicitis is a very operator-dependent study that can, in experienced hands, be accurate. In reality, the accuracy of this study is unlikely to surpass that of helical CT scanning, which does not suffer from the poor inter-operator reliability that plagues sonography. Ultrasonography may have a place in the evaluation of pregnant women, and for young children who may not lie still for the CT scan.

V. CT FINDINGS WITH APPENDICITIS; SHOULD CONTRAST BE GIVEN, AND HOW?

CT findings with appendicitis are appendiceal diameter of > 6 mm and periappendiceal inflammatory changes. An appendicolith can be seen in 40–50% of cases. Several studies[1-4] have examined the use of rectal contrast alone for the diagnosis of appendicitis and have found it to be very accurate. The sensitivity of helical CT scans with rectal contrast alone has ranged from 95%–98%.[3-4] Specificities were also good, ranging from 92%–100%. Advantages of this approach include the ability to perform the scan immediately after the contrast is administered (avoiding the 45–60 minute wait required with oral contrast), and lab testing of renal function is not necessary since IV contrast is not used. Other studies have found that CT scanning with no contrast whatsoever is also accurate.[5-10] These studies found the sensitivities of 90% to 96% while the specificities ranged from 85 %–99%. This still means that as many as 10% of those with appendicitis can be missed without contrast. The majority of studies utilizing CT for the diagnosis of appendicitis have used both IV and oral contrast.[4, 11-16] This approach has yielded a range of sensitivities of 91%–100%, the great majority demonstrate a sensitivity of ≥ 95%. Specificities ranged from 92%–98%. Several authors have examined the economic impact of CT scanning for appendicitis and found it to be a cost-effective test. Rao et al., reported that scanning all patients with possible appendicitis saved $447 per patient by reducing unnecessary hospitalizations and surgeries.[17] Another group found that CT scanning was cost-effective if the negative appendectomy rate was ≥ 13%;[12] most centers report a negative appendectomy rate of approximately 20%.

VI. DECISION MAKING WITH NEGATIVE, NONCONTRAST CT

In the case at hand, the noncontrast CT scan reportedly showed no evidence of appendicitis. This could have been a falsely negative CT scan, or it is possible that the reviewing radiologist looked only for ureteral stones since this was the indication. The CT interpretation stated: "unremarkable helical CT of abdomen and pelvis." It did not mention if the appendix was even seen. In these situations, it is important to discuss the case with the radiologist, explaining your concerns—additional information may make the difference between an accurate and inaccurate interpretation. If the radiologist still feels the CT is negative for appendicitis, the EP would have 2 options. If the index of suspicion for appendicitis was low, the EP might well decide that the negative noncontrast CT scan lowered the likelihood of appendicitis sufficiently to allow the patient to be discharged. Reexamination should then occur within the next 6–12 hours.

If the level of suspicion is high, a contrast-enhanced scan may be appropriate to improve the sensitivity. Some hospitals routinely perform abdomen/pelvic CT scans with and without contrast to improve accuracy, even though this doubles the radiation dose, to say nothing of the additional cost. In either case, while CT is very accurate, it is not infallible in diagnosing appendicitis. If the EP believes a patient has appendicitis despite an unremarkable CT scan, hospitalization or ED observation is prudent.

VII. CT DIAGNOSIS FOR OTHER INTRA-ABDOMINAL CONDITIONS—AORTIC ANEURYSM, DIVERTICULITIS, SMALL BOWEL OBSTRUCTION

CT scanning has proven valuable in evaluating a number of other conditions that cause abdominal pain. The imaging modality of choice today for ureteral calculi is noncontrast CT scan. CT is both sensitive and specific for this diagnosis. Even stones that have passed from the ureter are usually seen within the bladder. Stones seen within the renal parenchyma are generally not symptomatic, and other causes of pain should be sought in these patients.

Helical CT is also very accurate in diagnosing diverticulitis; it will demonstrate diverticula if they are present and will demonstrate inflammatory changes if diverticulitis is present. While helical CT can be falsely negative early in the disease process, several studies have demonstrated an accuracy of up to 99% when performed only with rectal contrast.[21,22] Traditionally, scans done to evaluate for diverticulitis are performed with oral and IV contrast.

Abdominal aortic aneurysm (AAA) can be rapidly fatal if not diagnosed quickly; the most rapid way to diagnose AAA is with a bedside ultrasound performed by the EP. It is clearly within the scope of EP practice to perform bedside ultrasound exams for evaluation of suspected AAA, abdominal trauma, first trimester pregnancy evaluation, pericardial tamponade, renal colic, and acute biliary disease.[23] When the aorta can be visualized from the diaphragm to its bifurcation, EPs have been found to be extremely accurate in diagnosing AAA in symptomatic patients.[24] The ultrasound exam can be completed in less than 5 minutes, while other interventions are being performed. If the EP cannot perform the ultrasound exam, radiology department ultrasound technicians can come to the ED to perform a bedside exam if they are immediately available. Ultrasound is not accurate in determining if the AAA has ruptured, but the primary question in this clinical setting is whether an aneurysm is present or not. Stable patients can undergo CT scanning, a very accurate method of diagnosing both the size and location of the aneurysm. Intravenous contrast will assist in determining the involvement of any branch vessels, but is not necessary to make the diagnosis of AAA. In emergent situations, when waiting for renal function studies may jeopardize the patient, an immediate noncontrast CT scan will quickly tell the EP whether the patient has an AAA.

CT is also extremely useful in diagnosing small bowel obstructions. The "obstruction series," consisting of an upright chest, upright abdomen and supine abdomen radiographs, has classically been used to rule in or rule out the diagnosis of a small bowel obstruction (SBO). Unfortunately, plain films are not nearly as accurate as many once believed they were; plain films have been found to be diagnostic in only 50% of SBO's.[25] CT findings include dilation of the bowel proximal to the obstruction and collapse of the bowel distal to the obstruction. When directly compared with plain films, CT has had a better sensitivity (93% vs. 77%) and specificity (100% vs. 50%), and is much more likely to identify the cause of the obstruction (87% vs. 7%).[26] CT scanning with oral and IV contrast should be considered for patients in whom you suspect a SBO but have nondiagnostic films, or whenever the differential includes another diagnosis that can be confirmed by CT (e.g., diverticulitis, AAA).

VIII. SUMMARY OF CASE

In the case presented, it is not clear whether the emergency physician gave serious consideration to the possible diagnosis of appendicitis. The unusual character of the patient's complaints (abnormal urinary stream, intermittent pain, radiation to the right groin) certainly were not typical of appendicitis, but did not remove it from the differential diagnosis. If ureterolithiasis was found, concurrent appendicitis would have been extremely unlikely, but with a negative scan, an explanation of the RLQ pain was still elusive. Given focal tenderness in the right lower quadrant, the emergency physician should have done one of the following: discharge the patient with scheduled reexamination within 6–12 hours, obtain surgical consultation, CT scan with GI and IV contrast, or admission.

TEACHING POINTS ABOUT CASE 2:

- Men with RLQ pain need to have an evaluation to specifically exclude appendicitis.
- CT scanning of the abdomen is a very accurate, but not perfect, test for appendicitis.
- When patients with continued RLQ pain are discharged, even after a negative CT scan, they need scheduled reexamination within 6–12 hours if the pain persists.
- When employed with the appropriate protocol, CT can be very helpful in diagnosing diverticulitis, AAA, small bowel obstruction, and ureteral lithiasis.

REFERENCES

1. American College of Emergency Physicians. ACEP emergency ultrasound guidelines–2001. Ann Emerg Med 2001; 38:470-81.
2. Balthazar EJ, Rofsky NM, Zucker R. Appendicitis: the impact of computed tomography imaging on negative appendectomy and perforation rates. Am J Gastroenterol 1998; 93:768-71.
3. Chen SC, Chen KM, Wang SM, et al. Abdominal sonography screening of clinically diagnosed or suspected appendicitis before surgery. World J Surg 1998; 22:449-52.
4. Choi YH, Fischer E, Hoda SA, et al. Appendiceal CT in 140 cases. Diagnostic criteria for acute and necrotizing appendicitis. Clin Imaging 1998; 22:252-71.
5. Ege G, Akman H, Sahin A, et al. Diagnostic value of unenhanced helical CT in adult patients with suspected acute appendicitis. Br J Radiol 2002; 75:721-5.
6. Hershko DD, Sroka G, Bahouth H, et al. The role of selective computed tomography in the diagnosis and management of suspected acute appendicitis. Am Surg 2002; 68:1003-7.
7. Kircher MF, Rhea JT, Kihiczak D, et al. Frequency, sensitivity, and specificity of individual signs of diverticulitis on thin-section helical CT with colonic contrast material: experience with 312 cases. AJR Am J Roentgenol 2002; 178:1313-8.
8. Kuhn M, Bonnin RL, Davey MJ, et al. Emergency department ultrasound scanning for abdominal aortic aneurysm: accessible, accurate, and advantageous. Ann Emerg Med 2000; 36:219-23.
9. Lane MJ, Katz DS, Ross BA, et al. Unenhanced helical CT for suspected acute appendicitis. AJR Am J Roentgenol 1997; 168:405-9.
10. Lane MJ, Liu DM, Huynh MD, et al. Suspected acute appendicitis: nonenhanced helical CT in 300 consecutive patients. Radiology 1999; 213:341-6.
11. Mullins ME, Kircher MF, Ryan DP, et al. Evaluation of suspected appendicitis in children using limited helical CT and colonic contrast material. AJR Am J Roentgenol 2001; 176:37-41.
12. Peck J, Peck A, Peck C. The clinical role of noncontrast helical computed tomography in the diagnosis of acute appendicitis. Am J Surg 2000; 180:133-6.
13. Pickuth D, Spielmann RP. Unenhanced spiral CT for evaluating acute appendicitis in daily routine. A prospective study. Hepatogastroenterology 2001; 48:140-2.
14. Raman SS, Lu DS, Kadell BM, Vodopich DJ, Sayre J, Cryer H. Accuracy of nonfocused helical CT for the diagnosis of acute appendicitis: a 5-year review. AJR Am J Roentgenol 2002; 178:1319-25.
15. Rao PM, Rhea JT, Novelline RA, et al. Helical CT combined with contrast material administered only through the colon for imaging of suspected appendicitis. AJR Am J Roentgenol 1997; 169:1275-80.
16. Rao PM, Rhea JT, Novelline RA, et al. Effect of computed tomography of the appendix on treatment of patients and use of hospital resources. N Engl J Med 1998; 338:141-6.

17. Rao PM, Rhea JT, Novelline RA, et al. Helical CT with only colonic contrast material for diagnosing diverticulitis: prospective evaluation of 150 patients. AJR Am J Roentgenol 1998; 170:1445-9.
18. Schuler JG, Shortsleeve MJ, Goldenson RS, et al. Is there a role for abdominal computed tomographic scans in appendicitis? Arch Surg 1998; 133:373-6; discussion 377.
19. Shrake PD, Rex DK, Lappas JC, Maglinte DD. Radiographic evaluation of suspected small bowel obstruction. Am J Gastroenterol 1991; 86:175-8.
20. Sivit CJ, Applegate KE, Berlin SC, et al. Evaluation of suspected appendicitis in children and young adults: helical CT. Radiology 2000; 216:430-3.
21. Skaane P, Schistad O, Amland PF, Solheim K. Routine ultrasonography in the diagnosis of acute appendicitis: a valuable tool in daily practice? Am Surg 1997; 63:937-42.
22. Suri S, Gupta S, Sudhakar PJ, et al. Comparative evaluation of plain films, ultrasound and CT in the diagnosis of intestinal obstruction. Acta Radiol 1999; 40:422-8.
23. Walker S, Haun W, Clark J, et al. The value of limited computed tomography with rectal contrast in the diagnosis of acute appendicitis. Am J Surg 2000; 180:450-4; discussion 454-5.
24. Wong SK, Chan LP, Yeo A. Helical CT imaging of clinically suspected appendicitis: correlation of CT and histological findings. Clin Radiol 2002; 57:741-5.
25. Yetkin G, Basak M, Isgor A, et al. Can negative appendectomy rate be decreased by using spiral computed tomography without contrast material? Acta Chir Belg 2002; 102:334-7.
26. Zielke A, Hasse C, Sitter H, Rothmund M. Influence of ultrasound on clinical decision making in acute appendicitis: a prospective study. Eur J Surg 1998; 164:201-9.

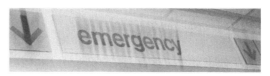

CASE 3

71 YEAR OLD MALE WITH BACK PAIN

Commentary:
Gregory L. Henry, MD, FACEP

CEO, Medical Practice Risk Assessment, Inc., Ann Arbor, Michigan
Clinical Professor, Department of Emergency Medicine
    University of Michigan Medical School, Ann Arbor, Michigan
Past President, American College of Emergency Physicians (ACEP)

Discussion:
M. Jacob Ott, MD

Ohio Chapter, American College of Emergency Physicians (ACEP)
    Ultrasound Instructor
Attending ED physician & ED Ultrasound Director
    Mt. Carmel St. Ann's Emergency Department
    Westerville, Ohio

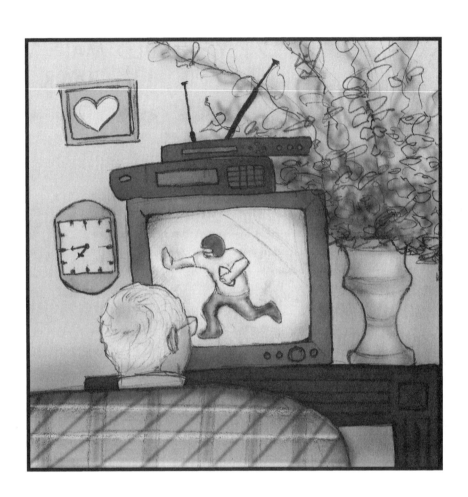

71 YEAR OLD MALE WITH BACK PAIN

—Initial Visit*—

*Authors' Note: The history, exam and notes are the actual documentation of the physicians and providers, including abbreviations (and spelling errors)

CHIEF COMPLAINT (AT 20:36): Back pain

VITAL SIGNS Time	Temp(F)	Pulse	Resp	Syst	Diast	Pos.	O2 sat	O2%	Pain scale
20:48	97.1(oral)	72	20	140	80	L			6
21:34		66	16	122	70	S		2L NC	
00:11		71	16	113	67	S	98	RA	2

HISTORY OF PRESENT ILLNESS (at 21:09): 71yo WM with h/o HTN reports was watching the game and it had just started overtime when felt a spasm and pain in left lower back. Denies any twisting/turning/lifting/trauma to the back. Reports lay down on the hard floor to help the pain, took 2 advil from his wife and placed a cool cloth on the back. Still with spasm and unable to get up off the floor, so called 911 for assistance to ED. Denies any known recent back injury. No prior illness. No cough/rhinorrhea/chest pain/ear ache/sore throat/dysuria/hematuria/urinary incontinence/numbness or tingling down extremities/bowel or bladder dysfunction/weakness in legs. Denies chest pain/abd. p., fever

PAST MEDICAL HISTORY/TRIAGE:

(RN): Pain started spontaneously while at home watching TV. Pain is a stabbing, pressure in the left lower back that does not radiate. Denies trauma. Denies pain, or burning with urination.

Medications, common allergies: Morphine (nausea)

Current meds: Prinivil

PMH: Hypertension, kidney stones

PSH: Lobectomy for TB in the 1960's

EXAM (at 21:10)

General: Alert and oriented X3, well-appearing WM in no acute distress; lying flat on his back on the bed; unable to sit upright, but can roll over on his side

Head: Normocephalic; atraumatic.

Resp: Normal chest excursion with respiration; breath sounds clear and equal bilaterally; no wheezes, rhonchi, or rales

Card: Regular rhythm, without murmurs, rub or gallop

Abd: Non-distended; Patient has some tenderness to palpation in left upper quadrant without guarding or rebound

Back: No c/t/l midline tenderness; +tenderness to palpation over left paraspinous area in lumbar region

Ext: 5/5 strength DF/PF at ankles/IS/HS/quads; nl sensation to light touch; patellar DTR's 2+ and symmetric bilaterally; neg SLR bilaterally; 2+ DP pulses bilaterally

Skin: Normal for age and race; warm and dry; no apparent lesions

ORDERS:

At 21:00: Demerol 50 mg IVP, Phenergan 12.5 mg IVP, .9NS – 1L bolus
At 23:39: Vicodin 2 PO, Vicodin 2 PO to go

RESULTS (Reviewed at 21:58):

Test	Flag	Value	Units	Ref. Range
WBC	H	15.3	K/uL	4.6-10.2
HGB	L	13.2	G/DL	13.5-17.5
PLT		175	K/uL	142-424

Test	Flag	Value	Units	Ref. Range
NA		135	MMOL/L	135-144
K		5.1	MMOL/L	3.5-5.1
CL		102	MMOL/L	98-107
CO2		26	MMOL/L	22-29
BUN	H	22	MG/DL	7-18
CREAT		1.3	MG/DL	0.6-1.3

LFT's, amylase/lipase: WNL

Urine dip stick: Protein; Results: Trace

PROGRESS NOTES (at 23:39): Abdominal exam benign with palpation although reports that abdomen sore with palpation of lower left side and upper left side. Still with some muscle spasm in the lower back, but able to walk and desires to go home. Counseled patient to return immediately for worsening abdominal pain, fevers, etc.

DIAGNOSIS: Spasm - muscle, back

DISPOSITION: The patient was discharged to Home ambulatory. Follow-up with primary care physician in 2 days. Prescriptions: Vicodin 5mg Twenty (20). Take 1-2 by mouth every 4-6 hours as needed. Released from the ED at 00:19.

Gregory L. Henry comments:

"Nothing in this history or physical exam defines muscular back spasm; this chart has nothing to defend it"

In this case a 71 year old man, with no history of back pain and no history of a lifting or traumatic injury, has a sudden onset of pain while watching television, symptoms which should never be attributed to muscular spasm. Don't forget that most patients with back pain have had a problem for years, and specific factors bring on the symptoms. Also, patients who have kidney stones generally have a history of kidney stones. The onset of sudden pain, without trauma, back pain history or kidney history, should immediately raise the possibility of aortic aneurysm.

Back pain is ubiquitous, but not in 71 year olds at rest. A 31 year old man lifting fertilizer bags who, at the end of the day, has severe back pain and abnormal physical findings, is a completely different entity than the patient in this case. Clinical judgment is important.

The evaluation and exam of this patient covers a considerable portion of his anatomy, yet the problem with this evaluation is the thought process. A physician who believes that abnormal urine is needed for a diagnosis of kidney stone has a core knowledge problem; urine positive for blood does not definitively diagnose a kidney stone. Hematuria can be seen with dissecting aneurysms if the aneurysm involves the renal arteries.

Nothing in this history or physical exam defines muscular back spasm; this chart has nothing to defend it.

- Thoroughness of Documentation: 7 out of 10.

- Thoroughness of Patient evaluation: 6 out of 10.

- Risk of Serious Illness Being Missed: High risk.

- Risk Management Legal Rating: High risk.

71 YEAR OLD MALE WITH
BACK PAIN

—Second Visit: 2 Days Later—

CHIEF COMPLAINT (at 21:09): Abdominal pain

```
VITAL SIGNS                                      O2
Time   Temp(F)  Pulse  Resp  Syst  Diast  Pos.  sat   O2%
21:16  96.1(T)  122    29    96    49     L     100   21NC
21:27           123    34    80    40     L     100   2LnC
```

HISTORY OF PRESENT ILLNESS (at 21:13): The patient is a 71-year-old male with a past history of hypertension who presents here today per squad. After he was on the toilet, he had the sudden onset of abdominal pain, which radiated through his back. The abdominal pain began suddenly. It is constant since that time, although the back pain has decreased. When I evaluated him, it had resolved. He had not received any medications for this. The back pain was severe and the abdominal pain was severe. After the pain beg. he called his primary doctor but did not hear back for 15 minutes so then called the squad. When the squad was called and they were transported him to the cart, he did have a syncopal episode. This incident occurred today about 15 minutes prior to calling the EMS. The patient denies any other complaints except he does have shortness of breath. He does deny runny nose, coughing, skin rash, chest pain, blood in the urine or stool.

PAST MEDICAL HISTORY/TRIAGE:

Per triage RN: Pt. called EMS with c/o severe back pain, sudden onset approx. 15 minutes prior to calling EMS. Upon EMS arrival pt. did have a syncopal episode, was and remains pale with low BP. After IV bolus per EMS pt. did arouse and is weak but able to answer questions at this time.

Allergies: Morphine (nausea)

Current meds: Prinivil/zestril and Vicodin

Social history: The patient said he was a smoker but stopped 40 years ago.

PHYSICAL EXAMINATION:

General: The patient is pale, diaphoretic; however, he was alert and responsive.

Lungs: The lungs are clear.

Cardiovascular: The heart is regular and tachycardic.

Abdomen: The abdomen does have voluntary guarding and it is moderately distended. He does have a pulsatile mass palpated in the left side of the abdomen.

Extremities: His femoral pulses were both present but slightly decreased. He did not have any peripheral edema on examination of the calf muscles.

HEENT: Examination of the eyes revealed round pupils but the palpebral conjunctiva was extremely pale.

Skin: As previously stated, his skin was pale. He was diaphoretic. His mental status was alert and oriented, although he did keep closing his eyes but when questioned he did seem to respond appropriately. He denied any headache or fever.

EMERGENCY ROOM COURSE:

21:09: This patient presented to the Emergency Department. I immediately evaluated the patient.

21:13: After the initial evaluation, a clinical diagnosis was made of ruptured aortic abdominal aneurysm, and the operating room was called to ready the operating room for emergency surgery and the vascular surgeon was also called.

21:16: The vascular surgeon called back. I informed him of this patient's condition and diagnosis and he said he would come in immediately for emergency surgery.

I did speak with him 2 other times during the patient's course; once when he called back to ensure that the surgical team was assembled, and I did tell him that we had made arrangements for that. In addition, the patient had O- blood, which was taken to the OR as the pt. was already there.

Also, I spoke with the surgical house officer just after speaking with the vascular surgeon and he immediately came down to evaluate the patient.

RESULTS:

Test	Flag	Value	Units	Ref. Range
WBC		10.1	K/uL	4.6-10.2
HGB	L	6.5	G/DL	13.5-17.5
PLT		185	K/uL	142-424

Test	Flag	Value	Units	Ref. Range
NA		135	MMOL/L	135-144
K		3.4	MMOL/L	3.5-5.1
CL		105	MMOL/L	98-107
AGAP		12.4	MMOL/L	6.0-18.0
CO2	L	21	MMOL/L	22-29

Test	Flag	Value	Units	Ref. Range
BUN		18	MG/DL	7-18
CREAT	H	1.4	MG/DL	0.6-1.3

Accudata (at 21:24): Fingertstick blood sugar-230

DIAGNOSIS: Acute ruptured AAA with hypotension and anemia

DISPOSITION (at 21:31) (Per RN notes): Pt. taken to surg. At this time, surg. House officer is here seeing the pt. Wife present and chaplin called per her request

HOSPITAL COURSE:

********** **Operative Report** **********

Preoperative Diagnosis: Ruptured abdominal aortic aneurysm.

Postoperative Diagnosis: Ruptured abdominal aortic aneurysm.

Operation: 1) Aorto-bi-iliac bypass with a 16x8 mm Hemashield graft.

  2) Reimplantation of inferior mesenteric artery.

Procedure: Upon entering, there was some free blood within the abdomen and a large retroperitoneal hematoma. The aorta was grasped and clamped. The aneurysm was then opened and back-bleeding lumbars were oversewn with interrupted 3-0 Prolene. Once hemostasis had been obtained, I chose a 16x8 mm Hemashield graft for the bypass. This sewn in end-to-end fashion to the proximal aorta. I then turned my attention to the left leg where I transected the common iliac artery and then sewed the graft in an end-to-side fashion to the iliac vessel. At that point, I inspected the sigmoid colon, which appeared somewhat dusky. It did not have good back-bleeding, so I reimplantated the inferior mesenteric artery. The patient was transferred to the Intensive Care Unit in stable condition

FINAL DIAGNOSIS: Ruptured abdominal aortic aneurysm.

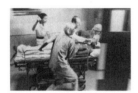

EVALUATION FOR ABDOMINAL AORTIC ANEURYSM, BEDSIDE ED ULTRASOUND

M. Jacob Ott, MD

I. INTRODUCTION

This patient unfortunately waited until his second visit to read the textbook. He returned to the emergency department with the classic triad of ruptured abdominal aortic aneurysm (AAA); hypotension, abdominal or back pain, and pulsatile abdominal mass. At this point in his presentation, it would be expected that his diagnosis be made immediately, without ancillary testing, and prompt resuscitation and surgical treatment initiated. This is exactly what occurred—he went straight to the operating room. Most patients are not kind enough to read the textbook, and recognition of the less common presentations, as well as a high index of suspicion, are absolutely necessary.

II. ABDOMINAL AORTIC ANEURYSM (AAA)

AAA is a common condition, and one which is likely to increase in prevalence as the population ages. The incidence is about 11% in men over 65. It is much more prevalent in men than in women (7:1 ratio), and is the cause of death of 1.2% of males in the US. Since 1970, there has been a 300% increase in the overall prevalence of AAA. To add insult to injury, most aneurysms are asymptomatic until they rupture, and once ruptured, the mortality is very high. Most asymptomatic aneurysms are detected as an incidental finding on CT scan or ultrasound of the abdomen, and usually patients who present with ruptured AAA have no prior known history of AAA, as occurred with our patient.

III. CLINICAL EVALUATION OF PATIENTS WITH SUSPECTED AAA

This patient presented initially with isolated lower back pain of sudden onset, without associated symptoms. This is one of many presentations of AAA. The most common presenting symptoms include syncope, abdominal pain, shock, back pain, or sudden death.[1] Unfortunately, most patients will present atypically, with only 1 or 2 of these symptoms; the classic triad of hypotension, abdominal or back pain, and pulsatile abdominal mass is present in less than 50% of patients.[1] AAA should be strongly suspected in patients age 55 or older with back pain, shock, or syncope of unknown etiology, and younger patients where multiple risk factors for atherosclerosis (such as hypertension or tobacco use) are present.[1,3] Our patient had several risk factors which should have raised concern: age (71), presence of hypertension, and sudden onset back pain. In addition, the history of tobacco use was elicited on the second visit, but was probably insignificant, since he quit several decades ago. His pain began the day of presentation, but longer duration of symptoms does not rule out AAA. Some patients can experience days to weeks of symptoms before seeking medical attention.[1]

The physical examination from the first visit documented tenderness to palpation over the lateral lower back and may have led the physician astray. Physical findings for AAA can be unreliable,[2] and can even point away from a diagnosis of AAA, as was the case here. For example, abdominal palpation has been reported to have a sensitivity of around 67%, with slightly higher sensitivity for larger aneurysms.[2] Femoral pulses frequently will be unaffected, even by aneurysm rupture, until shock is present. Cullen and Grey Turner's signs (periumbilical and flank ecchymosis indicating possible retroperitoneal hematoma) occur only rarely.[2,4] Obesity may also limit the physical exam, with regard to the abdomen. Other physical exam findings include flank tenderness due to the presence of retroperitoneal blood or an iliopsoas sign. To summarize, the absence of physical exam findings is not sufficient to rule out AAA.

On his second visit, the patient had several of the above mentioned physical signs, including abdominal tenderness, pulsatile mass, evidence of shock, and anemia. Careful evaluation of the primary presentation reveals several signs which could have led to the diagnosis, including left sided abdominal and left flank tenderness. Patients with musculoskeletal back pain should not have abdominal tenderness. Positive physical exam findings such as abdominal tenderness should be explored with additional history or some form of ancillary testing. If the pain cannot be explained, a plan should be made for further evaluation.

IV. THE ROLE OF ANCILLARY TESTING FOR AAA: LABS, X-RAY, CT

The diagnosis of ruptured AAA is often clinical. The presence of hypotension or instability should provoke action without ancillary testing; CT scanning is contraindicated in this case due to delay of definitive treatment and risk of an unstable patient leaving the ED. At the first visit, when the diagnosis was unclear, ancillary testing may have been of use. We will focus on those tests here.

Laboratory Evaluation: Blood tests, such as a CBC, electrolytes, and glucose, as well as BUN and creatinine, are rarely useful in the diagnosis of AAA. They may reveal, however, associated conditions, such as anemia from blood loss, or renal failure from involvement of the renal arteries, both are late findings. Other tests, such as lactate, CRP, or ESR, are of minimal value.

Radiologic Evaluation: Several radiographic studies may be of use in the evaluation of the aorta; each with advantages and disadvantages.

Plain Radiography: Plain radiography, including the upright abdominal film (KUB) and acute abdominal series (AAS), are the least useful modalities. They can identify AAA by the presence of calcifications in the mid abdomen. This is rather insensitive, however, showing the presence of AAA in only about 50% of patients. In addition, plain radiography is insensitive for leaking or rupture. The advantages of plain films over more sensitive modalities are speed and portability. As more sensitive and specific modalities are available, plain films are seldom used in this clinical setting.

CT Scan: CT scan with intravenous contrast is very sensitive for the detection of AAA. It is also very sensitive for ruptured or leaking AAA. It has the unique advantage of evaluating the retroperitoneum, where most aneurysms leak when they rupture. These advantages would seemingly make it an obvious choice for the evaluation of AAA, and it is a viable option in stable patients. The primary disadvantage is that the scanner is not portable, and the patient must be transported to the radiology department. This can be very limiting in evaluating unstable patients or those who may become unstable. Just as in the evaluation of trauma patients, transporting an unstable patient out of the ED, except to the OR, is inadvisable. As patients with ruptured AAA are likely to require emergent vascular surgery consultation and definitive management without the benefits of CT scan, portable modalities for the detection of AAA are essential.

V. EMERGENCY DEPARTMENT ULTRASOUND

Emergency Department ultrasound (EDUS) is an emerging technology, useful for a variety of clinical conditions[5] including diagnosis of AAA. It has several advantages over traditional imaging modalities, mostly the ability to use it at the bedside of even the most unstable patient. First, the diagnostic study can be performed while the patient is being stabilized, which saves valuable time in the resuscitation of hypotensive patients. Second, ultrasound is very sensitive and specific for the detection of AAA.[5,7,8,10] Third, if the aortic ultrasound examination is negative for AAA, other ultrasound examinations, including Focused Assessment with Sonography for Trauma (FAST scan), echocardiography, and venous Doppler, can be used to readily identify other causes of hypotension,[5,15] thus bedside ultrasound is rapidly becoming the test of choice for unstable patients. We will discuss the use of ultrasound in the diagnosis of AAA, and evaluate how it could have been applied to improve our patient's outcome.

Anatomy:

The abdominal aorta enters the retroperitoneum at the diaphragm, just to the left of the vertebral bodies, and courses through the abdomen to the level of the umbilicus, where it bifurcates into the common iliac arteries. Prior to bifurcation, the aorta gives off several branches, including the celiac artery, the superior and inferior mesenteric arteries, and left and right renal arteries. All of these branches can be easily visualized on ultrasound. Identification of the renal arteries is important, since aneurysms are defined by their relationship to these arteries (either infrarenal or suprarenal). The other branching arteries can be used as landmarks to help differentiate the aorta from the inferior vena cava.

Sonographic Findings:
The normal abdominal aorta is less than 3 cm in diameter at any point. It is widest when it enters the retroperitoneum at the diaphragm, and tapers distally, reaching a minimum width just prior to its bifurcation. Any dilatation greater than 3 cm is abnormal. The diameter of the common iliac arteries is maximally 1.5 cm in males, and 1.2 cm in females. The celiac trunk will be found just beneath the xiphoid process, running perpendicular to the aorta. The superior mesenteric artery, found several centimeters caudally, runs parallel to the aorta.

Anatomic landmarks or doppler should be used to differentiate the aorta from the inferior vena cava, which lies to the right of the vertebral body, in similar position to the aorta. If color flow Doppler is used, a pulsatile flow will be noted in the aorta (a pulsatile waveform with dicrotic notch will be seen if pulse Doppler is used). The presence of visual pulsations is not helpful, as transmitted pulsations can be seen in the vena cava.[3,5]

Once the aorta is identified, it should be followed from the xiphoid process all the way to the bifurcation. Any area which seems to be abnormally dilated should be measured. An aortic diameter greater than 3 cm is, by definition, an AAA. The aorta can also be viewed in long and short axes, to increase the detection of aneurysms. Aneurysms are most often fusiform, but can be bulbous, secular, dumbbell in shape[3,5,7]. No matter the shape of the aorta, the maximum normal measurement is 3 cm. Aneurysms can range in size from 3 to 14 cm, and are often readily visible. A mural thrombus will appear as heterogeneous gray matter in the lumen (figure 5). Dissection may also be present, but is rarely seen on ultrasound. Dissection can occur independently of AAA, and the presence of one does not imply the other.

Aortic rupture is the most feared complication of AAA. Blood is not usually seen on ultrasound[3,5], as most AAA's will rupture retroperitoneally, which is poorly visualized on ultrasound. If intraperitoneal rupture does occur, the blood will be visible on ultrasound. A FAST exam should be performed on all hypotensive patients with AAA[3]. Even if free intraperitoneal fluid is not found, all symptomatic and hypotensive patients with the presence of AAA should be assumed to have some degree of rupture, prompting surgical consultation.[9,10]

If the aorta is visualized from the xiphoid to the bifurcation, and is not dilated greater than 3 cm at any point, the aorta is normal. Time permitting, the iliac arteries should also be scanned since a significant proportion of patients with AAA will also have iliac aneurysms.

VI. CLINICAL UTILITY OF EDUS
Bedside ultrasound of the abdominal aorta, when performed by experienced operators, is essentially 100% sensitive for the detection of aneurysm,[8,9,13] with a miniscule rate of false positives.[12] Limiting factors on study quality include large body habitus and the presence of bowel gas. Certain techniques will decrease these limitations. The only major contraindication to bedside ultrasound is delay of definitive operative management. Due to the sensitivity in the detection of aneurysm, and availability and usefulness as an adjunct to the physical examination, EDUS should be considered in all patients with suspicion of abdominal aortic rupture.

Our patient is a perfect example of someone whose management would have improved by the availability of bedside ultrasound. Although his diagnosis was obvious on his second visit, requiring no confirmatory studies, the clinical picture during the first visit was not so clear. AAA is part of the differential diagnosis for anyone older than 55 with back pain; ultrasound could have been used to detect the presence of his AAA. Fortunately, the patient survived to his second visit, and the diagnosis was made; most patients are not so lucky.

VII. ULTRASOUND EVALUATION OF THE PATIENT WITH HYPOTENSION OF UNKNOWN ETIOLOGY

The evaluation of the patient with hypotension of unknown etiology can be very difficult. The differential diagnosis is broad, time to make a diagnosis is limited, and arrival at the correct diagnosis is essential since management of different etiologies vary widely. The symptoms of cardiogenic shock and hypovolemic shock can be similar, but the treatments are opposite; hypovolemic shock is treated with fluids or blood, while their use in cardiogenic shock could lead to a bad outcome. EDUS can differentiate between causes of hypotension and facilitate effective management. Hypovolemia can be evaluated with a FAST scan or US of the aorta, and limited cardiac ultrasonography and measurement of the inferior vena cava can diagnose cardiogenic shock. Findings include decreased wall motion and a larger than normal IVC which does not collapse with respirations[3,5]. In addition, the pericardium can be easily viewed to evaluate for pericardial effusion and cardiac tamponade.

In female patients of reproductive age, ultrasound of the uterus and adnexa can also find a ruptured ectopic pregnancy.[3] Although this was not in the differential diagnosis for our patient, it is an important cause of hypotension in pregnant women.

Combining these exams allows for a rapid screen for various causes of shock with more specific management, including prompt surgical consultation.

VIII. CONCLUSION

To summarize, our patient was a 71 year old male initially presenting with lower back pain with eventual diagnosis of a ruptured AAA, requiring operative management. Two important diagnostic failures occured in this case: first, the failure to think about AAA in an older patient with back pain, and second, failure to order a complete workup, including imaging examinations, when the diagnosis did not match the history and physical exam.

By the second presentation, the patient symptoms had become more "textbook," and his diagnosis was readily apparent. A high index of suspicion, and the liberal use of screening imaging tests such as bedside ultrasound, is absolutely essential to diagnosing AAA when the disease process is in its earliest stages.

TEACHING POINTS ABOUT CASE 3:

- Include AAA in the differential diagnosis of older patients with back pain or younger patients with risk factors.
- Positive physical exam findings, such as abdominal tenderness, need to be explored with history and ancillary testing, or addressed in a progress note with a plan for further evaluation.
- Bedside ultrasound of the abdominal aorta is essentially 100% sensitive for the detection of aneurysm.

Figure 1. Normal Sonographic Appearance of the Abdominal Aorta at the level of the renal arteries

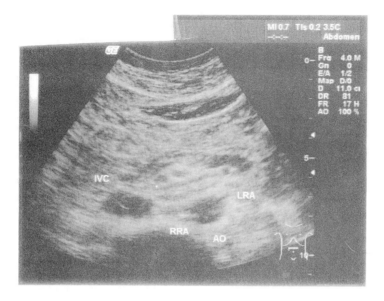

IVC = inferior vena cava; AO = Aorta; LRA = left renal artery; RRA = right renal artery

Figure 2. Normal Sonographic Appearance of the Common Iliac Arteries (at the bifurcation of the aorta)

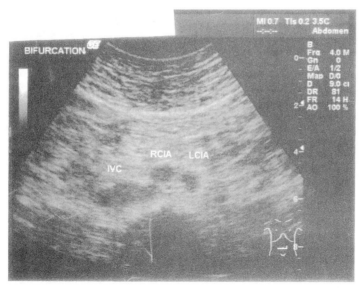

IVC = inferior vena cava; LCIA = left common iliac artery; RCIA = right common iliac artery

Figure 3. Long axis view of a normal aorta with Pulse Doppler Waveform

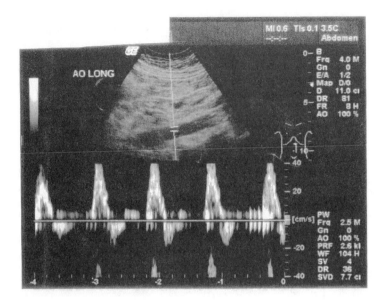

Figure 4. Abdominal Aortic Aneurysm with internal thrombus

Note the 7.68 cm aneurysm with internal thrombus

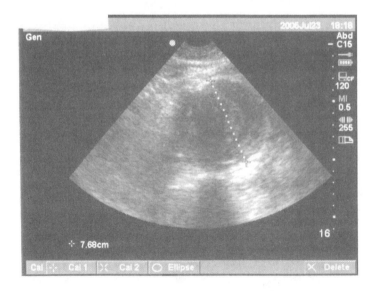

Figure 5. Abdominal Aortic Aneurysm with internal thrombus

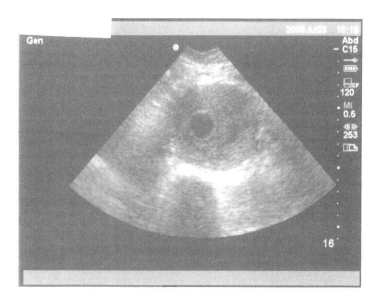

Figure 6. Free Intraperitoneal Fluid in Morrison's pouch on FAST Scan

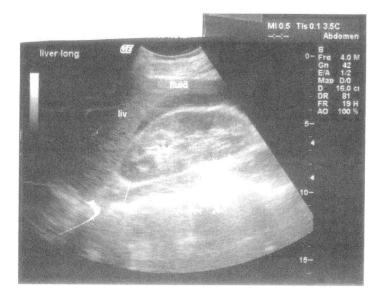

Figure 7. Free Intraperitoneal Fluid Above Liver and in Morrison's pouch (between liver and kidney)

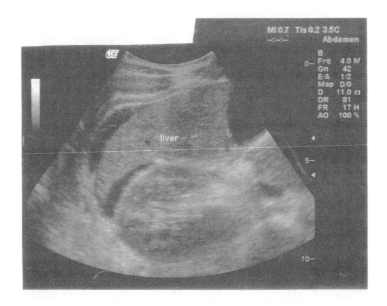

Figure 8. Pericardial Effusion on FAST Scan

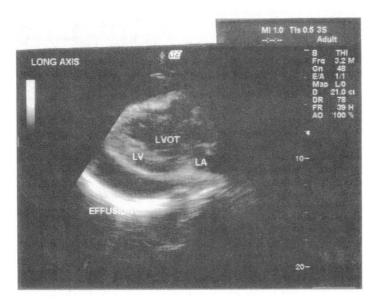

LV = left ventricle; LVOT = left ventricular outflow tract; LA = left atrium

REFERENCES

1. Tintinalli JE, ed. Emergency medicine, a comprehensive study guide. 5th ed. New York: McGraw Hill, 2000; 413-416.
2. Venkatasubramaniam AK, et al. The value of abdominal examination in the diagnosis of abdominal aortic aneurysm. Eur J Vasc Endovasc Surg 2004;27:56-60.
3. Jones, R. Emergency medical ultrasound. 2001 Ohio ACEP basic ultrasound syllabus. (Ch. 3: 1-24).
4. Niemann JT. The accuracy of physical examination to detect abdominal aortic aneurysm. Ann Emerg Med 2001; 37:3.
5. Ma O J, Mateer JR. Emergency ultrasound. New York: McGraw Hill, 2003; 128-41.
6. Norman, PE, et al. Population based randomized controlled trial on impact of screening on mortality from abdominal aortic aneurysm. BMJ 2004; 329(7477):1259.
7. Rogers RL, McCormack R: Aortic disasters. Emerg Med Clin North Am 2004;22:887-908.
8. Barkin AZ, Rosen CL. Ultrasound detection of abdominal aortic aneurysm. Emerg Med Clin North Am 2004; 22:675-82.
9. Hermsen K, Chong WK. Ultrasound evaluation of abdominal aortic and iliac aneurysms and mesenteric ischemia. Radiol Clin North Am 2004; 42:365-81.
10. Walker A, Brenchley J, Sloan JP, et al. Ultrasound by emergency physicians to detect abdominal aortic aneurysms: a UK case series. Emerg Med J 2004; 21:257-9.
11. Prisant LM, Mondy JS 3rd Abdominal aortic aneurysm. J Clin Hypertens (Greenwich) 2004; 6:85-9.
12. Lyon M, Brannam L, Ciamillo L, et al. False positive abdominal aortic aneurysm on bedside emergency ultrasound. J Emerg Med 2004;26:193-6.
13. Blaivas M, Theodoro D. Frequency of incomplete abdominal aorta visualization by emergency department bedside ultrasound. Acad Emerg Med 2004;11:103-5.
14. Salen P, Melanson S, Buro D. ED screening to identify abdominal aortic aneurysms in asymptomatic geriatric patients. Am J Emerg Med. 2003;21:133-5.
15. Hendrickson RG, Dean AJ, Costantino TG. A novel use of ultrasound in pulseless electrical activity: the diagnosis of an acute abdominal aortic aneurysm rupture. J Emerg Med 2001; 21:141-4.

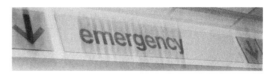

CASE 4

37 YEAR OLD FEMALE WITH HEADACHE & FLU-LIKE SYMPTOMS

Commentary:
Gregory L. Henry, MD, FACEP

CEO, Medical Practice Risk Assessment, Inc., Ann Arbor, Michigan
Clinical Professor, Department of Emergency Medicine
   University of Michigan Medical School, Ann Arbor, Michigan
Past President, American College of Emergency Physicians (ACEP)

Discussion:
Andy Jagoda, MD, FACEP

Professor and Vice Chair
   Department of Emergency Medicine
   Mount Sinai School of Medicine
   New York, New York
Chair, ACEP Clinical Policies Committee
Chair, ACEP Clinical Policy Subcommittee on Acute Headaches
Editor in Chief, Emergency Medicine Practice

John Bruns, Jr., MD

Assistant Professor
   Department of Emergency Medicine
   Mount Sinai School of Medicine
   New York, New York

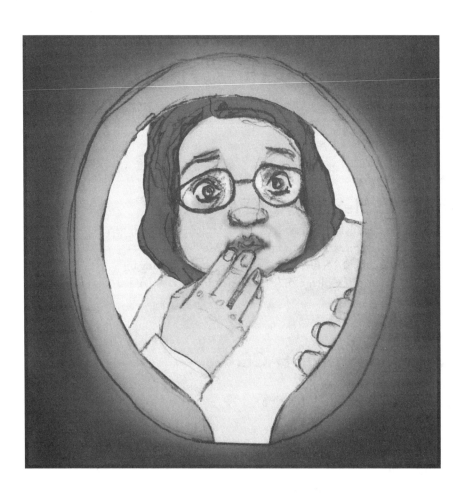

37 YEAR OLD FEMALE WITH
HEADACHE & FLU-LIKE SYMPTOMS

—Initial Visit*—

*Authors' Note: The history, exam and notes are the actual documentation of the physicians and providers, including abbreviations (and spelling errors)

CHIEF COMPLAINT (at 08:54): Flu-like symptoms

Time	Temp (F)	Rt.	Pulse	Resp	Syst	Diast	Pos	O2	sat O2%	Pain scale
08:57	97.8	Tym.	76	18	141	94	S			
09:12			59	20	126	37	S	100	100	8
11:19	97.3	Oral	88	16	120	70	S			4
12:00			68	20	108	56	S			2

HISTORY OF PRESENT ILLNESS (at 09:12): The patient presents with a spontaneous onset of a severe, sharp frontal headache that began gradually today at 6AM. The symptoms are constant and 8/10 in severity. She did have vomiting which beg. 3 hours ago. She did use Tylenol which was minimally effective. She does not have a history of headaches. Patient complains of photophobia. She denies, fever, rash, confusion, loss of consciousness, weakness of the extremities, slurred speech, vertigo, myalgias, diplopia or blurred vision, cough, rhinorrhea, facial pain, neck stiffness, lightheadedness, nausea/vomiting, or abdominal pain.

PAST MEDICAL HISTORY/TRIAGE:
Allergies: NKDA
Medications: Tylenol
PMH: None
PSH: None
Social history: No smoking, alcohol or drugs
Family history: Heart disease, HTN. No CA, DM, CVA.

PHYSICAL EXAM (AT 09:17):
General: Well-developed, well-nourished, poorly-hydrated individual in no acute respiratory distress.
Eyes: Pupils are equal, round and reactive to light. The extraocular muscles are intact. Fundoscopic exam is normal. Eyelids, conjunctiva, iris, and sclera are normal.
Ears: External ears are normal. The TM's are normal.
Nose: The nose is normal in appearance. There is no rhinorrhea.
Mouth/dental: The lips, gums, and teeth appear normal. There are no exudates or erosions on the buccal mucosa. The uvula is mid-line. The tonsils are not inflamed or erythematous. The posterior pharynx is free erythema and exudates.

Neck: The trachea is mid-line. The neck is supple and non-tender to palpation. There is no cervical lymphadenopathy. No masses or thyromegaly, no JVD.

Cardiovascular: The heart has a regular rate and rhythm. S1 and S2 are normal, no murmur, gallop, or rub. Apical impulse is normal. No JVD. Normal pulsations. No hepatojugular reflux or dependent edema. 2+ pulses bilaterally, no bruits, no mottling or cyanosis of the extremities. Brisk capillary refill. Radial, carotid and femoral pulses are normal. Bilaterally the lungs are clear and the abdominal exam is normal.

Respiratory: Respiratory rate and effort are normal. There is normal chest excursion with respiration. The lungs are clear to auscultation and percussion bilaterally.

GI: The abdomen is normal in appearance. Bowel sounds are normal and are heard in all four quadrants. There are no abdominal bruits. There is no pain with palpation. There is no evidence of spleen or liver enlargement. No masses were palpated.

Musculoskeletal: There are no deformities noted in all four extremities. There is full ROM with movement. The joints are non-tender to palpation.

Integumentary: The skin appears normal for age and race. It is warm and dry.

Neuro: Patient is alert and oriented to person, place, and time. Cranial nerves II-XII are intact. Sensory and motor functions are intact. Biceps, triceps, patellar, and achilles are equal and intact. Downward plantar reflexes are normal. Finger to nose is WNL. Grasp is equal bilaterally. The gait is normal.

ORDERS (at 09:17): Demerol 50mg IVP, Phenergan 12.5mg IVP. IV fluids NS 2 L bolus

RESULTS (results at 10:53):

Test	Flag	Value	Units	Ref. Range
WBC	H	13.1	K/uL	4.6-10.2
HGB	L	13.4	G/DL	13.5-17.5
PLT		254	K/uL	142-424

Test	Flag	Value	Units	Ref. Range
NA		136	MMOL/L	135-144
K		3.9	MMOL/L	3.5-5.1
CL		102	MMOL/L	98-107
CO2		28	MMOL/L	22-29
BUN		12	MG/DL	7-18
CREAT		0.8	MG/DL	0.6-1.3

Test	Flag	Value	Units	Ref. Range
CKH		233	U/L	21-232
CKMB	H	5.9	NG/ML	0.0-5.0
RELIND		2.5		0.0-4.0
TROPI		.06	NG/ML	.00-.27

Urine: Urine pregnancy – negative. Urine dip – WNL.

PROGRESS NOTES (at 11:57): Patient is feeling much better. The patient's condition is much improved. Patient is ready to go home. Spinal tap was discussed with the patient and her husband, but they refused, promising to return if fever, stiff neck, weakness, paralysis, or sensory loss.

RADIOLOGY: Unenhanced brain CT: Negative

DIAGNOSIS (at 11:58): Gastroenteritis, Cephalgia

DISPOSITION: The patient was discharged home. Follow with the PCP on call (she is given name and number) if not improved in 3-4 days. Aftercare instructions for gastroenteritis and headache. Prescriptions for Phenergan and Darvocet-N 100. Released at 12:26.

Gregory L. Henry comments:

"Normal examinations and benign histories do not, and should not, prompt further investigation"

Most people do not understand the flu. Headache and vomiting are not the flu. This patient's symptoms are very general and extremely common. With essentially normal vital signs and examination, minimal further evaluation is necessary for this patient.

The chief complaint and history discuss the gradual onset of headache and vomiting, without respiratory symptoms or cough. The physician has documented good review of systems which are all negative. In a patient with a new onset of headache, one must consider the condition of the furnace; documentation should include whether other members of the household have similar symptoms.

The evaluation of this patient seems reasonable. A good neurologic examination is performed. However, the laboratory workup is overkill—the only study of interest in this patient would be a carbon monoxide level. Instead, everything else (and the kitchen sink) is ordered. I have no idea what a set of electrolytes, CBC, or cardiac enzymes would show, and the justification for these labs is not well defended. The need for a pregnancy test is also questionable.

The most difficult study to rationalize is the CT scan. The plain CT scan, in a patient with a normal neurologic exam, generally shows nothing. In this case, the history and examination gave no indication of an intracranial bleed, mass lesion, or brain trauma. The un-enhanced CT scan for this type of problem should be outlawed; there is no bang for the buck. Normal examinations and benign histories do not, and should not, prompt further investigation. The patient was discharged on Phenergan, which is in no way inappropriate.

Documentation for this case is quite good.

- Thoroughness of documentation: 9 out of 10.
- Thoroughness of Patient Evaluation: 9 out of 10.
- Risk of Serious Illness Being Missed: Low risk.
- Risk Management Legal Rating: Low risk.

37 YEAR OLD FEMALE WITH HEADACHE & FLU-LIKE SYMPTOMS

—Second Visit: 3 Days Later—

CHIEF COMPLAINT (at 18:34): Numbness

```
VITAL SIGNS:
```

Time	Temp(F)	Rt.	Pulse	Resp	Syst	Diast	Pos	O2 sat
19:07	99.1	Tym.	77	18	162	84	S	
23:03			72	18	155	82	S	
23:23			78	20	158	78	S	99
01:31			88	16	150	91	S	98
02:11			81	19	165	75	L	100

HISTORY OF PRESENT ILLNESS (at 21:21): Pt. awoke from nap around 3:30 pm with left arm/hand numbness and weakness. Pt also felt that she had slurred speech when talking to her child. Pt. c/o intermittent headache and neck pains over past 4 days. Occasional blurred vision. Pt c/o neck pain currently but denies headache currently. Pt seen here a few days for headache and had negative head CT at that time. No previous hx of similar symptoms. She has not problems walking. No fever, unexplained weight change or malaise. No chest pain, SOB or edema. No cough or respiratory distress. No nausea, vomiting, diarrhea or abdominal pain. No dysuria, frequency or burning

EXAM (at 21:24):
General: Well-appearing; well nourished; A&O X 3, in no apparent distress.
Head: Normocephalic; atraumatic.
Eyes: PERRL; EOMI
Ears: TM's normal;
Nose: Normal nose; no rhinorrhea;
Throat: Normal pharynx with no tonsillar hypertrophy. Moist mucosa.
Neck: Supple; non-tender; no cervical lymphadenopathy.
Card: Regular rate and rhythm, no murmurs, rubs or gallops
Resp: Normal chest excursion with respiration; breath sounds clear and equal bilaterally; no wheezes, rhonchi, or rales.
Abd: Non-distended; soft and non-tender , without rigidity, rebound or guarding
Skin: Normal for age and race; warm and dry; no apparent lesions
Neuro/psych: Alert and oriented x3, cranial nerves II-XII intact, normal mentation. Upper and lower extremity strength weaker on left compared to right. Strenth 4/5 on left compared to 5/5. Biceps, patellar and achilles reflexes normal bilaterally. Coordination and gait are normal. Normal mood and mentation. Cerebellum testing OK.

ORDERS: Demerol 25mg IVP and phenergan 12.5mg IVP (21:18), phenergan 12.5mg IVP (22:50)

RESULTS (Resulted per physician at 00:17)

Test	Flag	Value	Units	Ref. Range
WBC		9.2	K/uL	4.6-10.2
HGB		13.5	G/DL	13.5-17.5
PLT		296	K/uL	142-424

Test	Flag	Value	Units	Ref. Range
NA		139	MMOL/L	135-144
K		3.9	MMOL/L	3.5-5.1
CL		101	MMOL/L	98-107
CO2		29	MMOL/L	22-29
BUN		7	MG/DL	7-18
CREAT		0.8	MG/DL	0.6-1.3

Test	Flag	Value	Units	Ref. Range
CKH		233	U/L	21-232
CKMB	H	5.9	NG/ML	0.0-5.0
RELIND		2.5		0.0-4.0
TROPI		.06	NG/ML	.00-.27

PT/INR/PTT - WNL

Urinalysis: WBC: 0-5, RBC: 10-25, Bacteria: Rare

RADIOLOGY: CT scan of the brain without contrast (ordered at 20:50 and results at 21:17): Indication: Left facial numbness. Left arm numbness for 1 day. Evaluate for CVA. CONCLUSIONS: No acute intracranial abnormality.

PROGRESS NOTES:

At 22:40 the patient is better with hand grip and foot strength on repeat exam. Pt with continued right sided neck pain up into occiput area requiring narcotics. Pt to be admittted for observation tonite. Pt still with what I think is slightly weaker grip in her left hand which is her dominant hand on repeat exams.

Lumbar puncture (ordered at 23:08 and procedure documented at 23:41):

Test	Value	Units	Ref. Range
CSF	Clear		Clear
CSF WBC CT	0	CMM	0-8
CSF RBC CT	1	CMM	0-8
CSFGLUC	64	MG/DL	40-75
CSFPROT	34	MMOL/L	15.0-45.0

GRAM STAIN: No polys, few mononuclear cells, no organisms seen

PROGRESS NOTES (continued):

At 23:23 (per RN) notes a sudden change of pat condition and physician given notice of pat. and noted incont of urine with right eye diff to right and left puple to left able to move gen. body with out cordinatioin. pat noted to have n/v.

At 23:46 (per MD) a CT of the neck was ordered.

At 01:35 follows some commands, grips with r hand, r eye deviated to r, perrl, spontaneous movement of r arm and leg, only slight movement of l side.

At 02:02 received a call from the radiologist. Patient noted to have an occluded Right ICA on Ct neck (see reading below). Spoke with the neurologist about possible intra-arterial TPA and was told that she's not a candidate because patient most likely has a carotid dissection. She reports that she puts these patients on heparin. Spoke with another neurologist about the results of CT scan and also about possibility of heparin. Patient had an LP approx 2.5 hours ago. Will begin patient on low dose heparin with careful checks of lower extremities and LP site. Patient can go to step down bed per neurologist as has remained stable for over 3 hours and no ICU bed available.

ENHANCED NECK CT: The findings are consistent with occlusion of the right internal carotid artery of unclear cause. Carotid dissection is a possibility. Further evaluation with a conventional angiogram could be obtained if clinically indicated. No neck masses or lymphadenopathy are present.

DIAGNOSIS (at 02:31):

1. Altered mental status
2. Left sided weakness/numbness – resolving
3. Neck pain
4. Hx of headaches
5. Vomiting episode in ED
6. Carotid artery occlusion

DISPOSITION: Disposition Admit the patient to stepdown unit. Left the ED at 03:06.

INPATIENT COURSE

MRI and MRA OF THE BRAIN WITH CONTRAST (ordered at 10:56 the next morning):

1. Findings are most consistent with a large right middle cerebral artery distribution infarct with edema in the right hemisphere and a small amount of subfalcine herniation.
2. Occlusion of the right internal carotid artery 1 cm from its origin. The etiology of the occlusion is not clear. A dissection would be in the differential.
3. I do not see any flow within the right internal carotid artery. There is flow within the right anterior cerebral artery that I suspect is due to communication through the anterior communicating artery. I believe there is a small amount of flow within the proximal right middle cerebral artery but minimal flow is present more distally. The left anterior circulation, as well as the vertebrobasilar system is unremarkable   .

********** **CT Report (the next day)************

CT-BRAIN W/O C: CT OF THE BRAIN – IMPRESSION: The findings suggest trans-falcine and transtentorial herniation of the infarcted right hemisphere in addition to a brainstem infarct.

********** **Nuclear Medicine Report** **********
CEREBRAL FLOW STUDY FOR BRAIN DEATH—IMPRESSION: Positive examination. No intracerebral flow is visualized on this exam. The finding is consistent with brain death as clinically suspected.

********** **Echocardiogram Report** **********
CONCLUSION: Essentially normal resting study with LVEF of 55 to 60%.

********** **Cardiovascular Report** **********
BILATERAL CAROTID DUPLEX IMAGING—same day
1. On the right side, velocities within the internal carotid artery are markedly diminished and the waveforms are severely blunted with no diastolic flow suggestive of a more distal stenosis or occlusion. The intracervical portion of the internal carotid artery appears widely patent and without evidence of stenosis.
2. On the left side, the internal carotid artery is patent and without significant plaque disease.
3. Both the right and left vertebral arteries demonstrate antegrade flow.

********** **Electroencephalogram Report two days after admission** **********
IMPRESSION: Electrical-cerebral inactivity consistent with brain death.

Physician note (2 days after admission): Patient is unresponsive with pupils fixed. No purposeful movements. BP is the 40's and HR 150's. She is now DNR CC. Extubated after EEG. Family aware and very reasonable. Continue supportive care. Prognosis terminal.

FINAL DIAGNOSIS: Carotid artery dissection.

Additional Gregory L. Henry comments:

Having now read the final outcome, let me just say that neurology is my field of interest and I would not have picked up on this case early on. The patient did return some three days later, and a question of a carotid artery occlusion was raised and she went on to stroke, and then herniated her brain. All the king's horses and all the king's men are not going to make this go away. She went from being awake and alert with some left-side weakness to being comatose within hours. There is no specific therapy for this problem and it is wrong for the emergency physician on the first visit to somehow blame him/herself for the outcome. There will be, once in your career, a case such as this and there is nothing you can do to prevent it. If every patient with a normal exam and a headache were admitted to the hospital for angiographic studies, we would hurt more people than we help. It is the nature of medicine that we will not diagnose all disease.

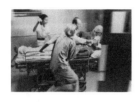

EVALUATION OF HEADACHES IN ADULTS AND DISCUSSION OF CAROTID ARTERY DISSECTION

Andy Jagoda, MD, FACEP
John Bruns, Jr., MD

I. INTRODUCTION

The patient was an otherwise healthy 37 year old female without prior headache history. She presented with an acute onset of severe sharp frontal headache (HA), nausea and vomiting (NV), and photophobia. The review of symptoms (ROS) was unremarkable except for noting that the patient did not have NV, which contradicted the history of present illness (HPI). There was no mention of trauma in the HPI and no mention of cervical bruits on the initial physical exam. If the neck had been auscultated, bruits may have been found, but this evaluation was not indicated during the initial encounter.

II. EVALUATION OF HEADACHES IN ADULTS

Headache is the chief compliant in 1 million ED visits per year, but only 3.8 % of these patients have a serious intracranial etiology.[1] HA can be divided by etiological classification into primary and secondary based on H&P. Etiologies of primary HA include tension (47%), migraine (31%), cluster (7%), rebound (narcotics or caffeine) and neuralgias (trigeminal, occipital). Etiologies of secondary HA are listed below (Table 1).

Table 1. Etiologies of Secondary or Symptomatic Headaches

Metabolic	Medications	Trauma
Hypoxemia	Nitrites	Head injury
Hypoglycemia	Indomethacin	Traumatic brain injury
Hypercarbia	Vasodilators	Subdural hematoma
Anemia		Subarachnoid hemorrhage
Hypertensive encephalopathy	**Toxins**	Spinal injury
Hypo/hyperthyroidism	Carbon monoxide	Facial injury
Hypoadrenalism	Lead	Carotid artery dissection
Altitude	Benzene	Post concussive syndrome
Coital headache	Insecticides	
	Nitrites	**Vascular**
Brain abnormality	Methanol	Temporal arteritis
Intracranial hemorrhage	MSG	
SAH		**Infectious**
ICH	**Ocular**	Meningitis
Stroke	Glaucoma	Encephalitis
Malignancy		Otitis/Mastoiditis
Tumor/Mass lesion	Idiopathic Intracranial	Pharyngitis/tonsillitis
	Hypertension	Zoster
Pregnancy		RMSF
Eclampsia/pre-eclampsia	**Psychiatric**	Ventriculoperitoneal shunt
Cerebral venous thrombosis	Psychological/psychiatric	malfunction/infection
	etiology	
Neuralgia		**Other**
Trigeminal		TMJ
Glossopharyngeal		

Adapted from Henry GL, et al. Neurological emergencies, a system oriented approach, 2nd ed. New York:McGraw-Hill, 2003.

For the patient presenting with new HA, or a HA different than their normal pattern, e\ character, intensity or duration, a cautious approach is prudent. Multiple categorization strat\ exist for secondary HA based on acuity of onset, character of pain, associated signs or sympt\ and patient demographics. An acute onset, severe HA has a particularly worrisome differential (Table 2). A thorough HPI, ROS, PMHx, Social and Medication history (including nonprescription and herbal preparations or their withdrawal) will typically narrow the differential diagnosis of secondary HA considerably.

Table 2. Differential Diagnosis of Atraumatic, Sudden Onset, Severe Headache

Subarachnoid Hemorrhage (SAH)
Carotid / Vertebral Artery Dissection
Cerebral Venous Thrombosis
Idiopathic Intracranial Hypertension

In this case, the acuity and severity of her symptoms, combined with an absence of an alternative diagnosis, warrant the acquisition of a head CT followed by an LP, looking for subarachnoid hemorrhage (SAH). A head CT is noninvasive and may reveal SAH or alternative etiology prior to LP.

The American College of Emergency Physicians (ACEP) recommends that patients presenting to the ED with HA and new neurological deficit or mental status changes, or presenting with acute sudden-onset HA, be considered for an emergent head CT. Additionally, patients over 50 years of age with a new type of HA should be considered for urgent neuroimaging, regardless of physical findings.[2]

Labs are usually unnecessary except for coagulation studies before lumbar puncture (LP) if indication of coagulopathy exists. Lumbar puncture should be performed for CSF analysis if CNS infection or SAH is suspected. Neuroimaging should be performed prior to LP in patients with papilledema, absent spontaneous venous pulsations on fundoscopy, altered mental status, or focal neurological findings. If SAH is suspected, head CT should precede LP. Patients with a thunderclap HA, normal head CT, normal opening pressure and normal CSF analysis do not need emergent angiography and can be discharged with appropriate follow up.[2]

In this case, head CT was negative and the patient declined LP. Feeling and looking well, she was appropriately discharged home on analgesics and in the company of a responsible adult. She declined LP, which prompts the medical-legal issue of discharging her against medical advice (AMA).

I disagree with the diagnosis of gastroenteritis. In the absence of a confident diagnosis, a symptomatic diagnosis would keep the differential diagnosis open, particularly for any subsequent medical encounters. In addition, given the differential diagnosis, lack of LP, and resultant diagnostic uncertainty, "three to four days" is a long time for follow up.

III. MANAGEMENT OF PRIMARY HEADACHES IN THE ED

In patients with a history of primary migraine, tension, or cluster HA, with a typical character and intensity of pain, symptomatic relief is usually all that is indicated. Most HA pharmacotherapy literature pertains to migraines and typically includes serotonin (5-HT) agonists. Since many HA patients have an idiosyncratic response to medications, my approach is to first utilize previously effective agents. Prochlorperazine (Compazine) and metaclopramide (Reglan) are good initial agents

HA, and sumatriptan (Imitrex) may be beneficial in migraines and cluster.
useful in cluster HA. NSAIDS, acetaminophen, or opiates are recommended

phenergan were administered in the ED. These medications did at least
her symptoms. According to the ACEP Clinical Policy regarding HA, pain response to
therapy should not be used as a diagnostic indicator of the underlying etiology of an acute headache.[2]

IV. DISCUSSION OF THE SECOND ED VISIT AND DIAGNOSIS OF CAROTID ARTERY DISSECTION

The second ED visit triage note stated that the patient had HA and neck pain for 4 days, and awoke 3 hr 37 min prior to ED presentation with left arm and hand numbness/weakness and slurred speech. The PE lacked a fundoscopic exam or assessment for a cervical bruit. Positive findings included left upper and left lower extremity weakness without facial involvement, miosis or oculosympathetic paresis. Upon presentation, I would have initiated consultation with interventional radiology and neurosurgery for an interdisciplinary approach to this patient with serious focal neurological findings. Initial labs should include metabolic and coagulation studies, toxicology screen, ESR, pregnancy test and ECG.

A differential diagnosis including carotid artery dissection (CAD), SAH, and spinal cord pathology should be considered. Presentations of CAD are highly varied (Table 3).[3] In CAD, an acute onset headache of varying character is typically ipsilateral and may include facial (maxillary and periorbital) pain and neck pain, particularly along the sternocleidomastoid muscle.[4] HA usually precedes a cerebral ischemic event by a median time of 4 days,[5] as in this case. TIAs may result from hemodynamic insufficiency, whereas strokes appear to be caused by embolization from carotid thrombus formation, and are found in 30–80% of presenting patients. Oculosympathetic paresis (Horner syndrome with miosis, ptosis, and facial anhydrosis), or more likely Raeder's syndrome (ptosis and miosis, but lacking anhydrosis), is present in up to 50% of CAD patients.[6] Cranial nerve deficits are present in about 10% of patients with extracranial CAD, as a result of aneurysmal dilatation or vascular supply compromise.

Table 3. Signs and Symptoms in Patients with Carotid Artery Dissection[6]

Sign or Symptom	Proportion of Patients %
Ipsilateral headache (slow onset, constant)	58-92
Cerebral ischemia	63-90
Oculosympathetic paresis	9-75
Neck pain	18-46
Subjective bruit / Pulsatile tinnitus	12-39
Scalp tenderness	8-27
ICA tenderness	8-19
CN Palsy	5-12
Syncope	11
Amaurosis Fugax	4-6
Neck swelling	3

Source: Zetterling M, Carlstrom C, Konrad P. Internal carotid artery dissection. Acta Neurol Scand 2000;101:1-7. Copyright 2000 Blackwell Publishing. Used with permission.

Head CT is typically the initial imaging study in patients with neurological signs. Head CT was ordered 103 minutes after the ED presentation; although this patient presented outside the 3 hour window for thrombolysis of ischemic stroke, neuroimaging should have occurred quicker. Stroke protocols can shorten the time to head CT acquisition—our institution has target times of door-to-CT completion and interpretation, of 25 minutes and 45 minutes respectively.

While the diagnostic accuracy for CAD has improved with neuroimaging techniques, head CT is an insensitive and unreliable screening technique since the neck is not evaluated. Therefore, with a high index of suspicion and a normal head CT, other imaging modalities such as MRI/ MRA of the head and neck should be pursued.

Etiological categorizations of stroke in young patients are presented below in Table 4.[7] In this case, CAD would have surfaced as a leading possibility. The US incidence of symptomatic CAD is 2.6 per 100,000 annually, and is a significant cause of stroke in patients younger than 45 years of age. Any of the cervical arteries may be affected, but internal carotid artery dissections (63%) are the most common, followed by the vertebrals (30%) and multi-vessel (7%). CAD often occurs in previously healthy individuals and develops either spontaneously, or following obvious or subtle injury. Obvious blunt trauma accounts for only 3—10% of CADs. Although trivial neck positioning or manipulation has been cited repeatedly in the literature, recall bias may have influenced this data. Antecedent infection, particularly URI, has been elicited as an independent risk factor,[8] but many CADs occur spontaneously.

Table 4. Causes of Stroke in Patients Less than Age 40

Cause	Patients (total 272)
Atherothrombotic	25
Cardioembolic	17
Non-atherosclerotic vasculopathy	17
Migraine 13 (29)	29
Dissection of extracranial arteries	20
Others	51
Hypercoagulable state	4
Cerebral venous thrombosis	1

Source: Varona JF, Bermejo F, Guerra JM, et al. Long-term prognosis of ischemic stroke in young adults. Study of 272 cases. J Neurol 2004; 51:1507-14. Copyright Steinkopff 2004. Used with permission.

Dissecting ICA aneurysms are the etiology of SAH in 0.3% of all SAH's, and in 3.1% of unverified cases of SAH.[9] In these cases, lumbar puncture results may be misleading, since xanthochromia may occur with rostral hematoma propagation. This finding may lead the physician to treat for SAH and neglect to perform further carotid work up. ECG and echocardiography may be performed to rule out a cardiac source of the emboli.

At 11:23 PM, the nursing records note acute neurological deterioration, anisocoria and NV. The patient rapidly deteriorates from this point secondary to massive cerebral edema, intracranial hypertension and transtentorial herniation.

A cervical CT was then ordered and read at 2:02 AM as "right ICA occlusion of uncertain etiology, no neck mass, consider carotid dissection." Cervical CT is currently a reliable screening technique for CAD, although helical CT may be used in the future.

MRI has surpassed angiography as the imaging study of choice for CAD. MRI proves dissection by direct viewing of the intramural hematoma with a hyperintense, crescent-shaped signal on T1 and T2 weighted images utilizing fat suppression.[10] MRI also depicts the degree of wall expansion and any effect on anatomically proximate structures. Magnetic resonance angiography (MRA) is performed noninvasively during an MRI study and allows multiplanar vessel imaging without intravenous contrast.[11] The combination of MRI and MRA is more sensitive for CAD diagnosis than either modality individually. Brain MRI and MRA were ordered at 10:56 the morning of admission, which revealed "a right middle cerebral artery infarct with edema and herniation, right ICA occlusion ...consider CAD." The diagnosis was inconclusive; however, the late night reader and (probable) use of teleradiology may have been suboptimal for CAD.

Previously the gold standard diagnostic study for CAD was contrast arteriography, which should still be strongly considered in patients with contraindications to MRI. Pathognomonic angiographic findings include a double lumen, intimal flap, a "string sign" with a long tapered narrowing, segmental stenosis or occlusion, or multiple scalloped narrowings. The disadvantage of angiography is its invasiveness; however, as part of therapeutic intervention with intra-arterial thrombolysis and stenting, the role of angiography will be evolving as endovascular therapies for CAD mature.

There are no pathognomonic sonographic findings for CAD. Although often nonspecific, abnormal flows are identified with up to 90% accuracy. It is quick, noninvasive, and can be performed early at the bedside to detect the characteristic pattern of dissection. Confirmatory MRI/MRA imaging is almost always indicated. The day following admission, bilateral carotid duplex imaging showed diminished velocities and blunted waveforms in the right ICA with normal cervical vasculature otherwise.

V. MANAGEMENT OF CAROTID ARTERY DISSECTION

The management of CAD is based on incomplete evidence and no treatment standards exist. It is imperative to consider any associated injuries, the anatomic location of the dissection, and the type of dissection before initiating treatment. Most dissections heal spontaneously, most aneurysms never rupture, and they infrequently cause delayed ischemic complications. Therefore, a medical approach is recommended for most pediatric and adult patients. Ischemic sequelae are thought to be due to embolic phenomenon from the thrombus.[12] Anticoagulation and/or platelet antiaggregant therapy are recommended as the initial treatment. After consultation with a second neurologist, heparin therapy was initiated at 2:30 AM, at low dose since the patient had previously had a LP performed. Unfractionated heparin therapy followed by coumadin to a target INR of 2.5 to 3 is the mainstay of medical management. Contraindications to anticoagulation include: 1) Large infarct with associated edema and mass effect; 2) infarction hemorrhagic transformation; 3) intracranial aneurysm; and 4) intracranial dissection extension. Low molecular weight heparin has not been studied.

Antiplatelet therapy may be considered in the absence of neurological ischemic symptoms. There is no evidence to support the use of platelet antiaggregates other than aspirin. A Cochran review of medical management in CAD found no randomized trials or reliable comparisons of antiplatelet drugs or anticoagulants with controls available. Twenty-six eligible studies comparing antiplatelet drugs with anticoagulants were included in the analysis. No significant difference in the odds of death or disability was found. Few intracranial hemorrhages (0.5%) were reported for patients on anticoagulants and none for patients on antiplatelets.[13]

Endovascular therapies have largely replaced surgery, and should be considered with failure of (or contraindication to) medical therapy. Intra-arterial thrombolysis of CAD with clot propagation to the MCA has been utilized with prompt symptom resolution.[14] Intra-arterial thrombolysis has also been employed in combination with endovascular stent placement.[15] While there is little data on the efficacy of intra-arterial thrombolysis in CAD, dissection itself is not an absolute contraindication to this therapeutic intervention. Percutaneous transluminal angioplasty and stenting without thrombolysis has been utilized with no procedure-related complications, and with significant clinical improvement within the first 24 hours and complete long-term recovery.[16] Aneurysms may require coil embolization or covered stent.

Surgical intervention is recommended for progressive or persistent ischemic symptoms despite optimal medical management in patients not amenable to endovascular interventions. If adequate collateral blood flow is present, carotid artery ligation or bypass can be performed, although risks of clot propagation and aneurysm formation do exist.[17] Decompressive craniectomy in stroke patients with severe cerebral edema is a reasonable consideration. Good outcomes have been demonstrated in patients with a pre-op Glasgow Coma Scale (GCS) > 7.[18]

The prognosis of CAD depends on the severity of the initial ischemic episode; extracranial is more favorable than intracranial dissection. Younger patients have a better prognosis, but the overall prognosis of extracranial CAD is good. The risk of recurrence is inversely related to age, with the greatest risk during the first month, and a 10-year recurrence rate of 11%.[19]

VI. FINAL DISCUSSION OF CASE AND SUMMARY

This unfortunate patient had a catastrophic outcome. I agree that the initial ED visit was managed and documented appropriately. During the second medical encounter, Dr. Henry comments on the rapidity with which the patient deteriorated. While this is true, an initial consideration of the differential diagnosis appears to be lacking. Head CT scan was ordered almost 2 hours after presentation, and while it may have been appropriate for initial screening, it fails to target the most likely diagnosis given the patient's symptoms, signs, and demographics. It's difficult to fully elucidate the sequence of events that took place. Documentation would have significantly helped this physician defend the sequence of events. For example, according to the nursing note, the patient deteriorates, but there is not a physician note documenting the event until 2 hours later. This note did not discuss any diagnostic or management interventions occurring.

Carotid artery dissection is infrequently encountered and no true standard of care exists. This is a perilous case that might have had a bad outcome regardless of what interventions were provided. However, an expedited acquisition of appropriate cerebral and cervical imaging and neurological and neurosurgical consultation may have altered the outcome for this patient, or at least provided an opportunity for such.

Lessons potentially learned from this case include: 1) a need for sequential neurological evaluations and documentation; 2) the use of protocols to facilitate triage and timely physician management; 3) the early use of consultants when they are available; 4) prioritization of oxygenation and perfusion in neuroresuscitation; and 5) early transfer to a center with neurological interventions when possible.

TEACHING POINTS ABOUT CASE 4:

- Etilogies of sudden onset severe HA include Subarachnoid Hemorrhage (SAH), Carotid / Vertebral Artery Dissection, Cerebral Venous Thrombosis, and Idiopathic Intracranial Hypertension.
- Per ACEP recommendations, pain response to therapy should not be used as a diagnostic indicator of the underlying etiology of an acute headache.
- Causes of stroke in patients less than 40 are different than in the elderly.
- The imaging study of choice for diagnosis of carotid artery dissection is MRI/MRA.

REFERENCES

1. Ramirez-Lassepas M, et al. Predictors of intracranial pathologic findings in patients who seek emergency care because of headache. Arch Neurol 1997;54:1506-9.
2. American College of Emergency Physicians. Clinical policy: critical issues in the evaluation and management of patients presenting to the emergency department with acute headache. Ann Emerg Med 2002; 39:108-22.
3. Zetterling M, Carlstrom C, Konrad P. Internal carotid artery dissection. Acta Neurol Scand 2000;101:1-7.
4. Fisher CM. The headache and pain of spontaneous carotid dissection. Headache 1982; 22:60-5.
5. Silbert PL, Mokri B, SchievinkWI. Headache and neck pain in spontaneous internal carotid and vertebral artery dissections. Neurology 1995;45:1517-22.
6. Murnane M, Proano L, Raeder's paratrigeminal syndrome: a case report. Acad Emerg Med 1996;3:864-7.
7. Varona JF, Bermejo F, Guerra JM, et al. Long-term prognosis of ischemic stroke in young adults. Study of 272 cases. J Neurol 2004; 51:1507-14.
8. Grau AJ, Brandt T, Buggle F, et al. Association of cervical artery dissection with recent infection. Arch Neurol 1999;56:851-6.
9. Ohkuma H, Nakano T, Manabe H, et al. Subarachnoid hemorrhage caused by a dissecting aneurysm of the internal carotid artery. J Neurosurg 2002; 97:576-83.
10. Kirsch E, Kaim A, Engelter S, et al. MR angiography in internal carotid artery dissection: improvement of diagnosis by selective demonstration of the intramural haematoma. Neuroradiology 1998; 40:704-9.
11. Cox LK, Bertorini T, Laster RE Jr, et al. Headaches due to spontaneous internal carotid artery dissection magnetic resonance imaging evaluation and follow up. Headache 1991; 31:12-6.
12. Lucas, C., et al., Stroke patterns of internal carotid artery dissection in 40 patients. Stroke, 1998; 29:2646-8.
13. Lyrer P, Engelter S. Antithrombotic drugs for carotid artery dissection. Stroke 2004; 35:613-4.
14. Sampognaro G, Turgut T, Conners JJ 3rd, et al. Intra-arterial thrombolysis in a patient presenting with an ischemic stroke due to spontaneous internal carotid artery dissection. Catheter Cardiovasc Interv 1999;48:312-5.

15. Abboud H, Houdart E, Meseguer E, Amarenco P, et al. Stent assisted endovascular thrombolysis of internal carotid artery dissection. J Neurol Neurosurg Psychiatry 2005; 76:292-3.

16. Bejjani GK, Monsein LH, Laird JR, et al. Treatment of symptomatic cervical carotid dissections with endovascular stents. Neurosurgery 1999;44:755-60; discussion 760-1.

17. Muller BT, Luther B, Hort W, et al. Surgical treatment of 50 carotid dissections: indications and results. J Vasc Surg, 2000; 31:980-8.

18. Reddy AK, Saradhi V, Panigrahi M, et al. Decompressive craniectomy for stroke: indications and results. Neurol India 2002; 50 Suppl:S66-9.

19. Gonzales-Portillo F, Bruno A, Biller J. Outcome of extracranial cervicocephalic arterial dissections: a follow-up study. Neurol Res 2002;24:395-8.

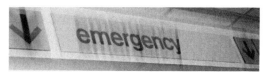

CASE 5

17 YEAR OLD MALE WITH FEVER & HEADACHE

Commentary:
Gregory L. Henry, MD, FACEP

CEO, Medical Practice Risk Assessment, Inc., Ann Arbor, Michigan
Clinical Professor, Department of Emergency Medicine
   University of Michigan Medical School, Ann Arbor, Michigan
Past President, American College of Emergency Physicians (ACEP)

Discussion:
Ann Dietrich, MD, FAAP, FACEP

Attending, ED physician, Columbus Children's Hospital
Associate Professor, The Ohio State University College of Medicine
   Columbus, Ohio
Editor-in-chief, Pediatric Emergency Medicine Reports
Editor-in-chief, Trauma Reports
ACEP, Pediatric Emergency Medicine Committee

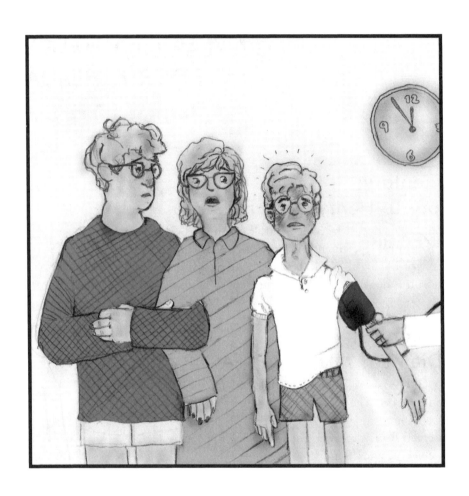

17 YEAR OLD MALE WITH FEVER & HEADACHE
—Initial Visit*—

*Authors' Note: The history, exam and notes are the actual documentation of the physicians and providers, including abbreviations (and spelling errors)

CHIEF COMPLAINT (at 23:39): Fever

VITAL SIGNS							Pain
Time	Temp	Pulse	Resp	Syst	Diast	O2 Sat	Scale
23:55	98.1	114	18	72	38	97%	5
01:21	99.0						

HISTORY OF PRESENT ILLNESS (at 00:19): Pt c/o headache and neck being sore. He c/o weakness in the arms and legs "like I have no energy in them" as described by the pt. He states they were numb earlier. He c/o a sore throat since yesterday and fever. He took Nyquil for the symptoms and temp at 7 pm was 104. He c/o bilateral ear pain. He vomited once today. He denies ill contacts.

PAST MEDICAL HISTORY/TRIAGE:
  Chief complaint/quote (Per triage RN): "fever headache legs and arms are numb" Pt. states he has had numbness in both arms and legs intermittently with stiff neck. Bilateral ear pain.
  Medication, common allergies: None
  PMH: Asthma
  PSH: None

EXAM (at 00:33):
  General: Well-appearing; well-nourished; in no apparent distress.
  Head: Normocephalic; atraumatic.
  Eyes: PERLA; EOM intact
  ENT: TM's normal; normal nose; no rhinorrhea; Throat is red, and mild exudates. Moist mucus membranes.
  Neck: Supple; nontender; no cervical lymphadenopathy. No meningeal signs
  Cardiovascular: Normal S1, S2; no murmurs, rubs, or gallops.
  Respiratory: Normal chest excursion with respiration; breath sounds clear and equal bilaterally; no wheezes, rhonchi, or rales.
  Abdomen: Normal bowel sounds; non-distended; nontender; no palpable organomegaly.
  Extremities: Normal ROM in all four extremities; nontender to palpation; distal pulses are normal and equal.
  Skin: Normal for age and race; warm; dry; good turgor; no apparent lesions or exudate.

ORDERS/RESULTS (at 01:17): Rapid strep—Negative

DIAGNOSIS (at 01:31): Unspecified viral infection

DISPOSITION: Disposition - Discharged: The patient was discharged to Home ambulatory. Follow-up with primary physician if not improved in 3 days.

"It is important to give the patient a specific follow-up time, but that time must be appropriate to the disease process at hand; in this case it was not."

The history as documented is unusual. Most 17 year olds do not want to come to the emergency department. In addition, the complaint of generalized numbness is concerning and should be taken seriously.

When one is approaching a headache patient, there are three questions on the table: a) Is there a bleed? b) Is there an infection? c) Is there a toxin, such as carbon monoxide, causing the headache? The combination of fever, headache, and stiff neck must raise the likelihood of an infectious process; meningitis is a common ED presentation, however, not everyone needs a work-up. The patient also complained of arm and leg numbness, definitely unusual symptoms for a young person. The only way to definitively diagnose meningitis is with a spinal tap.

Evaluation is problematic in this case. He presents with three neurologic complaints (headache, weakness, and numbness), raising the possibility of meningitis or encephalitis, and a neurologic examination is not documented. It is interesting that the exam notes extraocular movements, virtually never affected in an awake patient, but left out the funduscopic exam. If a patient presents with a severe headache, the fundi and condition of the optic disk should be documented. The loss of venous pulsations or papilledema would prompt a CT scan before a lumbar puncture. They have also commented that the patient is normocephalic, as if we would expect him to have a horn growing out of his head. Sensory testing, motor testing and gait observation are important considerations in a patient with a headache. The fact remains that the most important system in this patient was not examined.

Concerns about the disposition of this case are obvious. The vast majority of fever and headache patients will be sent out of the emergency department without testing, but a short interval follow up is the most important element. He was inappropriately advised to see a physician in 3 days; if such a patient is not feeling better in the next 12 hours, he should be re-examined. Symptoms, such as this patient's, tend to resolve or worsen in a fairly short period of time. It is important to give the patient a specific follow-up time, but that time must be appropriate to the disease process at hand; in this case it was not.

- Thoroughness of Documentation: 7 out of 10.

- Thoroughness of Patient Evaluation: 4 out of 10.

- Risk of Serious Illness Being Missed: High risk.

- Risk Management Legal Rating: High risk.

17 YEAR OLD MALE WITH FEVER & HEADACHE

—Second Visit: 16 Hours Later—

CHIEF COMPLAINT (at 17:55): Unresponsive

VITAL SIGNS					
Temp	Pulse	Resp	Syst	Diast	Sat O2
102.1	73	20	137	75	97%

HISTORY OF PRESENT ILLNESS (at 18:03): This is a 17-year-old white male who, according to the squad, was found unresponsive on a couch at noon on the day the patient came to the emergency department. He was at another ED on the evening prior to arrival according to his family and was sent home telling he had a viral infection. He has had a fever of 104 degrees for the last day. The family did not notice the rash yesterday or this morning, but when pointed out now, they stated that yes they did see one. They were unable to wake the patient up. They therefore called the squad. The family members indicate they did not notice any nausea or vomiting. They had indicated the patient was ill on the evening prior to arrival, complaining of fever, chills, headache, sore throat, and earaches. There has been no nausea or vomiting, and remainder of review of systems is unable to obtain secondary to the patient's obtundation.

EXAM (at 18:07):

General: The patient is obtunded. He does not appear in any acute distress, although he is moaning.

HEENT: His eyes are equal and reactive to light. He is anicteric. There is no conjunctival injection or drainage from his eyes. His pharynx is without erythema, edema, or exudates. Tympanic membranes are normal bilaterally.

Neck: The patient has nuchal rigidity. He has no thyromegaly.

Cardiovascular: Heart tones are S1 and S2 without murmur or rub. Regular rate and rhythm.

Respiratory: Normal effort, without stridor. Lungs are clear to auscultation.

Chest: The patient does not groan in pain when palpating his chest.

GI: Abdomen is soft. No tenderness, rebound, or guarding.

GU: No flank tenderness.

Lymphatic: He has no neck or groin lymphadenopathy.

Musculoskeletal: The patient has normal tone in all 4 extremities. He actively moves all 4 extremities.

Skin: Petechial rash on both upper and lower extremities, greater on the upper extremities than lower.

Neurological: The patient has motor tone in his extremities. He does withdraw to pain. He does have a normal gag reflex. Pupils do react to light.

RESULTS (at 18:48):

Test	Flag	Value	Units	Ref. range
WBC	H	12.4	K/uL	4.6-10.2
HGB	L	15.3	G/DL	13.5-17.5
PLT		143	K/uL	142-424
NA		139	MMOL/L	135-144
K	L	3.0	MMOL/L	3.5-5.1
CL		105	MMOL/L	98-107
CO2	L	21	MMOL/L	22-29
GLU	H	129	MG/DL	70-119
BUN		18	MG/DL	7-18
CREAT	H	1.4	MG/DL	0.6-1.3
PH		7.44		7.35-7.44
PCO2		33.5		35-45
PO2		128		70-100

PROGRESS NOTES: Upon the patients arrival in the emergency department, I immediately went to the patients bedside, saw the petechial rash, and noticed the nuchal rigidity along with his history and ordered Rocephin 2 gm IV stat (at 18:08). Respiratory precautions were undertaken at that point by all staff members. The patient was placed on the monitor, and Toradol as well as Decadron were given. I had spoken with infectious disease immediately upon seeing the patient as there was a concern regarding meningococcal meningitis. It was due to his recommendation that Decadron was given. The patient did receive a CT of his brain. He did not have a focal exam, but due to his obtundation, I was concerned about abscess or mass effect prior to spinal tap. CT of his brain did show an abnormality in the left dural sinus region (at 18:59). There is no evidence of contraindication to lumbar puncture. The patient had IV fluids and remained hemodynamically stable. His mental status did not improve. Also of note, the radiologist read pansinusitis disease but no evidence of acute sinusitis, and an MRI and MRV of the brain was recommended and obtained. Results were given to the critical care physician. Lumbar puncture was undertaken by myself (at 19:14). I did explain to the family the procedure, and they did agree to the risks associated with this. I did prep and drape his back in a sterile manner and anesthetized the L4-L5 interspace. I was unable to obtain CSF fluid. I went up 1 interspace, to L3-L4, and did obtain 4 cc of cloudy CSF. (See results below). The patient's initial Gram stain came back preliminary as gram positive, and Vancomycin and Acyclovir were added to his regimen. A final Gram stain did reveal the patient to have Gram-negative diplococci. Infection control had been aware of this patient since shortly after his arrival and were working on notifying the appropriate people and giving all exposures prophylaxis. Two blood cultures were sent off. Chest X-ray shows no infiltrate.

Test	Value	Units	Ref. Range
CSF	Cloudy		Clear
CSF WBC CT	11,194	CMM	0-8
CSF RBC CT	0	CMM	0-8
CSFGLUC	4	MG/DL	40-75
CSFPROT	539	MMOL/L	15.0-45.0
Differential: Segs 90%, lymphs 5%			
NO GROWTH AFTER 48 HOURS			

DIAGNOSIS (at 20:22):
1. Probable meningococcus meningitis.
2. Obtundation with altered level of consciousness.

DISPOSITION: The patient is admitted to medical service, with consults to infectious disease and the critical care physician. He is admitted to the ICU. Mental status did not change throughout the emergency department course, and the critical care time on this patient was 2 hours.

HOSPITAL COURSE:

********** **Consultation Report Infectious diseases************

GENERAL: 17-year-old fellow admitted to the hospital essentially with bacterial meningitis. He was in his otherwise state of stable health until about two days prior to admission when he developed generalized malaise, headache and fever. He was evaluated at a hospital emergency department last night and essentially, no obvious abnormalities were found. A throat swab was obtained because there was some sore throat and a question of Streptococcal disease was negative. He had a fever of 104. It was felt that he had a viral syndrome and he was released to home. However, this afternoon, he began to develop worsening lethargy and the squad was summoned. He was placed on IV Rocephin as soon as he entered the hospital. He has since received additional antibiotic therapy. He remained obtunded in the Emergency Department, however, this evening, he opens his eyes to me calling his name, and is moving his upper extremities. His lumbar puncture shows significant purulence. The gram stain on his CSF is preliminarily positive for gram-positive Diplococci.

IMPRESSION: I suspect he has bacterial meningitis and this is probably pneumococcal, given his presentation, his current appearance and perhaps even an early response to his antimicrobial therapy. Additionally, the gram stain suggests gram-positive Diplococci, again, more consistent with pneumococcal disease. At this point, I will continue broad spectrum IV antibiotic therapy, as we have begun, as well as Decadron for about 3-4 days and see how it goes.

FINAL DIAGNOSIS: Bacterial meningitis

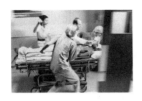

DISCUSSION OF FEVER WITHOUT A SOURCE & MENINGITIS IN CHILDREN

Ann Dietrich, MD, FAAP, FACEP

I. INTRODUCTION AND DISCUSSION OF CASE

Headaches and fever in children are common complaints; in the majority of patients they are not associated with a serious bacterial illness. Every child with a high fever may have a headache, and the majority of children will require only a careful history, thorough physical examination, and close follow up.

Our patient presented initally with symptoms concerning for meningitis: headache, fever and stiff neck. This was well documented in the nursing notes. The first two complaints were repeated in the physician HPI, and a sore neck is mentioned, but the documentation of *stiff* neck was not specifically addressed. Interestingly, the HPI is more of a listing of chief complaints than a true history. There are 7 complaints in all, including headache, sore neck, weakness and numbness of extremities, sore throat, fever, ear pain and vomiting. Unfortunately, only a few are discussed further. The numbness began "earlier," the "temp at 7PM was 104," Nyquil was used, and the ear pain was "bilateral." The other complaints were mentioned, but not discussed further.

The physical exam is more complete, with a good neck exam, but the sensitivity for excluding meningitis by neck exam is not even close to 100%! Was the exam believable? Was a child who was "found unresponsive on a couch" only 16 hours later really "well appearing" and "in no acute distress" at the initial visit?

Finally, it needs to be stressed that the responsibility on this physician was to prove that the patient did *not* have meningitis, not *to prove* that he had a "viral infection." If a lumbar puncture does not need to be done, this should be specifically addressed in a progress note. Follow up needs to be specific and obtainable. If the patient is not able to see a PCP in the recommended time, a return visit should be made to the ED.

This chapter will discuss diagnosis and management of meningitis, the role of lumbar puncture in suspected meningitis, and the evaluation of younger children with a fever without a source.

II. EVALUATION AND MANAGEMENT OF FEVER IN NEONATES AND CHILDREN LESS THAN 3 MONTHS OF AGE WITH FEVER

Fever is a common ED complaint and one that can challenge the clinician. The definition of a fever has been established as a rectal temperature of 100.4° F or higher. Any child who appears ill or has a history suggestive of serious illness (lethargy, altered response) should be aggressively evaluated. The probability of a child having a serious bacterial illness was estimated to be 7–9% in a non-toxic appearing febrile infant less than 3 months of age.[10]

The younger the child, the less likely they are to display the classic signs of meningitis. Children less than 3 months of age are particularly difficult and may present with a wide variety of nonspecific findings such as hyper- or hypothermia, irritability, lethargy, high-pitched cry, seizures or paradoxical irritability (quiet at rest, but cries when moved). The fontanelle of a child under 3 months of age should be carefully assessed for bulging (a sign of increased intracranial pressure).

In febrile neonates (a child< 28 days of age), the rule is a full sepsis evaluation to include CBC, blood culture, chest radiograph, lumbar puncture (LP), as well as initiation of antibiotic therapy and hospital admission. The most likely etiologic agents are Group B strep, L monocytogenes and E coli; antibiotic coverage should include Ampicillin (for L monocytogenes) and Gentamycin or ceftazidime (for Group B strep and E coli).

Children between 1–3 months of age should receive a complete sepsis evaluation, but outpatient management may be considered in a low-risk child. Low-risk infants, as defined by the Rochester criteria, are shown below (Table 1). Less than 1% of the infants that meet these criteria will have a serious bacterial illness.[11]

Table 1. Rochester criteria for low risk infants

1. Reliable parents and 24 hour follow up
2. Non-toxic-appearing, born full-term
3. Previously healthy, no current antibiotic use
4. WBC of 5,000-15,000 cells/mm³ with < 1500 bands
5. Stool WBC < 5 per high-power field (if diarrhea)
6. Normal chest radiograph (may not be necessary in all patients)
7. Normal urinalysis or urine Gram stain
8. Normal CSF

Discharge decisions in the 1 month to 3 month age group are the most controversial since these infants do not consistently show nuchal rigidity or other signs of meningeal irritation. Also, this group is at highest risk for developing occult bacteremia. Therefore, following a complete sepsis evaluation, the clinician must decide whether the child may go home, with or without a dose of antibiotics, or whether they should be admitted for observation. Children who meet the low-risk criteria may be considered for discharge with follow-up within 24 hours. If the child is sent home, some physicians administer a single intramuscular dose of ceftriaxone (50 mg/kg).

III. EVALUATION AND MANAGEMENT OF FEVER IN CHILDREN 3 TO 24 MONTHS

The majority of children who are bacteremic are between 6 and 18 months.[13] These children are at risk for occult bacteremia if they have no other source of fever (URI, positive RSV testing, diarrhea, etc). Approximately 60% of occult bacteremia is caused by S pneumoniae, although this incidence may change with the introduction of the pneumoococcal vaccine. Febrile females under 12 months of age have an approximate 8% incidence of UTIs and should have a urinalysis and urine culture obtained. In 1993, an expert panel developed very specific guidelines for the management of children under 36 months of age without a focus.[14] They recommended that non-toxic appearing children (male < 6 months and females < 2 years) with a temperature of 39° C (102.2° F) should have a urine culture obtained. Blood cultures and empiric antibiotic therapy (parenteral ceftriaxone 50 mg/kg IM or oral amoxicillin 60 mg/kg/day orally for 3 days) are recommended for all children or children with a WBC greater than 15, 000 cells/mm.³ Utilization of these guidelines is currently controversial, because this data was based on populations with a high incidence of H influenzae bacteremia and prior to introduction of the pneumococcal vaccine. Additionally, a meta-analysis found the incidence of meningitis following S pneumoniae bacteremia to be lower than previously reported.[15] Children over 24 months of age should be evaluated with a complete history and physical examination and diagnostic testing directed by the clinical appearance of the child and findings on physical examination.

Infections present in children with a headache and fever include streptococcal pharyngitis, viral illnesses and CNS infections, including meningitis. If the child lacks a fever, the differential of headache is substantially broader and includes toxic exposures, CNS structural disorders and trauma. Older children with meningitis are more likely to display the classic physical findings associated with meningitis, including a stiff neck and a positive Kernig's or Brudzinski's sign.

Neurologic complaints, as in this patient, are unusual, and a complete neurologic assessment and documentation of that assessment should be completed. A period of observation, with sequential examination and documentation, may be warranted, especially with complaints of a stiff neck and vague neurologic abnormalities.

IV. DISCUSSION OF MENINGITIS

In the United States the incidence of bacterial meningitis is 2–3 per 100,000. S pneumoniae has replaced H influenzae as the most common cause of bacterial meningitis in the United States, with a 1995 case fatality rate of 21%.[12] S pneumoniae is a gram-positive coccus that appears in pairs and chains in Gram stain samples; the nasopharynx is thought to be the primary site of human colonization. Neisseria meningitidis usually causes local outbreaks among young adults, and has an increased incidence in the late winter or early spring. Group B streptococci meningitis may occur in newborns and Listeria monocytogenes may occur in newborns, elderly or the immunocompromised. S pneumoniae has the highest mortality rate (26.3–30%) and Neisseria meningitidis has the lowest mortality rate (3.5–10.3%). Up to 30% of children have neurologic sequelae, with S pneumoniae having the highest rate of complications.

Vital signs are important objective markers of a patient's status. Abnormalities in vital signs should be recognized, repeated, and a note written with justification for action or inaction. This patient's systolic blood pressure of 72 is clearly abnormal. Discharging a patient who has substantially abnormal vital signs can be risky when the quality of care needs to de defended.[16]

V. LUMBAR PUNCTURE IN SUSPECTED MENINGITIS

Most patients with fever, headache and menigismus do not require a brain CT scan prior to LP. Pediatric indications for performing a CT prior to LP include evidence of head trauma, altered mental status, focal neurologic findings, papilledema or inability to complete a fundoscopic or neurologic exam.[7] In adults, CT indications prior to LP include a history of immunocompromise, CNS disease, abnormal mental status, inability to answer two consecutive questions correctly or to follow two consecutive commands, gaze palsy, abnormal visual fields, facial palsy, arm drift, leg drift, abnormal language or a seizure within 1 week prior to presentation.[6] In addition, an hemodynamic instability would be an indication to delay the LP until the patient has been stabilized. In all cases the decision to delay the LP should not delay the administration of antibiotics. A blood culture should be obtained prior to the initiation of antibiotics.

Antibiotic therapy should be initiated as soon as the diagnosis of meningitis is suspected. Ideally, empiric therapy should be started within 30 minutes, with or without a lumbar puncture (LP). If an LP is performed, the diagnosis is based on CSF findings (Table 2). Aronin, et al., reported that an adverse clinical outcome was more common in patients with meningitis who became progressively ill in the ED prior to the administration of initial antibiotic.[1]

Table 2. Normal CSF Findings

	Newborn	Infant/child
Pressure	<110 mmH20	<200 mmH20 Lateral recumbent
WBC Cell count	0-22 WBCs/mm3 (61% PMNs)	0-7 WBCs/mm3 (0% PMNs)
Glucose	34-119 mg/dL	40-80 mg/dL
Protein	20-170mg/dL	5-40 mg/dL

Empiric antibiotic administration prior to lumbar puncture has received much attention to determine the time interval for diagnostic testing that would still definitively identify the etiologic agent and antibiotic sensitivity. A retrospective study attempted to answer the question: how long after antibiotic administration was the etiologic agent recoverable from the CSF? The pathogens that infected the 128 study patients included: Streptococcus pneumoniae (49), Neisseria meningitidis (37), group B Streptococcus (21), Haemophilus influenzae (8), other organisms (11), and undetermined (3). Thirty-nine patients (30%) had first LPs after initiation of parenteral antibiotics, and 55 (43%) had serial LPs before and after initiation of parenteral antibiotics. After a dose of a third-generation cephalosporin (greater or equal to 50mg/kg), 3 of 9 LPs in meningococcal meningitis were sterile within 1 hour, occurring as early as 15 minutes, and all were sterile by 2 hours. With pneumococcal disease, the first negative CSF culture occurred at 4.3 hours, with 5 of 7 cultures negative from 4 to 10 hours after initiation of parenteral antibiotics. Reduced susceptibility to beta-lactam antibiotics occurred in 11 of 46 pneumococcal isolates. Group B streptococcal cultures were positive through the first 8 hours after parenteral antibiotics. Blood cultures were positive in 74% of cases without pretreatment and in 57% to 68% of cases with negative CSF cultures. This study demonstrates that CSF sterilization may occur more rapidly after initiation of parenteral antibiotics than previously suggested, with complete sterilization of meningococcus within 2 hours and the beginning of sterilization of pneumococcus within 4 hours.[9]

In a 10-year retrospective study of all children who had cerebrospinal fluid latex agglutination testing for bacterial antigens performed at 1 tertiary care urban children's hospital, of the 176 patients with culture-negative meningitis who were pretreated with antibiotics before lumbar puncture, none had a positive latex agglutination study (0 of 176; 95% confidence interval, 0–2%). Latex agglutination studies identified no additional cases of bacterial meningitis beyond those identified by culture in pretreated patients.[8]

VI. MANAGEMENT OF MENINGITIS—ANTIBIOTICS AND STEROIDS

In the emergency department, the pathogen and its susceptibility patterns are unknown, and therefore broad-spectrum antibiotic coverage should be initiated. Based on the age of this patient and the petechiael rash, initial antibiotic coverage should be for S pneumoniae and N meningitidis. Because of alterations in penicillin-binding proteins, penicillin susceptibility for S pneumoniae is no longer the rule. Currently in the US, 14%–22% of tested pneumococci have intermediate resistance to penicillin. In contrast, more than 90% of these strains remain sensitive to a third-generation cephalosporin, such as ceftriaxone. Many studies have reported the geographic variation in the proportion of drug-resistant pneumococci. In areas where the drug resistant S pneumoniae (DRSP) is > 2%, the recommendation from infectious disease specialists is cefotaxime (pediatric dose 50 mg/kg IV q 6hr) or ceftriaxone (pediatric dose: 75 mg/kg, adult dose: 2g IV q 12h) plus vancomycin (pediatric dose 15 mg/kg IV q 6h) The Committee on Infectious Diseases (COID) of the American Academy of Pediatrics has recommended that vancomycin be administered routinely in combination with ceftriaxone or cefotaxime to all children over 1 month of age with probable or definite bacterial meningitis.[4,5] Vancomycin monotherapy is not recommended because of unpredictable CSF penetration (particularly in the presence of dexamethasone) and reported clinical failures.

The use of adjunctive dexamethasone therapy in patients with bacterial meningitis is controversial. In 1995 Wald, et al., reported a study conducted at six large children's hospitals designed to determine if children treated with ceftriaxone and dexamethasone had less hearing loss or other neurologic abnormalities than those receiving ceftriaxone alone. Auditory brainstem responses were made within 24 hours of admission. Analysis of their data reveals a very favorable effect of dexamethasone on patients with H influenza type b meningitis who had bilateral moderate to severe hearing loss on final audiologic evaluation.[17] A meta-analysis in 1997 of all controlled trials of dexamethasone from 1988 to November 1996 found that, for meningitis caused by H influenzae type b, the use of dexamethasone was associated with a reduction in severe hearing loss overall (combined odds ratio, 0.31; 95% CI, 0.14 to 0.69) The data suggested a possible benefit with pneumococcal meningitis, but only if used early. Based on this data, the COID states that dexamethasone should be recommended for infants and children with H influenzae type b meningitis and should be considered for pneumococcal meningitis in children over 6 weeks of age.[5] DeGans and colleagues published a study in 2002 that showed a very beneficial effect of early dexamethasone therapy for adults with bacterial meningitis, particularly that caused by Streptococcus pneumoniae. Dexamethasone should not be used in children under 6 weeks of age or those with "partially treated" meningitis or aseptic meningitis. It should be started as soon as possible in the course of the disease in a dose of 0.15 mg/kg/dose intravenously every 6 hours for no more than 4 days.[3]

TEACHING POINTS ABOUT CASE 5:

- Periods of observation may be beneficial in pediatric patients with fever and neurologic complaints.
- A systolic pressure of 72 was present at the initial visit. Grossly abnormal vital signs need to be addressed, and if no action is taken, should be discussed in a progress note.
- The follow-up program should correlate with the disease process at hand.
- Antibiotics should be administered as soon as meningitis is suspected.
- The first dose of dexamethasone should be given with the first dose of antibiotics.

REFERENCES

1. Aronin SI, Peduzzi P, Quagliarello VJ. Community-acquired bacterial meningitis: risk stratification for adverse clinical outcome and effect of antibiotic timing. Ann Intern Med 1998;129:862-9.
2. Feigin RD, Watson JT, Gerber SI. Use of corticosteroids in bacterial meningitis. Pediat Infect Dis J 2004; 23: 355-7.
3. DeGans J, Van de beck D. European dexamethasone in Adulthood bacterial meningitis Study Investigators. Dexamethasone in adults with bacterial meningitis. N Engl J Med 2002; 347:1549.
4. Pickering LK,ed. Red Book: 2003 report of the Committee on Infectious Diseases. 26th ed. Elk Grove Village, IL: American Academy of Pediatrics 2003:293, 493.
5. American Academy of Pediatrics, Committee on Infectious Disease Therapy for Children with invasive pneumococcal infections. Pediatrics 1997;99:289-99.
6. Hasbun R, Abrahams J, Jekel J, Quagliarello VJ. Computed tomography of the head before lumbar puncture in adults with suspected meningitis. N Engl J Med 2001;345:1727-33.
7. Gopal AK, Whitehouse JD, Simel DL, et al. Cranial computed tomographybefore lumbar puncture: a prospective clinical evaluation. Arch Intern Med 1999; 159:2681-5.
8. Nigrovic LE, Kuppermann N, McAdam AJ, et al. Cerebrospinal latex agglutination fails to contribute to the microbiologic diagnosis of pretreated children with meningitis. Pediatr Infect Dis J 2004; 23:786-8.
9. Kanegaye JT, Soliemanzadeh P, Bradley JS. Lumbar puncture in pediatric bacterial meningitis: defining the time interval for recovery of cerebrospinal fluid pathogens after parenteral antibiotic pretreatment. Pediatrics 2001;108:1169-74.
10. Baraff LJ, Oslund SA, Schriger DL, et al. Probability of bacterial illness in febrile infants less than 3 months of age: a meta-analysis. Pediatr Infect Dis J 1992;11:257-65.
11. Baker MD, Bell LM, Avner JR. Outpatient management without antibiotics of fever in selected infants. N Engl J Med 1993;329:1437-41.
12. Schuchat A, Robinson K, Wenger JD, et al bacterial Meningitis in the United States in 1995. N Engl J Med 1997;337:970-6.
13. Sinkinson CA, Pichichero ME. Occult bacteremia in children: what are the odds? Emerg Med Rep 1991;12:1-10.
14. Baraff LJ, Bass JW, Fleischer GR, et al. Practice guidelines for management of infants and children 0–36 months of age with fever without source. Pediatrics 1993;92:1-12.
15. Rothrock SG, Green SM, Clark M. Do oral antibiotics prevent meningitis in children with occult bacteremia? A meta-analysis. Acad Emerg Med 1995;2:A.
16. Henry GL. Emergency medicine risk management: a comprehensive review. 2nd ed. Dallas, TX:American College of Emergency Physicians, 1997.
17. Wald ER, Kaplan SL, Mason EO Jr, et al. Dexamethasone therapy for children with bacterial meningitis. Pediatrics 1995;95:21-8.

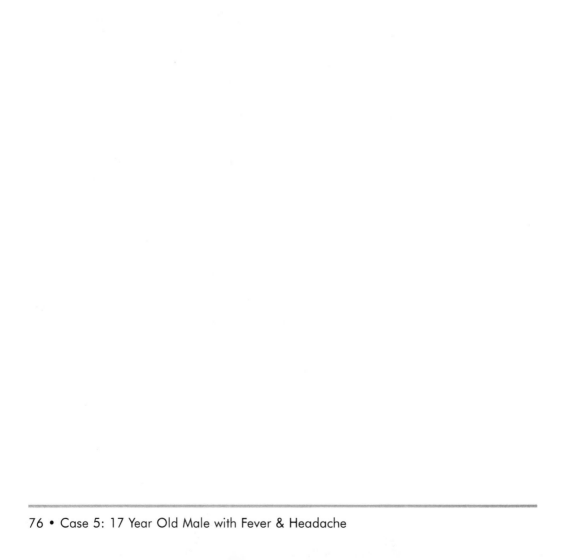

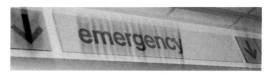

CASE 6
24 YEAR OLD MALE WITH ABDOMINAL PAIN

Commentary:
Gregory L. Henry, MD, FACEP

CEO, Medical Practice Risk Assessment, Inc., Ann Arbor, Michigan

Clinical Professor, Department of Emergency Medicine
   University of Michigan Medical School, Ann Arbor, Michigan

Past President, American College of Emergency Physicians (ACEP)

Discussion:
Stephen A. Colucciello, MD, FACEP

Associate Chair, Department of Emergency Medicine
   Carolinas Medical Center, Charlotte, North Carolina

Adjunct Professor, Department of Emergency Medicine
   University of North Carolina at Chapel Hill, Chapel Hill, North Carolina

Former Member, ACEP Clinical Policies Committee

Former Member, ACEP Clinical Policies Subcommittee on Abdominal Pain

Chair (1998-2000), ACEP Clinical Policies Subcommittee on Syncope

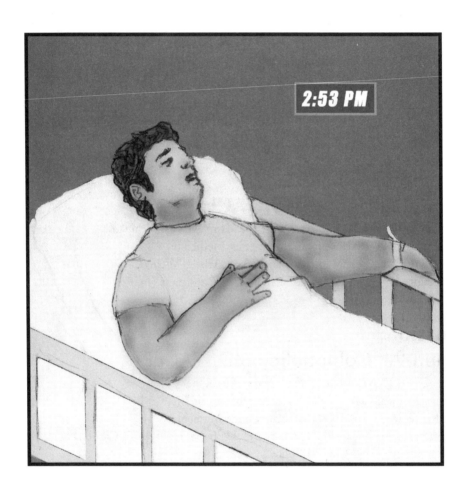

2:53 PM

24 YEAR OLD MALE WITH ABDOMINAL PAIN

—Initial Visit*—

*Authors' Note: The history, exam and notes are the actual documentation of the physicians and providers, including abbreviations (and spelling errors)

CHIEF COMPLAINT (at 14:23): Abdominal pain

```
VITAL SIGNS
Time   Temp(F) Rt. Pulse  Resp  Syst  Diast  Pos.  Pain scale
14:53  97.8    Tym. 102    18    145   90     S     6
15:51            76         20    145   86     S     0
```

HISTORY OF PRESENT ILLNESS (at 15:08): 24 y/o male c/o abdominal pain and n/v/d x 1 day. States he had a temperature yesterday and began to have stomach upset. States he began throwing up this am x 5 and admits to diarrhea today. States pain is in the top part of his abdomen. Denies bloody urine or stool. States he has not been able to keep any liquids down today. Denies radiation of pain. Rates pain 6/10. Denies fever, chest pain, SOB, cough, rhinorrhea, dysuria or hematuria.

PAST MEDICAL HISTORY/TRIAGE:

Chief complaint/quote: (Per triage nurse): Pt. states he have severe lower abd. pressure pain vomiting also lower back pain. Complains of nausea, vomiting, diarrhea and flank pain. Pt c/o difficulty urinating. No private physician.

Allergies: No known allergies.

Medications: The patient is not taking medications at this time.

Past medical history: No significant medical history. No significant surgical history.

EXAM (at 15:26)

General: Alert and oriented X3, obese, well appearing, in no apparent distress

Head: Normocephalic; atraumatic.

Eyes: PERRL

Nose: The nose is normal in appearance without rhinorrhea

Resp: Normal chest excursion with respiration; breath sounds clear and equal bilaterally; no wheezes, rhonchi, or rales

Card: Regular rhythm, without murmurs

Abd: Non-distended; tender over RUQ, Epigastrium and LUQ, soft, without rigidity, rebound or guarding

Skin: Normal for age and race; warm and dry; no apparent lesions

ORDERS (at 15:40): Demerol 25mg IVP, Pheneran 12.5mg IVP, .9NS 1 L bolus

PROGRESS NOTES (at 16:22) When the patient was ready to leave, he mentioned that the last time he had a stool, he saw some blood in it. I ordered levaquin 500mg X 1 in the ED and prescribed levaquin 500mg QD for 3 days in case this was bacterial in origin as there is good data to support a decrease in duration of symptoms with quinolone therapy. Patient is feeling better.

DIAGNOSIS: 1. Gastroenteritis, 2. Vomiting - and nausea

DISPOSITION (at 17:03): The patient was discharged to Home ambulatory. Given name and number of PCP for follow up if not improved in 3-4 days. Prescriptions for Phenergan 25mg PO and suppositories. After care instructions for nausea, vomiting and diarrhea.

Gregory L. Henry comments:

"The principal test with abdominal pain is the test of time"

Generalized abdominal pain is one of the most common complaints in the emergency department, and requires a unified approach. Most importantly, the principal test with abdominal pain is the test of time; in short order, a patient usually gets better or worse. My discussion, as with all cases I have commented upon, was done without looking at the final presentation, but some important points need to be made.

The history documented is adequate. We know that the patient has been ill for the past day, with both vomiting and diarrhea, but documentation of hematemesis was not included. The patient does comment that he cannot keep down fluids, and the denial of fever or urinary symptoms is also useful to note.

The patient is adequately evaluated. Standard examination of head, ears, eye, nose, throat, heart, and lungs was accomplished. The abdominal examination does not comment on the presence or absence of bowel sounds, but this is a minor issue; there has not been a paper published in which bowel sounds have been used to decide if a patient has a surgical abdomen. One area of criticism is that a rectal exam might have been worthwhile, to check for heme positive stool.

A decision is made in this case to use Levaquin for the diarrhea, assuming a bacterial cause. Evidence does not suggest that Levaquin or any other antibiotic is useful in a patient with a viral irritation of the bowels. It is hard to understand why an antibiotic was used.

The administration of pain medication for abdominal pain prior to diagnosis used to be considered an anathema. We now know that pain relief has essentially no adverse effect on diagnosis. I am personally not a Demerol fan and have stopped using it, but the suppression of the patient's pain was appropriate and in no way affected the outcome of this case.

The diagnosis and disposition need some comment. Gastroenteritis is a disease entity that should not be used as a "diagnosis" in emergency medicine. Vomiting and diarrhea are both symptoms, which are acceptable "impressions" to use in emergency medicine cases. Gastroenteritis is a term found on the charts of more malpractice cases than any other diagnosis in emergency medicine—it is the refuge of the intellectually destitute. It is perfectly fine to reassure the patient that the exact etiology is not known, but that careful follow up will be done.

The principal concern here is the follow up time. Most abdominal pains and diarrhea should resolve quickly. A follow-up time of 3–4 days in a patient with abdominal pain is simply too long —a more reasonable time frame would be to see the patient back the next morning to see how he is progressing. The exact nature of the patient's problem is not clear, which is perfectly acceptable in emergency medicine—we must get used to dealing with some degree of uncertainty. Almost half the patients who present to the emergency department with abdominal pain do not have a specific diagnosis at the time of discharge. This is not only acceptable, but also quite appropriate. Most problems resolve themselves; the follow up interval is the key issue.

- Thoroughness of Documentation: 8 out of 10.

- Thoroughness of Patient Evaluation: 7 out of 10.

- Risk of Serious Illness Being Missed: Low risk.

- Risk Management Legal Rating: Medium risk.

24 YEAR OLD MALE WITH ABDOMINAL PAIN

—Second Visit: Early Next Morning (About 8 Hours Later)—

CHIEF COMPLAINT (at 00:38): Vomiting

```
VITAL SIGNS
Time     Temp(F)     Rt.     Pulse    Resp    Syst    Diast    Pos
00:42     95.2       Tym.      80      28      100      60       S
```

HISTORY OF PRESENT ILLNESS (at 00:46): 24 yo WM returns to the ED with c/o vomiting and mid-epigastric abdominal pain. Patient reports that he has had persistant vomiting for a couple of days with fever yesterday. Now with continuous vomiting and bloody stool. No fever today. No fevers/cough per patient. No ear ache/sore throat per patient. No fever, chills, hematemesis, chest pain, cough, sore throat.

PAST MEDICAL HISTORY/TRIAGE (per triage nurse):
Patient arrived by stretcher via EMS transport from Home. Complains of abdominal pain. Pain Index: 10; frowning, moaning, and holding a painful area. There is a severe stabbing pain located in the epigastric area. Pain became more severe around 22:00.
Medication, common allergies: No known allergies.
Current meds: Phenergan
Past medical/surgical history: No significant medical history. No significant surgical history.

EXAM (at 00:48)
General: Alert WM who appears uncomfortable and c/o nausea with vomiting
Head: Normocephalic; atraumatic.
Eyes: PERRL
Nose: The nose is normal in appearance without rhinorrhea
Oropharynx: Dry mucous membranes
Resp: Normal chest excursion with respiration; breath sounds clear and equal bilaterally; no wheezes, rhonchi, or rales
Card: Regular rhythm, without murmurs, rub or gallop
Abd: Non-distended; + tenderness to palpation mid-epigastrium, soft, without rigidity, rebound or guarding
Ext: 2+ radial pulses bilaterally; no peripheral edema
Skin: Normal for age and race; warm and dry; no apparent lesions

ORDERS (at 00:47): Dilaudid 1mg IVP, Phenergan 12.5mg IVP, .9NS-500cc bolus then to 125cc/hour

ED COURSE: (Per RN): At 01:00 IV was changed to warmed fluids for bolus administration. The patient was given a warm blanket. The patient was repositioned to a position of comfort. At approx. 01:05 patient brother came to ask what med the patient was given, stating, "I don't think he's breathing." I was outside patient room and immediately went into room. Pt was cyanotic in face, took an agonal breath, no pulse palpated carotid. Code blue called and patient moved to trauma room for resuscitation.

PROGRESS NOTES per MD: Patient was noted to be apneic and pulseless in the room. A "code blue" was called at approx 01:09 throughout the hospital and the patient was immediately moved to a trauma room. The patient was immediately intubated and chest compressions were begun while being attached to the monitor. Patient was found to be initially in v-fib and was shocked at 200J. Patient then went into PEA. A Right femoral triple lumen CVP was placed by a second ED physician who had come in to assist. The patient continued to alternate between v-fib and PEA. The patient was given narcan, glucose, bicarb x2, calcium chloride, magnesium, and several rounds of epinephrine and atropine per the med sheet. Chest compressions and bagged respirations were continued throughout the code except during the defibrillatory shocks. The patient's wife was initially in the room when the patient became apneic and pulseless. The patient's wife was escorted immediately into a family consultation room by staff. I asked the patient's family if they would like to be present in the room and the patient's wife and brother accompanied me back into the trauma room. The code continued as per the med sheet with family present. The patient was coded for an hour without return of a pulse despite multiple medications and shocks. The code was ended with agreement by staff at 02:09. The patient's brother was in the room at the time.

RESULTS:

Test	Flag	Value	Units	Ref. Range
NA		135	MMOL/L	135-144
K	H	5.8	MMOL/L	3.5-5.1
CL	H	108	MMOL/L	98-107
CO2	C	5	MMOL/L	22-29
BUN		15	MG/DL	7-18
CREAT	H	2.5	MG/DL	0.6-1.3
ALB	L	1.9	G/DL	3.2-4.6

Test	Flag	Value	Units	Ref. Range
TP	L	4.7	GM/DL	6.4-8.2
BILT		.5	MG/DL	0-1.0
BILD		0.2	MG/DL	0.0-0.3
BILI		.3	MG/DL	.0-1.0
ALT	H	105	U/L	22-65
ALP		81	U/L	42-144
AST	H	56	U/L	10-34

(continued on next page)

Test	Flag	Value	Units	Ref. Range
AMY	L	20	U/L	25-115
LIP		159	U/L	114-286
GLUC	C	548	MG/DL	70-110
ACET		NEGATIVE		NEGATIVE

Test	Flag	Value	Units	Ref. Range
pH	C	6.956		7.350-7.450
PCO2	L	24.7	MMHG	32.0-48.0
PO2	H	128.0	MMHG	83.0-108.0
HCO3	L	5.2	MMOL/L	21.0-28.0
FI O2		100.00		
O2 SAT		95.8	%	95.0-99.0

DISPOSITION: The patient was pronounced by the Emergency Department physician at 02:09.

FINAL DIAGNOSIS (by autopsy): Infarction of small bowel, mesenteric vein thrombosis, multiple other sites of thrombi including several small PE's

Additional comments by Gregory L. Henry:

Having seen the final diagnosis on this case, I believe nothing could have been done on the first visit to come up with this diagnosis. This is less than a one in a million kind of case and no emergency physician could have been expected to make such a diagnosis on the first visit.

The follow up time interval is the critical question, and recommending re-evaluation in 12 hours may have been preferable, but the patient returned before this time. It is inappropriate and unrealistic for anyone to believe that the average, competent emergency physician is going to make a diagnosis of infarction of the small bowel and mesenteric vein thrombosis on a 24 year old.

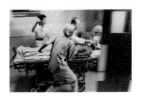

EVALUATION AND DIAGNOSIS OF ABDOMINAL PAIN IN ADULTS

Stephen A. Colucciello, MD, FACEP

I. INTRODUCTION

Abdominal pain is one of the most common complaints seen in the Emergency Department, and accounts for almost 10% of visits.[1] The spectrum of disease ranges from life-threatening to benign. Pain may be secondary to either intra-abdominal or extra-abdominal pathology. It is more important for the emergency physician to exclude "badness," in particular acute surgical disease, than to make an accurate diagnosis. However, this task is not always accomplished in one ED visit.

II. HISTORY

The history should target high risk conditions, including older age, pain that migrates to the right lower quadrant, and severe or progressive pain. In addition, women of childbearing potential (ectopic pregnancy), and the immunosuppressed (intra-abdominal infections) are at higher risk of serious disease. In the present case, our patient had no high-risk factors, with the possible exception of rectal bleeding. While ischemic bowel, peptic ulcer disease, Meckel's diverticulum, aorto-enteric fistula, diverticulitis, and other serious conditions can cause abdominal pain and rectal bleeding, most rectal bleeding in a young person is due to either hemorrhoids or simple enteritis.

Past medical history may be revealing. Asking if the patient has ever had a similar (or better yet, identical) attack in the past is useful; peptic ulcer disease, biliary colic, pancreatitis, and inflammatory bowel disease are notoriously recurrent. Prior surgeries are associated with a higher likelihood of obstruction, while vascular disease and arrhythmias predispose to ischemic bowel. Once again, our patient did not report any significant past medical history.

III. PHYSICAL EXAMINATION

Extremes of vital signs can alert the physician to serious disease, but many patients with abdominal pain will have normal or near-normal parameters. While fever piques the interest of a surgical consultant, patients with surgical disease are often afebrile, while those with medical illness may have high fever. At our patient's initial visit, the only significant abnormality was mild tachycardia, with a heart rate of 102, which had resolved on recheck.

With abdominal pain, the physical examination drives much of the ED evaluation. From the doorway, determine how uncomfortable the patient is. Is the patient writhing in pain, as occurs in colic, or curled up in a ball, as occurs with peritoneal pain? Our patient had 6 out of 10 pain but appeared "in no acute distress." Abdominal distention should alert the physician to the possibility of bowel obstruction or an ileus. While the presence or absence of bowel sounds and their character is rarely diagnostic, high-pitched, tinkling bowel sounds should prompt a search for bowel obstruction, particularly in those with a history of abdominal surgery.

Palpation provides a roadmap for further investigation. While topographical localization of pain can direct further work-up, be aware of "extra-quadrant" disease; e.g., appendicitis causing either right upper or left lower quadrant pain. Our patient had diffuse upper abdominal pain, a finding that did not significantly narrow the differential diagnosis.

Peritoneal signs are important predictors of surgical disease. While some patients with serious intra-abdominal conditions may initially present with a benign examination, the presence of voluntary guarding should elicit concern; involuntary guarding is especially worrisome. Peritoneal signs also include rebound tenderness, when the patient complains of significant pain when an examining hand is taken off the belly. Other ways to determine peritonitis include "cough and shake" peritoneal signs and eliciting abdominal pain with heel tap (banging the hand on the patient's heel provokes pain or grimace). Our patient had a soft abdomen without rigidity, rebound or guarding.

In this case, no rectal examination was performed on either visit. Traditional indications for a rectal examination include the presence of a patient with a rectum and the presence of a physician with a finger! The actual utility of the digital rectal exam is less clear. It is certainly useful in the detection of blood and rectal foreign bodies, however several studies show that it rarely provides any information beyond that revealed by abdominal examination in patients with right lower quadrant pain.[2,3] Despite this evidence, it is interesting to note that the failure to perform a rectal exam is a recurring theme in the malpractice literature.[4] If a rectal exam had been performed on the first visit, and had revealed blood, it would have been unlikely to have changed the management, since the physician probably would have assumed the blood was a consequence of bacterial enteritis, and not ischemic bowel.

IV. DIAGNOSTIC TESTING—OVERVIEW
Clearly not every patient with abdominal pain needs diagnostic studies. The need for further study is often driven by high risk findings and the severity or persistence of pain. High risk findings include advanced age, significantly altered vital signs, intractable vomiting, severe tenderness or distention, peritoneal findings, involuntary guarding, and right lower quadrant tenderness in the absence of previous appendectomy. Persistent and significant localized tenderness in any quadrant apart from the left upper quadrant may prompt imaging; e.g., ultrasound for RUQ tenderness, or CT scan for right and left lower quadrant tenderness if appendicitis or acute diverticulitis is suspected. Women of childbearing potential should routinely be tested for pregnancy.

In one study of adults presenting to the ED with non-traumatic abdominal pain, the treating physicians believed that the most useful tests were the abdominal CT scan (31%) and the urinalysis (17%). The CBC was listed as most useful by 14% (these physicians were clearly delusional) and only 7% listed plain x- rays.[5]

V. DIAGNOSTIC TESTING—LABORATORY STUDIES
The nature of the first visit did not mandate laboratory testing, (no, not even a CBC). In fact, the most insidious investigation in the patient with abdominal pain is the CBC. The medical and legal literature is rife with cases where the physician is mislead by the white blood cell count and differential. Patients with abdominal catastrophes may have normal white counts, while others with simple gastroenteritis may have elevated counts with a dramatic left shift. One famous study in women with abdominal pain showed that providing the results of a CBC to an examining physician was more likely to change management in the **wrong** direction (inappropriate discharge or unnecessary

admission).[6] Fortunately, surgeons no longer ask for the results of the CBC when consulted for possible appendicitis. Instead they ask, "What does the CT show?"

The lack of significant localized tenderness in our patient argues against the need for amylase, lipase, or liver function tests. A urinalysis is similarly low yield in a male with diffuse upper abdominal pain.

VI. DIAGNOSTIC TESTING—IMAGING STUDIES

Plain films of the abdomen are generally unhelpful in the assessment of abdominal pain.[7] Apart from the occasional foreign body, they are most useful in two discrete circumstances; clinically suspected viscus perforation (sudden severe pain, rigid abdomen, absent bowel sounds) and clinically suspected obstruction (prior abdominal surgery, intractable vomiting, abdominal distention, and tinkling bowel sounds). This patient did not fit either picture.

In diffuse upper abdominal pain in a young male, imaging of the biliary system would be a low-yield investigation, especially without a positive Murphy's sign. The question at hand is, "Did this patient deserve an abdominal CT scan?"

The CT scan has achieved supremacy as the diagnostic study of choice to rule out most abdominal surgical conditions. While less accurate than ultrasound for evaluation of biliary or adnexal disorders, it is the study of choice in detecting appendicitis, diverticulitis, gut perforation, intra-abdominal abscesses, AAA (in stable patients), and possibly ischemic bowel. CT scans may decrease the rate of unnecessary surgery and hospital admissions while increasing the rate of early appropriate surgery.[8] The problem is determining the appropriate candidate for this study. Currently, there are no good evidence-based guidelines describing who should be scanned. However, the best candidates are probably those likely to have serious disease, including the elderly and patients with significantly abnormal examinations, especially if pain is localized to one of the lower quadrants.

VII. MEDICATIONS IN PATIENTS WITH ABDOMINAL PAIN

There are a variety of interventions to control abdominal pain. The patient's response to some of these, such as H2 blockers, GI cocktails, antacids, and antispasmodics may provide diagnostic information. Non-steroidal anti-inflammatory drugs, in particular parenteral ketorolac, are useful for presumed biliary or renal colic; however, it is poor form to give them in the setting of peptic ulcer pain.

Until recently the use of narcotics to control abdominal pain was discouraged under the assumption that they would mask serious pathology. Several studies have successfully challenged this assumption.[9,10,11,12] In nearly all studies, administration of narcotic pain medication did not adversely affect the physician's ability to identify surgical disease, and in many cases enhanced it. However, in one prospective observational study (non-randomized), the authors found an association between administration of opioids and adverse outcome in patients with abdominal pain. They hypothesized that since patients with worse pain are more likely to be given opioids, pain severity might be a marker of poor prognosis.[13] Another paper noted the association between opioid administration and successful litigation in ruptured appendicitis.[14]

The studies are hard to compare since they used a wide variety of narcotics; some PO, others IM or IV (and some of the opioids are not even available in the US). In general, I use 4–8 mg of IV morphine in adults (or 25–50 mg of IV Demerol) to start, and then titrate up as needed. If given with Phenergan to a nauseated patient, these relatively small doses do the trick in most patients. If someone obviously has a surgical abdomen with severe pain, I have no problem giving 10 mg of IV morphine right from the start.

I reserve narcotics for those with significant abdominal pain and tenderness. I do not routinely give it for minor cramping or typical gastritis/PUD pain. I also have a general rule to scan patients who require parenteral narcotics, unless they have a chronic pain-type diagnosis such as previously CT or US-diagnosed biliary colic or recurring pancreatitis with typical presentation and no peritoneal signs.

In our patient, there are several minor concerns regarding the use of pain medication. First, there was no attempt to use non-narcotic interventions, such as a GI cocktail (which generally contains an antacid, lidocaine, and an antispasmodic). Second, a repeat abdominal examination was not documented. While the progress note states the patient felt better after the narcotic administration, it would have been prudent to actually palpate the abdomen again prior to discharge. Documentation of serial examinations of the patient with abdominal pain remains a cornerstone of patient care (and risk management). Finally, the question remains, should a patient with undifferentiated abdominal pain severe enough to require parenteral narcotics get an abdominal CT scan? While I personally think that the answer is "Yes," this question has not been adequately answered by the literature.

VIII. FOLLOW UP FOR ABDOMINAL PAIN
Abdominal pain (and in particular, missed appendicitis) remains a leading cause of malpractice litigation in Emergency Medicine. Patients who present to the ED with abdominal pain are well-served by a mandatory recheck in 8–12 hours. While many argue that this does not represent a national standard of care, it remains an important risk management strategy. Routine instructions may include, "Please return to the ED for a recheck in 8–12 hours; sooner if you get worse."

IX. SUMMARY OF THE CASE
If this patient had been a 75 year old vasculopath with atrial fibrillation and pain out of proportion to physical findings, the diagnosis of ischemic gut would have been first on the list. However, the pretest probability of mesenteric thrombosis in a previously healthy 24 year old with abdominal pain is astronomically small. In retrospect, this patient must have had a severe undiscovered coagulation disorder (protein C deficiency, antiphospholipid syndrome, antithrombin III deficiency, etc.) responsible for his calamitous decline.

TEACHING POINTS ABOUT CASE 6:
- While rectal bleeding is a red flag for serious disease, most rectal bleeding in a young patient is due to hemorrhoids or simple enteritis.
- Caution should be used in using the term "gastroenteritis" as a diagnosis. Consider using "vomiting" or "vomiting and diarrhea" instead.
- Administration of small amounts of narcotic medication to patients with abdominal pain does not adversely affect the ability to diagnose surgical disease.
- Repeat abdominal examinations prior to discharge are prudent.
- Follow up in patients with abdominal pain should be within 8–12 hours.

REFERENCES

1. Powers RD. Guertler AT. Abdominal pain in the ED: stability and change over 20 years. Am J Emerg Med 1995; 13:301-3.
2. Manimaran N, Galland RB. Significance of routine digital rectal examination in adults presenting with abdominal pain. Ann R Coll Surg Engl 2004 86:292-5.
3. Dixon JM, Elton RA, Rainey JB, et al. Rectal examination in patients with pain in the right lower quadrant of the abdomen.[see comment]. BMJ 1991; 302(6773):386-8
4. Rusnak RA, Borer JM, Fastow JS. Misdiagnosis of acute appendicitis: common features discovered in cases after litigation.[see comment]. Am J Emerg Med 1994; 12:397-402.
5. Nagurney JT, Brown DF, Chang Y, Sane S, et al. Use of diagnostic testing in the emergency department for patients presenting with non-traumatic abdominal pain. J Emerg Med 2003; 25:363-71.
6. Silver BE, Patterson JW, Kulick M, et al. Effect of CBC results on ED management of women with lower abdominal pain. Am J Emerg Med 1995; 13:304-6.
7. Ahn SH, Mayo-Smith WW, Murphy BL, et al. Acute nontraumatic abdominal pain in adult patients: abdominal radiography compared with CT evaluation. Radiology 2002; 225:159-64.
8. Rosen MP, Siewert B, Sands DZ, et al. Value of abdominal CT in the emergency department for patients with abdominal pain. Eur Radiol 2003; 13:418-24.
9. Pace S, Burke TF. Intravenous morphine for early pain relief in patients with acute abdominal pain. [see comment]. Acad Emerg Med 1996; 3:1086-92.
10. Kim MK, Strait RT, Sato TT, et al. A randomized clinical trial of analgesia in children with acute abdominal pain. Acad Emerg Med 2002; 9:281-7.
11. Thomas SH, Silen W, Cheema F, et al. Effects of morphine analgesia on diagnostic accuracy in emergency department patients with abdominal pain: a prospective, randomized trial. [see comment]. J Am Coll Surg 2003; 196:18-31.
12. LoVecchio F, Oster N, Sturmann K, et al. The use of analgesics in patients with acute abdominal pain. J Emerg Med 1997; 15:775-9.
13. Lee JS, Stiell IG, Wells GA, et al. Adverse outcomes and opioid analgesic administration in acute abdominal pain. Acad Emerg Med 2000; 7:980-7.
14. Rusnack RA, Borer JM, Fastow JS. Misdiagnosis of acute appendicitis: common features discovered in cases after litigation. Am J Emerg Med 1994; 12:397-402.

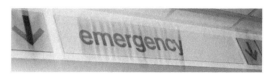

CASE 7
38 YEAR OLD MALE WITH CHEST PAIN

Commentary:
Gregory L. Henry, MD, FACEP

CEO, Medical Practice Risk Assessment, Inc., Ann Arbor, Michigan
Clinical Professor, Department of Emergency Medicine
   University of Michigan Medical School, Ann Arbor, Michigan
Past President, American College of Emergency Physicians (ACEP)

Discussion:
Amal Mattu, MD, FAAEM, FACEP

Associate Professor and Residency Director
   Emergency Medicine Residency Program
   University of Maryland School of Medicine
   Baltimore, Maryland
Author, *ECG's for the Emergency Physician*
Consulting Editor, Emergency Medicine Clinics of North America
Section Editor for Best Practices in Emergency Medicine, Journal of Emergency Medicine
American Academy of Emergency Medicine (AAEM) Young Educator of the Year, 2002

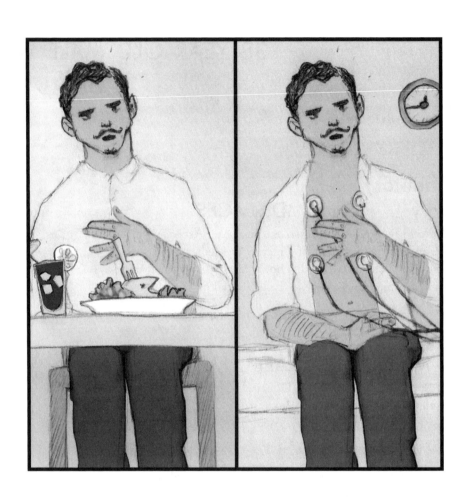

38 YEAR OLD MALE WITH CHEST PAIN

—Initial Visit*—

*Authors' Note: The history, exam and notes are the actual documentation of the physicians and providers, including abbreviations (and spelling errors)

CHIEF COMPLAINT (at 21:59): Chest pain

```
VITAL SIGNS
Time      Temp     Pulse    Resp     Syst     Diast    O2 Sat
22:03     98.9     103      16       122      69       99%
```

HISTORY OF PRESENT ILLNESS (at 22:47): Pt. 38 year old male with a PMH of myocarditis and pericarditis in 1983 and 1991,who ate dinner at 6:30 (salad, french onion soup and fish) and began feeling pressure across his anterior chest while watching TV at 7:30 PM. - it felt like "some was sitting on my chest". Associated SOB and radiation into his shoulder and left hand "tingling". He has had heartburn but this felt different. Took baking soda (which he normally takes for his heartburn) and this did not help. No syncope, nausea, vomiting, fever, RUQ pain or history of food intolerances. He did have some viral symptoms 2 weeks ago (nonproductive cough, sinus HA and PND which has all resolved.) No orthopnea, PND, relation of pain to exercise, chest trauma, pleuritic component

PAST MEDICAL HISTORY/TRIAGE:
Medication, common allergies: None
PMH: Myocarditis/Pericarditis
PSH: None
SocHx: Non-smoker
FamHx: Positive for CAD with 52 year old sibling with MI, father CABG at 53

EXAM (at 22:52):
General: Well-appearing; well-nourished; in no apparent distress.
Head: Normocephalic; atraumatic.
Eyes: PERLA; EOM intact
ENT: TM's normal; normal nose; no rhinorrhea; Throat is red, and mild exudates.. Moist mucus membranes.
Neck: Supple; nontender; no cervical lymphadenopathy. No meningeal signs
Cardiovascular: Normal S1, S2; no murmurs, rubs, or gallops. No reproducible chest wall tenderness
Respiratory: Normal chest excursion with respiration; breath sounds clear and equal bilaterally; no wheezes, rhonchi, or rales.

Abdomen: Normal bowel sounds; non-distended; nontender; no palpable organomegaly.

Extremities: Normal ROM in all four extremities; nontender to palpation; distal pulses are normal and equal.

Skin: Normal for age and race; warm; dry; good turgor; no apparent lesions or exudate

PROGRESS NOTES: (at 23:12) he received 2 baby aspirin and SL NTG with relief of chest discomfort. He then had 1 inch of Nitropaste placed. At 00:44 his pain returned and his ECG was repeated. He was given 15mg Maalox without improvement then ½ inch more NTP which did relieve the discomfort.

RESULTS:

EKG 1: Flattened T waves inferior and in V2-V6.

EKG 2: No changes

Note: Actual ECG's are no longer available

LABS:

Test	Flag	Value	Units	Ref. Range
WBC		7.3	K/uL	4.6-10.2
HGB		13.9	G/DL	12.0-16.0
PLT		284	K/uL	142-424

Test	Flag	Value	Units	Ref. Range
NA		139	MMOL/L	135-144
K		4.3	MMOL/L	3.5-5.1
CL		97	MMOL/L	98-107
CO2		26	MMOL/L	22-29
BUN	H	21	MG/DL	7-18
CREAT		1.1	MG/DL	0.6-1.3

Test	Flag	Value	Units	Ref. Range
CKMB		0.2	NG/ML	0.0-5.0
TROPI		0.0	NG/ML	.00-.27

CXR: Negative

DIAGNOSIS (at 01:57): Chest pain, history of myocarditis

DISPOSITION (at 02:02): The patient was admitted to telemetry for serial enzymes and cardiology evaluation. Pt. discharged from the ED at 02:48.

HOSPITAL COURSE:

Pt. underwent serial enzymes and repeat ECG in the morning. He ruled out for MI and was released. A subsequent stress ECHO was negative after exercising for 12.5 minutes with no chest discomfort or ECG changes.

Gregory L. Henry comments:

"Positives may lead toward a diagnosis of myocardial disease, but there are almost no negatives that rule it out"

When an emergency physician is presented with a 38 year old male with chest pain, diaphoresis may be present in both the patient and the physician. The most expensive litigation in emergency medicine involves chest pain patients. It is important to understand that positives may lead toward a diagnosis of myocardial disease, but there are almost no negatives that rule it out.

The history in this case is reasonably well taken. The history of myocarditis and pericarditis are important, but should not deter the physician from thinking of coronary artery disease as a diagnosis. It is interesting that this patient gave the classic story of "someone sitting on my chest". Most people actually have never had someone sit directly on their chest and the sensation is difficult to reproduce.

No single history or constellation of historical features definitively rules out coronary artery disease. The story of pain radiating into the left shoulder and arm is of interest, but does not have to be present in acute coronary syndrome.

The patient has a previous history of heartburn, but the difference between heartburn and angina are so subtle that any relief of pain with heartburn-type medication cannot be used to make the patient's diagnosis. Similarly, the paternal history of MI at age 53 does raise suspicion. Cardiac risk factors, i.e., hypertension, smoking, diabetes, dyslipidemia, obesity, etc. are useful for counseling in primary care; they are not useful in an emergency department for ruling out myocardial disease.

The evaluation of this patient is perfectly reasonable. The usual physical examination is undertaken; a normal chest exam does not rule in or out cardiac disease. Frequently patients with significant myocarditis or pericarditis will have no findings on auscultation. The neck is commented upon, but jugular venous distention is not mentioned; if restrictive pericarditis is being considered, this might be useful to include. The standard laboratory studies were obtained, as well as EKG and chest x-ray. This patient was treated in a manner that can be considered "standard" in emergency departments at this time. Flattened t-waves have little significance, but would not be found in patients with pericarditis. One can say only that this early ECG is equivocal. Initial laboratory studies are also equivocal, and do not rule in or out a disease process.

The documentation on this chart is excellent—I would be pleased to have this level of documentation on all of the cases that I review.

The physician had the proper concerns; he/she was not going to be led astray by equivocal findings. If we learned anything from Euclidian geometry, it is that two points determine a line, and three points a plane. This type of thinking is required to rule out an acute coronary syndrome. The patient was appropriately admitted for repeat ECGs, enzymes, and subsequently had a stress echocardiogram, which was negative. The real question then becomes "what is the most appropriate test to continue to evaluate this patient's myocardial status?" The emergency medicine handling of this case is completely acceptable.

- Thoroughness of Documentation: 9 out of 10.
- Thoroughness of Patient Evaluation: 10 out of 10.
- Risk of Serious Illness Being Missed: Low risk.
- Risk Management Legal Rating: Low risk.

38 YEAR MALE WITH CHEST PAIN

—Second Visit: 7 Weeks Later—

CHIEF COMPLAINT (at 19:50): Chest pain and shortness of breath

VITAL SIGNS					
Time	Temp	Pulse	Resp	Syst	Diast
19:52	97.9	91	18	129	71

HISTORY OF PRESENT ILLNESS (at 20:25): 38 year old with PMH significant for pericarditis in 1982 and 1990 (first in Canton, OH then in Germany where he was stationed – no etiology found) and seen at our ED 6 weeks ago. Subsequently had stress echocardiogram which was negative. Saw primary doctor last week and diagnosed with reflux and given Prilosec. Today presents with chest tightness and dyspnea, which is worse with exertion and after a meal. Has not eaten much in last few days because of this. Woke up last night with pain, took a Prilosec, and it did seem to improve the pain. Is sleeping propped up in bed as this does improve the symptoms. Was in Mexico last week and did not have much pain there. Not having a lot of stress in his life. No radiation, diaphoresis, fever, cough, peripheral edema, calf muscle pain.

TRIAGE AND PAST HISTORY:
  Medications: Prilosec and an antibiotic
  PMH: Myocarditis/Pericarditis, GERD
  PSH: None
  SocHx: Non-smoker
  FamHx: Positive for CAD with 52 year old sibling with MI, father CABG at 53

EXAM (at 20:30):
  General: Well-appearing; well-nourished; in no apparent distress.
  Head: Normocephalic; atraumatic.
  Eyes: PERLA; EOM intact
  ENT: TM's normal; normal nose; no rhinorrhea; Throat is red, and mild exudates. Moist mucus membranes.

Neck: Supple; nontender; no cervical lymphadenopathy. No meningeal signs

Cardiovascular: Normal S1, S2; no murmurs, rubs, or gallops. No reproducible chest wall tenderness

Respiratory: Normal chest excursion with respiration; breath sounds clear and equal bilaterally; no wheezes, rhonchi, or rales.

Abdomen: Normal bowel sounds; non-distended; nontender; no palpable organomegaly.

Extremities: Normal ROM in all extremities; nontender to palpation; distal pulses are normal and equal.

Skin: Extensive sunburn noted over back, arms, and legs

PROGRESS NOTES: (At 20:51) he received aspirin 325mg. SL NTG was given, but his pain was already completely resolved by the time it was given. Later received Tylenol for a nitro headache. Lopressor 5mg IV. PO. Lovenox 90mg SQ, NTP 1 ½ inches, and Lopressor 50mg PO.

RESULTS:

EKG: NSR and T wave inversion in aVL and Q waves in V1 and V2 and nonspecific ST changes. Note: Actual ECG is no longer available

Test	Flag	Value	Units	Ref. Range
WBC		7.7	K/uL	4.6-10.2
HGB		14.3	G/DL	12.0-16.0
PLT		198	K/uL	142-424

Test	Flag	Value	Units	Ref. Range
NA		143	MMOL/L	135-144
K		4.2	MMOL/L	3.5-5.1
CL		101	MMOL/L	98-107
CO2		27	MMOL/L	22-29
BUN		18	MG/DL	7-18
CREAT		0.9	MG/DL	0.6-1.3

Test	Flag	Value	Units	Ref. Range
CK		313	NG/ML	
CKMB	H	23.1	NG/ML	0.0-5.0
TROPI	H	5.9	NG/ML	.00-.27

CXR - Negative

DIAGNOSIS (at 23:11): Acute MI

DISPOSITION (at 23:16): Patient was admitted to ICU and evaluated by cardiology.

HOSPITAL COURSE:

The next day, he was transferred for a cardiac catheterization and was found to have coronary artery disease. PTCA was performed and a stent was inserted. He tolerated the procedures well.

FINAL DIAGNOSIS: Acute myocardial infarction

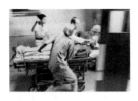

EVALUATION OF CHEST PAIN AND DIAGNOSIS OF ACUTE CORONARY SYNDROME

Amal Mattu, MD, FAAEM, FACEP

I. EVALUATION OF THE PATIENT WITH CHEST PAIN

Chest pain is the presenting complaint for more than 5% of the patients in Emergency Departments (EDs) in the United States. The evaluation of the patient with chest pain is a tremendous challenge, largely due to the broad differential diagnosis for chest pain, but also because of the risk associated with misdiagnosis. Amongst the most rapidly fatal conditions in emergency medicine are acute coronary syndrome (myocardial ischemia and infarction), aortic dissection, pulmonary embolism, pericarditis with cardiac tamponade, myocarditis, tension pneumothorax, and esophageal rupture. All of these conditions tend to manifest with chest pain, and they all should be considered early in the evaluation of the patient with chest pain.

Table 1. Rapidly Life-Threatening Diagnoses Presenting with Chest Pain

Acute coronary syndrome (myocardial ischemia and infarction)
Aortic dissection
Pulmonary embolism
Pericarditis with cardiac tamponade
Myocarditis
Tension pneumothorax
Esophageal rupture

It is the responsibility of the emergency physician to evaluate these patients with the list of potential life-threats at the top of the differential diagnosis (see Table). A detailed history, physical examination (with focus on cardiac, pulmonary, and vascular examinations), and basic testing information (e.g., electrocardiogram, chest radiograph) can often rapidly rule out these life-threats with reasonable accuracy. However, in cases where this initial rapid assessment fails to rule out one of the deadly diagnoses, further ED or in-hospital workup is warranted.

Many of the potential life-threats that present with chest pain are described elsewhere in this book. The focus of the discussion in this section is the acute coronary syndrome (ACS).

II. PRESENTATION OF THE PATIENT WITH ACS: CLASSIC VS. ACTUAL PRESENTATIONS

Most textbooks and teachings to students and junior physicians describe a typical or "classic" presentation of ACS as follows: the patient presents with gradual onset of midsternal and/or left-sided chest pain; the pain usually radiates to the left side, including the left arm, left neck, or left jaw; the pain is described as a pressure or squeezing sensation; the pain is brought on by and worsened with exertion; and associated symptoms include nausea, dyspnea, and diaphoresis.

Although this "classic" presentation may occur in some patients, multiple authors have demonstrated that the "actual" presentation is often very different.[1-9] The *onset* of pain in more than half of patients is a sudden onset rather than gradual, which may lead to misdiagnoses or delays in diagnoses as the treating physician focuses the workup on pulmonary embolism, aortic dissection, or other typically "sudden" causes of chest pain. Up to 20% of patients will report that the *location* of the pain is in the upper abdomen rather than the chest. Other common sites of isolated pain include the left arm, anterior neck/jaw, and upper back. Of even greater concern, up to one-third of patients have completely painless presentations. Most of those patients will instead present with an alternative "anginal equivalent," including dyspnea, vomiting, diaphoresis, generalized weakness, etc. Painless presentations occur most commonly in the elderly, diabetics, and women.

Radiation of the pain is common, but in up to 40% of cases, the pain radiates to the right side of the torso or to the right arm instead of the left side. In fact, radiation of the pain to right side of the body may be even more *specific* for cardiac pain than radiation of the pain to the left side. Pain may also radiate bilaterally, a finding that carries an even higher specificity for cardiac pain. (see table below) The *character* of the pain is described as classic "pressure" or "squeezing" in less than one-third of patients. Instead, 10–15% of patients describe the pain as a mild ache, and an additional 15–20% describe the pain as "sharp" or "stabbing" in nature. In 20% of cases, patients report a "burning" or "indigestion" type of pain, often leading to a misdiagnosis of reflux. The most common factor that is associated with onset or *worsening of pain* is moderate-to-heavy activity (physical stress). However, cardiac ischemia has also been noted to be brought on by emotional stress in 7% of cases. In 15% of cases, the chest pain of cardiac ischemia is worsened with direct palpation, and the pain is completely reproduced with direct palpation in 6–7%. Associated symptoms in ACS are common, especially nausea, dyspnea, and diaphoresis. However, increased belching is also common, present in up to half of all cases, and this may lead to a misdiagnosis of reflux or some other GI condition.

Table 2. Clinical Features That Increase the Probability of a Myocardial Infarction in Patients Presenting with Acute Chest Pain

Clinical Feature	Likelihood Ratio (95% Confidence Interval)
Pain in chest or left arm	2.7*
Chest pain radiation	
Right shoulder	2.9 (1.4–6.0)
Left arm	2.3 (1.7–3.1)
Both left and right arm	7.1 (3.6–14.2)
Chest pain most important symptom	2.0*
History of myocardial infarction	1.5–3.0†
Nausea or vomiting	1.9 (1.7–2.3)
Diaphoresis	2.0 (1.9–2.2)
Third heart sound on auscultation	3.2 (1.6–6.5)
Hypotension (systolic blood pressure ≤80 mm Hg	3.1 (1.8–5.2)
Pulmonary crackles on auscultation	2.1 (1.4–3.1)

* Data not available to calculate confidence intervals.
† In heterogeneous studies the likelihood ratios are reported as ranges.

Source: Panju AA, Hemmelgarn BR, Guyatt GH, et al. The rational clinical examination. Is this patient having a myocardial infarction? JAMA 1998;280:1256-63, 1261 (references omitted). Copyright © 1998. American Medical Association. Used with permission.

Table 3. Clinical Features That Decrease the Probability of a Myocardial Infarction in Patients Presenting with Acute Chest Pain

Clinical Feature	Likelihood Ratio (95% Confidence Interval)
Pleuritic chest pain	0.2 (0.2–0.3)
Chest pain sharp or stabbing	0.3 (0.2–0.5)
Positional chest pain	0.3 (0.2–0.4)
Chest pain reproduced by palpation	0.2–0.4†

† In heterogeneous studies the likelihood ratios are reported as ranges.

Source: Panju AA, Hemmelgarn BR, Guyatt GH, et al. The rational clinical examination. Is this patient having a myocardial infarction? JAMA 1998;280:1256-63, 1261 (references omitted). Copyright © 1998. American Medical Association. Used with permission.

It is interesting to note that the patient described in this case presented to the ED on two separate occasions with presentations that could easily have been misdiagnosed as reflux esophagitis or an alternative GI condition. On his first visit, he reported that he had been eating just prior to the onset of pain. He also described his pain as "heartburn." The treating physician must have given at least some consideration to this diagnosis because he chose to treat the patient with Maalox at one point. Fortunately there was no response, and the physician admitted the patient for a cardiac workup. After hospital discharge, the patient saw his primary care doctor and was diagnosed with reflux and given Prilosec. On his second visit to the ED, he reported that his chest pain was worse with eating, improved with Prilosec, and improved with sleeping propped up in bed. This scenario could easily be misattributed to reflux. Fortunately, the treating physician obtained an ECG and cardiac biomarkers, both of which were positive for ACS. If these tests had been normal, as they often are in the setting of cardiac ischemia, this patient could easily have been sent home from the ED and had a disastrous outcome … disastrous for the patient *and the physician.*

Reflux esophagitis is the most common misdiagnosis in cases of missed ACS. In reviewing the data above, it's no wonder why many patients with proven ACS present complaining of burning or indigestion, many patients will have an increase in belching, 8% of patients will have onset of pain while eating,[3] and nearly 30% will have relief of their pain with antacids.[10] Emergency physicians should beware the "pseudo-reflux ACS" and always think twice before writing "reflux" on the chart of a patient with chest pain!

III. RISK FACTOR ASSESSMENT

The treating physician should always consider cardiac risk factors (CRFs) when risk-stratifying the patient with chest pain for ACS. However, although the presence of any of these CRFs should increase one's suspicion for ACS, their absence should not dissuade one from pursuing the workup. In other words, even in the absence of any CRFs, a concerning history or ECG is still highly predictive of ACS.

The 7 "classic" CRFs identified in the Framingham studies are: male gender, age > 55 years old, diabetes mellitus, cigarette smoking, family history of early CAD, hypertension, and hyper-cholesterolemia. Additionally, several additional independent cardiac risk factors have been identified in recent years, including cocaine use, systemic lupus erythematosus, human immunodeficiency virus, and chronic renal disease. These will be discussed as well.

A few important considerations regarding gender, age, and diabetes mellitus should be made at this point. Although it is true that males are at greater risk of cardiac disease and ACS, women are at greater risk of misdiagnosis of ACS and poor outcome. Up to 20% of women with ACS lack chest pain, presenting instead with isolated arm or abdominal pain, nausea/vomiting, dyspnea, or diaphoresis.[11-13] Additionally, pain is noted to radiate to the right side more frequently than in men. Even when women have chest pain, they are less likely to have an ECG performed, and the ECGs are more likely to demonstrate nonspecific or subtle abnormalities than in men.[14] Women are also more likely to have false-negative stress tests and are less likely to receive thrombolytics and invasive therapies than men.[15] Many of these factors lead to a higher mortality in women, even young women, with ACS.[16]

Elderly patients are another high-risk group for atypical presentations of ACS and misdiagnosis. Painless presentations of ACS are present in 40% of patients > 65 years old and in 60–70% of patients > 85 years old. In these patients, the most common anginal equivalent is dyspnea, but diaphoresis, vomiting, and neurologic abnormalities (confusion, lethargy, generalized weakness, stroke symptoms, syncope) are common as well.[17,18] As a general rule, ECG testing should be rapidly obtained on any elderly patient with one of these presentations, regardless of whether or not the patient reports chest pain. Atypical presentations and concerns regarding complications of treatment have led physicians to undertreat elderly patients with ACS. The elderly are less likely to receive thrombolytics as well as percutaneous coronary interventions, even when other contraindications are not present. Although the complication rates in elderly patients receiving these treatments are higher than in younger patients, the relative mortality benefit is higher as well, and aggressive treatment of elderly patients with ACS is recommended.

Young patients (< 45 years old) represent another group at high risk for misdiagnosis of ACS, primarily because of a tendency on the part of physicians to underestimate cardiac risk in young patients. Up to 10% of myocardial infarctions in the US occur in patients < 45 years old, the majority of which are related to atherosclerotic heart disease. Atherosclerotic disease was noted in 17% of teenagers in one study,[19] and multivessel disease noted in 20% of young adults (avg. age 26 years old) in an autopsy study of victims of inner city violence.[20] A recent ED study found that 5.4% of patients 24–39 years old presenting with chest pain ruled-in for ACS, and 2.2% had an adverse cardiac event (defined as death, MI, need for percutaneous coronary intervention or cardiac bypass surgery) within 30 days.[21] Although the overall incidence of ACS is lower in young patients, physicians should not discount a concerning HPI purely based on a patient's age.

Diabetes mellitus (DM) represents another high-risk condition in terms of potential for misdiagnosis of ACS. Patients with DM are prone to painless presentations when they have cardiac ischemia. Atypical presentations (e.g., dyspnea, confusion, emesis, fatigue) occur in up to 40% of cases. Diabetic patients are also more likely to have adverse outcomes from ACS.[22] One study, in fact, demonstrated that diabetic patients with ACS and negative cardiac biomarkers have the same risk of adverse outcomes as non-diabetic patients with ACS and *positive* biomarkers.[23] Treating physicians must therefore not rely on typical presenting complaints to initiate a cardiac workup in diabetic patients, nor should they rely on positive cardiac biomarkers to prompt an aggressive approach to treatment in these patients.

Cocaine use must be considered an additional independent risk factor for atherosclerotic heart disease and MI, even in young patients. Some authors estimate that cocaine accounts for up to 25% of acute MIs in patients < 45 years old.[24] Acute use of cocaine can induce coronary vasoconstriction, increased platelet aggregation, and/or adrenergic stimulation that leads to dysrhythmias and ischemia. Chronic use of cocaine is associated with MI, as well, causing markedly accelerated atherogenesis and subsequent early MI. Its use is also associated with contraction band necrosis of myocytes which, over the course of years, leads to the development of cardiomyopathies.[25] Overall, cocaine users have a 7-fold increased risk of MI.[24] It is estimated that 6% of cocaine users presenting to the ED with chest pain will rule-in for myocardial infarction.[26]

Systemic lupus erythematosus (SLE) is a significant but underappreciated risk factor for early atherosclerosis and myocardial infarction. Young patients with SLE are estimated to have a nine-fold increased risk of early MI.[27-29] Women, < 45 years old in particular, are at increased risk, with estimates of increased risk of early MI as high as 50-fold.[30,31] The cause of premature atherosclerosis in SLE is likely multifactorial, but largely related to co-existing systemic inflammation and dyslipidemias.

Human Immunodeficiency Virus (HIV) infection has recently been identified as an independent risk factor for premature atherosclerosis as well. Evidence suggests that HIV infection causes endothelial injury to coronary vessels, initiating an inflammatory cascade leading to atherosclerotic lesions.[32] The finding of premature atherosclerosis is especially prominent in patients with later stages of HIV infection (CD4 count ≤ 200).[33] The medication regimens that are currently used in treating HIV (protease inhibitors) also exacerbate the risk of early atherosclerosis. These medications may cause insulin resistance, elevations of triglyceride levels, and elevations of low-density lipoprotein levels.[34] Overall, HIV patients with ACS present at an age that is more than 10 years younger than non-HIV patients.[35]

Chronic renal disease (CRD) has also recently been identified as an independent risk factor for accelerated atherosclerosis. Several metabolic abnormalities have been directly linked to CRD, including dyslipidemias, homocysteinemia, and elevated levels of lipoprotein (a).[36] Each of these abnormalities is directly associated with atherogenesis. In addition, CRD is associated with chronic inflammation[36] and increased platelet aggregation.[37] These factors, combined with an increased prevalence of concomitant conventional risk factors, produce a disproportionately high risk of cardiac events in these patients.[36]

IV. DIAGNOSTIC TESTING IN THE PATIENT WITH SUSPECTED ACUTE CORONARY SYNDROME

There is considerable literature pertaining to the topic of diagnostic testing in patients with chest pain and suspected ACS. The most common and important tests used in evaluating patients for ACS are electrocardiography, cardiac biomarkers, stress testing, and coronary angiography. For brevity's sake, the discussion that follows will focus on some risk management issues pertaining to these diagnostic tests.

Most patients presenting to the ED with a complaint of chest pain should receive prompt electro-cardiography. The most recent guidelines of the American College of Cardiology/American Heart Association (ACC/AHA)[38] state that a 12-lead ECG should be obtained and shown to an experienced emergency physician within 10 minutes of ED arrival for all patients with symptoms suggestive of ST-segment elevation MI (e.g., chest pain). The primary utility of the ECG, however, is to risk stratify patients being admitted for ACS and determine the type of care. For example, the physician should use the ECG to determine whether the patient warrants emergent reperfusion therapy (thrombolytics, PCI) vs. ICU admission vs. floor admission, etc. The ECG should *not* be used to rule out ACS, since up to 50% of patients with cardiac ischemia or infarction will have a non-specific or normal ECG.[39] Serial ECGs can increase the diagnostic yield for confirming the presence of ACS in patients with ongoing symptoms, and they are recommended under the ACC/AHA Guidelines when the initial ECG is non-diagnostic but a strong suspicion of ACS remains. However, serial ECGs cannot rule out ischemia or infarction, and they have limited utility once the symptoms have resolved.

Much like the ECG, cardiac biomarkers are useful when they are positive but have limited utility when they are normal. Serial biomarker testing over the course of 6–12 hours has become a routine protocol in many EDs and has excellent sensitivity for detecting evidence of MI. However, biomarkers cannot be relied upon to rule out cardiac ischemia. If the HPI is suggestive of ACS, patients should not be discharged from the ED based on negative biomarkers. Physicians should also be wary of obtaining a single set of biomarkers prior to discharge, since this may actually increase the liability of the emergency physician if an adverse outcome occurs.[40] The bottom line is that, if there is a significant enough concern for biomarker testing, the patient usually requires hospital admission, not simply discharge after a negative test.

Stress testing and coronary angiography are being used more commonly early in the evaluation of patients with chest pain to rule in ACS. Although a negative stress test or angiogram is associated with a *lower* risk of underlying CAD, neither test can definitively *rule out* ACS or the presence of significant underlying coronary thromboses. The majority of stress testing modalities detect evidence of significant coronary lesions with only 85–95% sensitivities.[41,42] Coronary angiography is also an imperfect test; false negative angiography interpretations are not uncommon in the presence of diffuse disease, eccentric plaques, "flush" occlusions, branch ostial lesions, overlapping side branches, and even when lesions are present within the left main coronary artery.[43] Further compromising the reliability of these tests is data indicating that the majority of MIs occur from occlusions within arteries that were previously < 50% obstructed before the infarct occured.[44-47] These types of lesions are usually associated with negative stress tests or "non-significant" angiograms if the tests are done prior to infarct. As a result, physicians should be wary of discharging a patient with a concerning HPI purely because of a recent "negative" stress test or coronary angiogram.

V. SUMMARY
The evaluation of chest pain and possible ACS in the ED is a high-risk endeavor. The decision to pursue a "full cardiac workup" should primarily be based on a thorough HPI. Physicians should be aware of the frequency of atypical presentations, especially in women, elderly, and diabetic patients. Young patients also deserve special consideration, as their risk is often underappreciated. Several new independent cardiac risk factors have been identified in recent years which warrant extra attention, including cocaine use, systemic lupus erythematosus, human immunodeficiency virus, and chronic renal disease. Diagnostic testing in the ED consists of electrocardiography, helpful to rule in ACS, but not to rule out the diagnosis, and cardiac biomarker testing, which is also primarily useful when

positive. The single set of biomarkers, when obtained in the ED, has limited utility and may actually increase medicolegal risk to the emergency physician. Finally, the negative stress test or angiogram is very helpful at stratifying patients to a low risk of ACS and CAD, but physicians should remember that they do not definitively *rule out* the diagnosis.

TEACHING POINTS ABOUT CASE 7:

- A negative stress test does not exclude a possibility of cardiac disease.
- In 20% of cases, patients report indigestion-type discomfort, often leading to a misdiagnosis of reflux.
- 30% of patients with ACS will have pain relief with antacids. Reflux esophagitis is the most common misdiagnosis in cases of missed ACS. Relief of discomfort with antacids does not exclude a diagnosis of cardiac disease.

REFERENCES

1. Canto JG, Shlipak MG, Rogers WJ, et al. Prevalence, clinical characteristics, and mortality among patients with myocardial infarction presenting without chest pain. JAMA 2000; 283:3223-9.
2. Coronado BE, Pope HJ, Griffith JL, et al. Clinical features, triage, and outcome of patients presenting to the ED with suspected acute coronary syndromes but without pain: a multicenter study. Am J Emerg Med 2004; 22:568-74.
3. Culic V, Eterovic D, Miric D. Meta-analysis of possible external triggers of acute myocardial infarction. Int J Cardiol 2005; 99:1-8.
4. Disla E, Rhim HR, Reddy A, et al. Costochondritis. A prospective analysis in an emergency department setting. Arch Intern Med 1994; 154:2466-9.
5. Goodacre S, Locker T, Morris F, et al. How useful are clinical features in the diagnosis of acute, undifferentiated chest pain? Acad Emerg Med 2002;9:203-8.
6. Goodacre SW, Angelini K, Arnold J, et al. Clinical predictors of acute coronary syndromes in patients with undifferentiated chest pain. Q J Med 2003;96:893-8.
7. Gupta M, Tabas JA, Kohn MA. Presenting complaint among patients with myocardial infarction who present to an urban, public hospital emergency department. Ann Emerg Med 2002; 40:180-6.
8. Lusiani L, Perrone A, Pesavento R, et al. Prevalence, clinical features, and acute course of atypical myocardial infarction. Angiology 1994:45:49-55.
9. Panju AA, Hemmelgarn BR, Guyatt GH, et al. The rational clinical examination. Is this patient having a myocardial infarction? JAMA 1998; 280:1256-63.
10. Teece S, Crawford I. Towards evidence based emergency medicine: best BETs from the Manchester Royal Infirmiry. Antacids and diagnosis in patients with atypical chest pain. Emerg Med J 2003; 20:170-1.
11. Milner KA, Vaccarino V, Arnold AL, et al. Gender and age differences in chief complains of acute myocardial infarction (Worcester heart attack study). Am J Cardiol 2004;93:606-8.
12. Patel H, Rosengren A, Ekman I. Symptoms in acute coronary syndromes: Does sex make a difference? Am Heart J 2004; 148:27-33.
13. Rosengren A, Wallentin L, Gitt AK, et al. Sex, age, and clinical presentation of acute coronary syndromes. Eur Heart J 2004; 25:663-70.

14. Arnold AL, Milner KA, Vaccarino V. Sex and race differences in electrocardiogram use (the national hospital ambulatory medical care survey). Am J Cardiol 2001; 88:1037-40.
15. Heer T, Schiele R, Schneider S, et al. Gender differences in acute myocardial infarction in the era of reperfusion (the MITRA registry). Am J Cardiol 2002; 89:511-7.
16. Vaccarino V, Parsons L, Every NR, et al. Sex-based differences in early mortality after myocardial infarction. N Engl J Med 1999; 341:217-5.
17. Canto JG, Fincher C, Kiefe CI, et al. Atypical presentations among medicare beneficiearies with unstable angina pectoris. Am J Cardiol 2002; 90:248-53.
18. Kalbfleisch N. Acute myocardial infarction. In: Sanders AB (ed.). Emergency care of the elder person. St. Louis: Beverly Cracom Publications, 1996.
19. Tuzcu EM, Kapadia SR, Tutar E, et al. High prevalence of coronary atherosclerosis in asymptomatic teenagers and young adults: evidence from intravascular ultrasound. Circulation 2001; 103:2705-10.
20. Joseph A, Ackerman D, Talley JD, et al. Manifestions of coronary atherosclerosis in young trauma victims—an autopsy study. J Am Coll Cardiol 1993; 222:459-67.
21. Marsan RJ Jr., Shaver KJ, Sease KL, et al. Evaluation of a clinical decision rule for young adult patients with chest pain. Acad Emerg Med 2005; 12:26-32.
22. Fergus TS, Fazel R, Fang J, et al. Presentation, management, and outcomes of diabeteic patients compared to non-diabetic patients admitted for acute coronary syndromes. Heart 2004; 90:1051-2.
23. Fazel R, Fang J, Kline-Rogers E, et al. Prognostic value of elevated biomarkers in diabetic and non-diabetic patients admitted for acute coronary syndromes. Heart 2005; 91:388-90.
24. Qureshi AI, Suri MF, Guterman LR, et al. Cocaine use and the likelihood of nonfatal myocardial infarction and stroke: data from the Third National Health and Nutrition Examination Survey. Circulation 2001; 103:502-6.
25. Kloner RA, Rezkalla SH. Cocaine and the heart. N Engl J Med 2003; 348:487-8.
26. Weber JE, Chudnofsky CR, Boczar M, et al. Cocaine-associated chest pain: how common is myocardial infarction? Acad Emerg Med 2000; 7:873-7.
27. D'Agate DJ, Kokolis S, Belilos E, et al. Premature coronary artery disease in systemic lupus erythematosus with extensive reocclusion following coronary artery bypass surgery. J Invasive Cardiol 2003; 15:157-63.
28. Hahn BH. Systemic lupus erythematosus and accelerated atherosclerosis. N Engl J Med 2003; 349:2379-80.
29. Rahman P, Urowitz MB, Gladman DD, et al. Contribution of traditional risk factors to coronary artery disease in patients with systemic lupus erythematosus. J Rheumatol 1999; 26:2363-8.
30. Manzi S, Meilahn EN, Rairie JE, et al. Age-specific incidence rates of myocardial infarction and angina in women with systemic lupus erythematosus: comparison with the Framingham Study. Am J Epidemiol 1997; 145:408-15.
31. Ward MM. Premature morbidity from cardiovascular and cerebrovascular diseases in women with systemic lupus erythematosus. Arthritis Rheum 1999; 42:338-46.
32. Varriale P, Saravi G, Hernandez E, et al. Acute myocardial infarction in patients infected with human immunodeficiency virus. Am Heart J 2004; 147:55-9.
33. Hsue PY, Lo JC, Franklin A, et al. Progression of atherosclerosis as assessed by carotid intima-media thickness in patients with HIV infection. Circulation 2004; 109:1603-8.

34. Carr A, Samaras K, Thorisdottir A, et al. Diagnosis, prediction, and natural course of HIV-1 protease-inhibitor-associated lipodystrophy, hyperlipidaemia, and diabetes mellitus: a cohort study. Lancet 1999; 353:2093-9.

35. Hsue PY, Giri K, Erickson S, et al. Clinical features of acute coronary syndromes in patients with human immunodeficiency virus infection. Circulation 2004; 109:316-9.

36. Yerkey MW, Kernis SJ, Franklin BA, et al. Renal dysfunction and acceleration of coronary disease. Heart 2004; 90:961-6.

37. Aggarwal A, Kabbani SS, Rimmer JM, et al. Biphasic effects of hemodialysis on platelet reactivity in patients with end-stage renal disease: a potential contributor to cardiovascular risk. Am J Kidney Dis 2002; 40:315-22.

38. Antman EM, Anbe DT, Armstrong PW, et al. ACC/AHA guidelines for the management of patients with ST-elevation myocardial infarction—executive summary: a report of the American College of Cardiology/American Heart Association Task Force on Practice Guidelines (Writing Committee to Revise the 1999 Guidelines for the Management of Patients With Acute Myocardial Infarction). Circulation 2004; 110:588-636.

39. Brady WJ, Aufderheide TP, Chan T, et al. Electrocardiographic diagnosis of acute myocardial infarction. Emerg Med Clin North Am 2001; 19:295-320.

40. Henry GL. Specific high-risk medical-legal issues. In: Henry GL, Sullivan DJ (eds.). Emergency Medicine Risk Management, 2nd ed. Dallas: American College of Emergency Physicians, 1997.

41. Ioannidis JPA, Salem D, Chew PW, et al. Accuracy of imaging technologies in the diagnosis of acute cardiac ischemia in the emergency department: a meta-analysis. Ann Emerg Med 2001; 37:471-7.

42. Lateef F, Gibler WB. Provocative testing for chest pain. Am J Emerg Med 2000; 18:793-801.

43. Schwartz L, Gourassa MG. Evaluation of patients with chest pain and normal coronary angiograms. Arch Int Med 2001; 161:1825-33.

44. Giroud D, Li JM, Urban P, et al. Relation of the site of acute myocardial infarction to the most severe coronary arterial stenosis at prior angiography. Am J Cardiol 1992; 69:729-32.

45. Hackett D, Davies G, Maseri A. Pre-existing coronary stenoses in patients with first myocardial infarction are not necessarily severe. Eur Heart J 1988;9:1317-23.

46. Hackett D, Verwilghen J, Davies G, et al. Coronary stenoses before and after acute myocardial infarction. Am J Cardiol 1989; 63:1517-8.

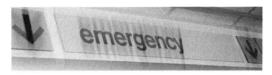

CASE 8
38 YEAR OLD FEMALE WITH ABDOMINAL PAIN

Commentary:
Gregory L. Henry, MD, FACEP

CEO, Medical Practice Risk Assessment, Inc., Ann Arbor, Michigan
Clinical Professor, Department of Emergency Medicine
   University of Michigan Medical School, Ann Arbor, Michigan
Past President, American College of Emergency Physicians (ACEP)

Discussion:
William Mallon, MD, FACEP, FAAEM

Associate Professor of Clinical Emergency Medicine
   Keck School of Medicine at USC
Director, Division of International Emergency Medicine
   Los Angeles County + USC Medical Center, Los Angeles, California
American Academy of Emergency Medicine (AAEM) Program Director of the Year, 2004

Jan M. Shoenberger, MD, FAAEM

Assistant Professor of Clinical Emergency Medicine
Director of Medical Student Education
Assistant Program Director
   Keck School of Medicine at USC
   Los Angeles County + USC Medical Center, Los Angeles, California

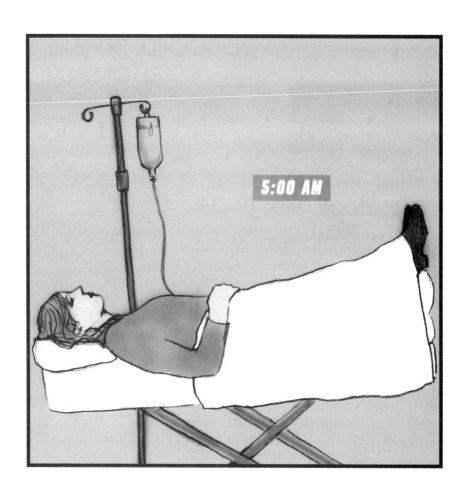

38 YEAR OLD FEMALE WITH
ABDOMINAL PAIN

—Initial Visit*—

*Authors' Note: The history, exam and notes are the actual documentation of the physicians and providers, including abbreviations (and spelling errors)

CHIEF COMPLAINT (at 02:43): Abdominal pain

VITAL SIGNS

Time	Temp(F)	Pulse	Resp	Syst	Diast	Pain Scale
02:49	99.0	100	18	110	80	8
04:36		92	19	101	63	0

HISTORY OF PRESENT ILLNESS (03:19): Last night at 19:30 pt had a sudden onset of sharp, RLQ pain. She has had nausea and vomiting 3 times. She did have a syncopal episode. She is currently undergoing fertility therapy. She has never been pregnant. LMP 23 days ago. She had some spotting last week and saw her GYN who did a pelvic. She has a history of endometriosis. No history of kidney stones, although there is a family history. No fever, rigors, dysuria, frequency or hematuria. No vaginal discharge or history of STDs. No rash. She has had an inguinal herniorrhaphy but no other abdominal or pelvic surgeries. No DM or other chronic illness, cough, dyspnea, or back pain. Appetite is good.

PAST MEDICAL HISTORY/TRIAGE (02:45):
  Allergies: No known allergies.
  Meds: The patient is not taking medications at this time
  PMH: Endometriosis
  PSH: Herniorrhaphy
  Family history: Kidney stones

EXAM (03:23)
  General: Pale-appearing; well-nourished; awake and alert
  Head: Normocephalic; atraumatic
  Eyes: No icterus, no conjunctival pallor
  Nose: The nose is normal in appearance without rhinorrhea
  Neck: No JVD or distended neck veins
  Resp: Normal chest excursion with respiration; breath sounds clear and equal bilaterally
  Card: Regular rhythm, without murmur
  Abd: Non-distended; tender to both LQs, +obturator and heel tap, otherwise soft, without rigidity, rebound or guarding, no pulsatile mass. Negative bilateral Lloyd's sign

Skin: Normal for age and race; warm and dry without diaphoresis ; no apparent lesions
Extremities: Pulses are 2 plus and equal times 4 extremities, no peripheral edema or calf muscle pain
GU: External genitalia normal. Pelvic exam: cervix with blue hue and scant clear discharge at the os but appears to be closed. +CMT. +exquisite R adnexal tenderness. No masses palpated.

ORDERS (03:12): Dilaudid 1mg IVP, phenergan 12.5mg IVP

PROCEDURES (03:13): Urine pregnancy test (ordered in triage and performed by RN in ED) is positive.

RESULTS: *Reviewed and resulted by the physician at 03:58*

Test	Flag	Value	Units	Ref. Range
WBC	H	22.5	K/uL	4.6-10.2
HGB		13.0	G/DL	12.0-16.0
PLT		325	K/uL	142-424
SEGS		84%		40-85
BANDS		5%		
BLOOD TYPE		OPOS		

Test	Flag	Value	Units	Ref. Range
NA		137	MMOL/L	135-144
K		3.7	MMOL/L	3.5-5.1
CL		100	MMOL/L	98-107
CO2		27	MMOL/L	22-29
BUN		13	MG/DL	7-18
CREAT		0.9	MG/DL	0.6-1.3

Test	Flag	Value	Units	Ref. Range
HCGQUANT	H	196	mIU/ML	0-6

Urinalysis—WNL except WBC=5-10, bacteria=rare. RBC=0-5

Wet prep: Negative for trichomonas and yeast

PROGRESS NOTES:
- **At 04:15** I paged an OB/GYN for consultation
- **At 04:19** I spoke with the OB attending for hospital admission
- **At 04:22** I spoke with OB house officer and they will come to the ED to see the patient.
- **At 04:30** The OB house officer did come down to the ED and evaluated the patient and discussed the case with the attending and feels this is appendicitis and a surgeon should be consulted.

Second half of ED visit follows...

Gregory L. Henry comments:

"There is a name given to women who use the date of their last menstrual period to predict ovulation—it's called mommy!"

Women of childbearing age are pregnant until proven otherwise. I am essentially an anti-test doctor, but the urine pregnancy test is incredibly useful. A positive urine pregnancy test can never be ignored. If the test says a patient is pregnant, she is pregnant with 99.7% accuracy. The fact that the woman has not been sexually active should make no difference. Questions regarding sexual activity are almost useless; I do not really care if a woman is sexually active. I just want to know if she is pregnant. There is a name given to women who use the date of their last menstrual period to predict ovulation—it's called mommy!

The main causes of sudden onset of abdominal pain are rupture of a hollow viscous or vascular structure and the sudden obstruction of a tube. Appendicitis rarely has a sudden onset. Most importantly, a patient with a positive pregnancy test and no intrauterine pregnancy should be considered to have an ectopic pregnancy until proven otherwise. The lack of tachycardia does not mean the patient is not going into shock. Studies documenting bradycardia due to blood against the peritoneal reflection are well known. Bradycardia is the paradoxical response until the patient is considerably shocky. The physician should not be dissuaded by the initial heart rate, blood pressure, or hemoglobin.

The fact that an OB resident disagreed with the emergency physician should not impede in the appropriate management of this patient. Residents are children. If there is a difference of opinion, the ED physician needs to speak to the attending directly. With a positive pregnancy test, to believe that the abdominal pain is due to appendicitis is folly.

The documentation on this case is really quite good. We do know that the OB house officer evaluated the patient and when important events occurred. However, it is not documented that the emergency physician disagreed with the plan or if the OB attending appeared in the emergency department. Whenever there is a conflict between the emergency physician and the attending physician, the attending physician needs to either acquiesce to the emergency physician's opinion, or come to the department and evaluate the patient. Failure to do so spells disaster. Everyone wants to sail the ship in fair weather. When the storm blows (the patient goes into shock), it will always be the emergency physician's fault, unless he clearly insisted and properly documented his concerns and expectations for the specialist.

- Thoroughness of Evaluation of Patient: 9 out of 10.

- Thoroughness of Documentation: 9 out of 10.

- **Risk of Serious Illness Being Missed:** High risk.

- **Risk Management Legal Rating:** High risk. This is the problem of too many cooks spoiling the soup. A resident should never stand in the way of intelligent medical care.

38 YEAR OLD FEMALE WITH ABDOMINAL PAIN

—Continuation of Same ED Visit: ED Course—

RESULTS: Ultrasound (*results at 04:49*): No intrauterine pregnancy is seen. There is a large amount of inhomogeneous hypoechoic material in the pelvis, which could represent blood or complicated fluid. This is not specific, but the possibility that this could be related to a ruptured ectopic pregnancy should be strongly considered. Clinical correlation is suggested.

VITAL SIGNS									
Time	Temp(F)	Pulse	Resp	Syst	Diast	Pos.	O2	Sat O2%	Pain Scale
05:12		88	20	79	55	S			0
05:16		86		91	55	L			0
05:36		90	20	86	45	L	100	ra	
06:09		76	20	105	70	L			2
06:28		76	22	112	56	L			2

PROGRESS NOTES per physician unless otherwise specified (continued):
- (Time not given) The patient's condition has changed and she is now hypotensive and I have asked the OB house officer to go back into the room to re-examine the patient. They did re-examine and felt that she looked worse, but disagreed about the diagnosis of ectopic as her quant was too low, menses was only 3 weeks ago and her WBC was too high. They asked for a surgery consultation to evaluate for appendicitis.
- **At 05:14** (per RN) - Pt. placed in trendelenburg, is increasing pale, denies lightheadedness but states that she is having trouble staying awake. OB residents present and aware. Pt. continues to deny pain.
- **At 05:26** I spoke with the surgeon to discuss case and I spoke with surgical house officer and they will come to the ED to evaluate the patient.
- **At 05:28** I spoke with the OB attending to discuss case and told them that the BP had dropped and they recommended recheck CBC and if the Hb has dropped (see below) they would take to OR. They felt that she wasn't tachycardic and Hb wasn't low enough to be a ruptured ectopic.
- **At 05:32** (per RN) - Pt. remain in trendelenburg position. Multiple attempts to obtain another IV access have failed. The doctor is aware. Surg. Resident here and aware of pt's condition. Husband remains at bedside and updated.
- **Re-exam at 05:39** – Pt. with increased pallor. Abdomen appears normal. Abdomen is firm, tender RLQ and pelvis with some voluntary guarding.
- **At 06:47** I again spoke with the OB attending and the OB house officer and related my concerns for ectopic or hemorrhagic cyst and the need for lap ASAP. Pt's pain has worsened but her exam is unchanged. Her VS are stable with a room air sat of 100%.

```
CBC (drawn at 05:36)
  Test     Flag  Value    Units     Ref. Range
  WBC       H     18.6     K/uL       4.6-10.2
  HGB       L     11.2     G/DL      12.0-16.0
  PLT             306      K/uL      142-424
```

DIAGNOSIS:
1. Pelvic pain
2. Pregnancy
3. Leukocytosis
4. Anemia

DISPOSITION: Patient assigned to OR bed. She did have a lap at 7:15 AM with a post op diagnosis of ruptured tubal pregnancy. She did well post-op and left the hospital without complications.

FINAL DIAGNOSIS: Ruptured tubal pregnancy

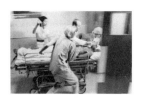

DISCUSSION OF ECTOPIC PREGNACY WITH A RISK MANAGEMENT FOCUS

William Mallon, MD, FACEP
Jan M. Shoenberger, MD, FAAEM

I. EVALUATION OF ABDOMINAL PAIN

Abdominal pain is a common ED presentation which can be particularly vexing from a diagnostic and management standpoint. In most ED series of unselected patients with abdominal pain (i.e., no referral bias), the final diagnosis in one-third was "non-specific abdominal pain" or "abdominal pain of unknown etiology." While most of these patients do well, and indeed, most with a defined etiology are also managed as outpatients, there is a subset of patients with abdominal pain who will require immediate surgical care.

The mantra of emergency medicine is "think worst first." Focusing on surgical diseases which need immediate intervention is an important part of the ED thought process. Since **early** surgical intervention is desirable in many of these entities, **time** is an important feature. Failure to get to the operative suite in a timely fashion allows the surgical condition to worsen with resultant life-threatening problems (Table 1).

Table 1. Outcomes of Delayed Diagnosis of a Surgical Abdomen

	SURGICAL ENTITIES	TIME RELATED OUTCOME
1.	Ectopic (± ruptured)	Hemorrhagic shock
2.	Ovarian torsion	Ovarian death & loss of reproductive capability
3.	Ruptured ovarian cyst	Hemorrhagic shock
4.	Ruptured AAA	Hemorrhagic shock
5.	Ischemic bowel	Septic shock
6.	Testicular torsion	Testicular death & loss of reproductive capability
7.	Diverticulitis	Perforation
8.	Cholecystitis	Septic shock
9.	Incarcerated hernia	Ischemic bowel→sepsis
10.	Appendicitis	Septic shock
11.	Perforated ulcer	Pancreatitis, sepsis

When this list is further reviewed, it can be cross-referenced with the patient's demographics (age, gender) and historical features. The salient elements of our patient are: female, young, afebrile, with a sudden onset of pain, severe enough to cause syncope. These historical features help to narrow our differential (from the table above) to ectopic pregnancy, ovarian torsion, ruptured ovarian cyst, and ruptured AAA.

II. THE URINE PREGNANCY TEST AND USE OF QUANTITATIVE β-HCG LEVELS

Several features in her history should immediately point to the need for a pregnancy test. She saw her gynecologist recently, she is undergoing infertility treatment, and she is still menstruating. This 38 year old who is G? P? (a big hole in the history) who has a history of endometriosis and is trying to be pregnant.

Early in her care, a bedside pregnancy test is done and found to be positive. Ectopic pregnancy is now a diagnosis that is really in play. The sensitivity of a bedside test for pregnancy is 99% and the specificity is 99%. The quantitative β-hCG adds to delay and is often irrelevant, although specialists will request it. The quantitative test can be a vehicle for errors and delay.

ERROR 1 ✘ Waiting for it to be done

ERROR 2 ✘ Holding up the ultrasound for a β-hCG in the discriminatory zone

ERROR 3 ✘ Failure to recognize that abnormal pregnancies produce abnormally low amounts of β-hCG

In every series of patients with ectopic pregnancies, many are identified with β-hCG levels well below the discriminatory zone (β-hCG level of 1,200). While the quantitative β-hCG might help with interpretation of the ultrasound by indicating that an intrauterine pregnancy should be visible, a low β-hCG in no way rules out ectopic pregnancy. In Rick Bukata's essay on the topic, he says:

> "It is important to note that as many as a third of patients with ruptured ectopic pregnancies will have β-hCG levels below 100 mIU/mL and that β-hCG levels do not correlate well with the potential for rupture. It has been suggested that serial levels should <u>not</u> be obtained when the diagnosis of ectopic pregnancy is likely and that, when they are performed, it should be done in consultation with a gynecologist who will follow the patients and interpret the results."[1]

How should the quantitative β-hCG be used? First, if the β-hCG is greater than 1200, it is above the discriminatory zone and an IUP should be visible on ultrasound if present. Second, serial β-hCGs may be followed serially. If a β-hCG is decreasing rapidly (by more than 50%) over 24–48 hours, it is unlikely to be an ectopic pregnancy and miscarriages are much more common. If the β-hCG is increasing significantly (more than 66%) over 24–48 hours, this is strongly suggestive of a normal pregnancy. If the rate of change is between these two, ectopic may be present. The risk of an ectopic with an empty uterus by transvaginal ultrasound and a positive β-hCG (**regardless** of the magnitude of the quantitative vale) is great (odds ratio 24.8!).[2] In this case, a quantitative β-hCG has almost no role in the determination of diagnosis because the ultrasound is positive for free fluid, not indeterminate. Serial β-hCG testing is of most utility when the ultrasound is "indeterminate" (see VII. Ultrasound below).

III. VITAL SIGNS AND SYNCOPE

In every series of patients with ectopic pregnancy, syncope is found as a presenting symptom. The disproportionate amount of syncope relates to the fact that patients with ruptured ectopics and hypovolemia fail to manifest tachycardia. This "inappropriate" bradycardia is another source of errors, falsely reassuring clinicians that the "low-ish" blood pressure cannot be hemorrhagic shock because the pulse rate is "too low" to be shock. One explanation for this "paradoxical bradycardia" involves increased vagal tone.[3,4] The essential fact to remember is that syncope occurs if you have hemorrhage without compensatory tachycardia. Our patient's syncopal episode, in the setting of a positive pregnancy test, further points to ectopic pregnancy (although ruptured AAA can cause syncope and bradycardia—a very unlikely diagnosis for our patient!). This scenario is so well known as to be a standard oral exam case.

The shock index is the Heart Rate/Systolic Blood Pressure, with a normal range of 0.5–0.7. It has been proposed to help compensate for the poor pulse rate response in cases of ruptured ectopic pregnancy.[5] Our patient has a positive shock index (0.9) at presentation, which rises throughout her ED course to a maximum of 1.1. While the sensitivity here is low (28%), the specificity is high (96%).

IV. PHYSICAL EXAM

The physical examination is usually a device to confirm clinical suspicions and indicate pace and aggressiveness of therapy. In our patient the key features are:

1. Bilateral lower quadrant tenderness
2. Peritoneal signs (Positive heel tap)
3. Blue cervix (Chadwick's sign)
4. Positive cervical motion tenderness
5. Extreme right adnexal tenderness

This exam is stating loud and clear that the right adnexa is the source of the problem. Ovarian torsion, ruptured cyst, tubo-ovarian abscess (TOA) and ectopic are all possible; however, the presentation does not fit with TOA as the patient was afebrile with a sudden onset of pain. At this time, we have narrowed the diagnosis down to the following possibilities:

1. Intrauterine pregnancy with torsion of right ovary
2. Ectopic, right fallopian tube
3. Intrauterine pregnancy with heterotopic ectopic
4. Ruptured ovarian cyst

Speculum examination in cases of ectopic pregnancy has been shown to be of little to no value and only adds to delay in treatment.[6] One study has suggested that the physical exam is unreliable as a means to diagnose ectopic pregnancy, and that ultrasound should be done in any case where ectopic is in the differential.[7] In any event, our patient's examination should be completed with haste, since time is important in all of the above scenarios.

V. LABORATORY RESULTS

The quantitative β-hCG is below the discriminatory zone, but the white blood cell count (WBC) is quite high at 22.5. This is extremely non-specific, although it is non-specifically bad. In an afebrile patient, leukocytosis may not point to infection, but may be due to demargination and adrenergic surge. The electrolytes are all normal. Urinalysis is negative.

Whenever repeat labs are requested, it should hint that "lab trending" is taking the place of action. The repeat CBC drawn at 05:36 (for the consultant) shows that the hemoglobin has fallen almost 2 points, equaling a hematocrit fall of about 5%. The WBC is still elevated at 18.6. Many articles confirm the low utility of WBC counts in this context; all indicate that the WBC count is much less important than the clinical features of the case. Nagurney et al. noted that the CBC was of low utility in patients with non-traumatic abdominal pain.[9] In reference 8, the CBC affected patient management in only 2% of cases. In one of those cases, the diagnosis was erroneously changed to appendicitis due to an elevated WBC, identical to what occurred in this case. The WBC count is as often misleading as it is helpful.

Other laboratory tests that should be mentioned include creatine kinase and serum progesterone. Serum creatine kinase (CK) is not helpful in this diagnosis.[10, 11] Serum progesterone levels are not generally available in most EDs, with a turnaround time that is helpful to the physician. Despite this, a growing body of literature exists to suggest a single serum progesterone may be helpful in those cases with an indeterminate ultrasound (not our patient). The best series, which includes a validation set, suggests a cutoff of 22ng/mL, which would have a high sensitivity (100%) but low specificity for ectopic pregnancy.[12]

VI. HETEROTOPIC PREGNANCY

Heterotopic pregnancy (co-existing intrauterine and ectopic pregnancy) is often considered to be so rare (1:20,000–30,000 pregnancies)[13] as to be irrelevant. In this case, though, the incidence is much higher since she is undergoing "fertility therapy." In one study of a patient population undergoing in vitro fertilization (IVF), the rate of ectopic pregnancy was 5.4% over a 10-year period.[14] The medical record has some significant historical gaps here which would help quantify her increased risk for ectopic or heterotopic pregnancy. First, her parity and gravidity are totally absent from the record. Secondly, what type of "fertility treatment" is she undergoing? The possibilities are:

1. Ovarian stimulation (with clomiphene)
2. Embryo transfer
3. In vitro fertilization (IVF)
4. Intracytoplasmic sperm injection (ICSI)

Of these, ovarian stimulation with clomiphene (Clomid, Serophene) carries the highest risk for heterotopic pregnancies. The documentation of "no meds" does not exclude clomiphene therapy in the recent past. With infertility treatment and assisted reproduction, heterotopic pregnancy rates can be as high as 1/100![15,16] This possibility must be kept in mind. Early attending involvement is important because the patient has usually already invested $10–20,000 in this pregnancy, and will want their specialist involved. Residents in Ob-Gyn are not endocrine and infertility specialists.

VII. THE ULTRASOUND

Bedside transvaginal ultrasound by the emergency physician is fast and very sensitive for intrauterine pregnancy, starting at around 5½ weeks.[17,18] It can also identify free fluid when an ectopic has ruptured. Had a bedside ultrasound been performed in this case, free fluid would have been detected in under an hour and an alarm call would have gone out. This would have occurred well before she became hypotensive at 05:12 (approximately 2½ hours into her visit). If a formal ultrasound is obtained (still standard in most community EDs), it needs to be done quickly. Presentation was at 02:49 and the ultrasound result was available at 04:49. This time frame is typical of many EDs, but the 2 hours involved make further delays less tolerable.

Any assertion in this case that the ultrasound is indeterminate fails to acknowledge the free fluid. Free fluid is the most important finding when evaluating for ectopic pregnancy because it suggests hemorrhage, especially when the free fluid is heterogenous and has some echogenic material (blood clots) within it. When the ultrasound is truly indeterminate (no IUP, no adnexal mass, no free fluid) the other ultrasonographic findings can allow subclassification of these patients and stratify them for risk of ectopic pregnancy. Ectopic pregnancy risk is lowest when there is echogenic intrauterine material but no IUP, and highest when there is truly an empty uterus.[19]

Transvaginal ultrasound is clearly superior to transabdominal ultrasound and will identify intrauterine pregnancy earlier. The transvaginal probe uses higher frequency (better resolution) and has greater proximity to the pathology (ectopic or cyst) when it is present. Further refinement can be made by adding color flow Doppler because ectopic pregnancies have a distinctive vascularization pattern known by ultrasonographers as the "ring of fire." In one series, the addition of color flow Doppler to transvaginal ultrasound was credited with decreasing the rate of ectopic pregnancy rupture from 78% to 20%.[20] Doppler can also help with identification of ovarian torsion.

VIII. ENTER THE CONSULTANTS

The OB resident offers up all of the classic errors; the quantitative β-hCG is too low (error 1), menses was 3 weeks ago (error 2), the WBC is too high (error 3), and (error 4) ruling out appendicitis in an afebrile patient with a sudden onset of lower abdominal pain! The attending is not much better, stating she isn't tachycardic enough (error 5) and her hemoglobin isn't low enough (error 6) for an ectopic! A general surgeon should never have been called or involved in this case. None of the consultants seem to hear that there is a **large volume** of fluid in the pelvis that is **not** contained in any anatomically appropriate space (bladder, intestines, cyst walls, etc.). This ultrasound finding, combined with syncope, an abnormal shock index, and a falling hemoglobin screams ectopic! The fluid is heterogeneous—i.e., clotted blood—and has a fairly distinctive appearance as compared with ascites or the fluid from ovarian hyperstimulation syndrome (OHSS). The suggestion of appendicitis in the presence of a large volume of free fluid and a positive β-hCG is ridiculous, and should not have been entertained.

The EP is often unpopular in these situations, but a more appropriate response must be obtained. This woman's life is hanging by a thread and the consultants are stating falsehoods from a distance. This is all too common between midnight and 5 AM, when consultants loathe the ED call. The obstetrics attending, or the chief of that service, must immediately come in. Suggesting that the chief be called will often get action—no compromise can occur. When an ED doc is popular with everybody, somebody loses, and that somebody is the patient. Tell the resident to go home (and read these references), and tell the attending to come in now! Call the blood bank for a couple of units of packed red cells. Call the OR. Call another OB and ask for a favor. The ongoing delay is now compounding the problem like interest on a credit card. At 05:26, the patient has pallor, hemorrhagic shock and her physiologic choices are becoming limited. Which organs should fail first—the kidneys or the brain?

IX. AGGRESSIVENESS AND TEMPO

One of the oft-noted elements of ED care is the matching of clinical aggressiveness with disease progression. Diseases which occur slowly should be corrected slowly. Our patient is suffering from severe tempo mismatch. Diagnosis was a little slow and the consultant response was snail-like, despite the fact that she has a suddenly ruptured ectopic with ongoing hemorrhage. Her reproductive ability is critically important to her (she has already invested in I&E—Infertility and Endocrinology therapy). This therapy is expensive and usually not covered by insurance. This adds pressure to the case, because she may lose an ovary with this ectopic.

TEACHING POINTS ABOUT CASE 8:
- Positive β-hCG and abdominal pain equal ectopic until proven otherwise—even with a low quant, normal hemoglobin, and normal blood pressure!
- Bedside transvaginal ultrasound is a winner (consider Doppler if done in radiology).
- Heterotopic pregnancy must be considered with I&E treatments.
- Match your response to the disease tempo; compounded delays are unacceptable.
- Syncope and inappropriate bradycardia go hand in hand with ectopic pregnancy.
- The CBC is very nonspecific.
- You can't always be nice to consultants and their resident trainees.

REFERENCES
1. Bukata WR. Emerg Med Acute Care Essays. Nov 11, 2000; 24.
2. Dart RG, Mitterando J, Dart LM. Rate of change of serial β-hCG values as a predictor of ectopic pregnancy in patients with indeterminate transvaginal ultrasound findings. Ann Emerg Med 1999; 34:703-10.
3. Jansen RP. Relative bradycardia: A sign of intraperitoneal bleeding. Aus NZ J Obstet Gyn 1978; 18:206-8.
4. Adams SL, Greene JS. Absence of a tachycardic response to intraperitoneal hemorrhage. J Emerg Med 1986; 4:383-9.
5. Birkhan RH, Gaeta TJ, Van Deusen SK, et al. The ability of traditional vital signs and shock index to identify ectopic pregnancy. Am J Obstet Gyn 2003;189:1293-6.
6. Hoey R, Allan K. Does speculum examination have a role in assessing bleeding in early pregnancy? Emerg Med J 2004; 21:461-3.
7. Dart RG, Kaplan B, Varaklis K. Predictive value of history and physical examination in patients with suspected ectopic pregnancy. Ann Emerg Med 1999; 33:283-90.
8. Silver BE, Patterson JW, Kulick M, et al. Effect of CBC results on ED management of women with lower abdominal pain. Am J Emerg Med 1995; 13:304-6.
9. Nagurney JT, Brown DF, Chang Y, et al. Use of diagnostic testing in the emergency department for patients presenting with non-traumatic abdominal pain. J Emerg Med 2003; 25:363-71.
10. Plewa MC, Ledrick D, Buderer NF, et al. Serum CK is an unreliable predictor of ectopic pregnancy. Acad Emerg Med 1998; 5:300-3.

11. Vandermolen DT, Borzelleca JF. Serum creatine kinase does not predict ectopic pregnancy. Fertil Steril 1996; 65:916-21.

12. Buckley RG, King KJ, Disney JD, et al. Serum progesterone testing to predict ectopic pregnancy in symptomatic first trimester patients. Ann Emerg Med 2000; 36:95-100.

13. Duce MN, Ozer C, Egilmez H, et al. Heterotopic pregnancy: case report. Abdom Imaging 2002; 27:677-9.

14. Ng EH, Yeung WS, So WW, et al. An analysis of ectopic pregnancies following in vitro fertilization treatment in a 10-year period. J Obstet Gynaecol 1998; 18:359-64.

15. Hulvert J, Mardesic T, Voboril J, et al. Heterotopic pregnancy and its occurrence in assisted reproduction. Ceska Gynekol 1999; 64:299-301 (article in Czech).

16. Ahove OI, Sotiloye OS. Heterotopic pregnancy following ovulation stimulation with clomiphene: a report of three cases. West Afr J Med 2000; 19:77-9.

17. Garcia CR, Barnhart KT. Diagnosing ectopic pregnancy: decision analysis comparing six strategies. Obstet Gyn 2001; 97:464-70.

18. Mateer JR, Valley VT, Aiman EJ, et al. Outcome analysis of a protocol including bedside endovaginal sonography in patients at risk for ectopic pregnancy. Ann Emerg Med 1996; 27:283-9.

19. Dart RG, Howard K. Subclassification of indeterminate pelvic ultrasonogram: stratifying the risk of ectopic pregnancy. Acad Emerg Med 1998; 7:313-9.

20. Emerson DS, Cartier MS, Altieri LA, et al. Diagnostic efficacy of endovaginal color Doppler flow imaging in an ectopic pregnancy screening program. Radiology 1992; 183:413-20.

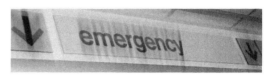

CASE 9

34 YEAR OLD MALE WITH LEG PAIN

Commentary:
Gregory L. Henry, MD, FACEP

CEO, Medical Practice Risk Assessment, Inc., Ann Arbor, Michigan
Clinical Professor, Department of Emergency Medicine
    University of Michigan Medical School, Ann Arbor, Michigan
Past President, American College of Emergency Physicians (ACEP)

Discussion:
Jeffrey A. Kline, MD, FACEP

Research and Fellowship Director, Department of Emergency Medicine
    Carolinas Medical Center
Adjunct Professor of Biology, Faculty, PhD Program, Biomedicine and Biotechnology
    University of North Carolina, Charlotte
Member ACEP Subcommittee on Suspected Pulmonary Embolism
Member ACEP Subcommittee on Suspected Lower-Extremity DVT
Member ACEP Subcommittee on MI and Unstable Angina
Board of Directors, Society for Academic Emergency Medicine

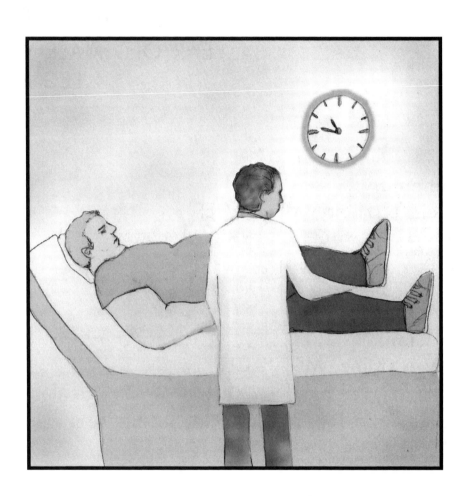

34 YEAR OLD MALE WITH
LEG PAIN

—Initial Visit*—

*Authors' Note: The history, exam and notes are the actual documentation of the physicians and providers, including abbreviations (and spelling errors)

CHIEF COMPLAINT (at 10:38): Leg pain

```
VITAL SIGNS
Time    Temp    Pulse   Resp    Syst    Diast   Pulse Ox
11:21   95.8    67      20      140     94      99%
```

HISTORY OF PRESENT ILLNESS (at 11:42): Pt is 34 year old male who indicates for the last week has had right calf pain that is worsened with palpation and walking and he has noticed over the last few days some exertional shortness of breath. He has had no chest pain and denies leg trauma. He saw his primary care physician today who referred him to the ED for evaluation. Pt notes he has been hospitalized for DVT and cellulitis at least 2 times in the past, at least 5 years ago. He indicates this does not feel quite the same as it did with previous DVT, he has noticed no swelling. Pt. started having SOB on Monday when walking from car to a building, now SOB is constant when pt ambulates. Saw PCP today and he recommended that pt come to ER for possible blood clot in right leg. No vomiting, chest pain, diaphoresis, palpitations, syncope, edema, hemoptysis, or cough.

PAST MEDICAL HISTORY/TRIAGE: Chief complaint/quote (per RN): "I might have a blood clot in my right lower calf, I was sent into ER by my doctor"
Medications: Ziac
Allergies: No known allergies.
PMH: HTN, DVT
PSH: None

EXAM (at 11:46):
  General: Well-appearing; well-nourished; pt. appears morbidly obese. A moderate sized panniculus is present. A&O X 3, in no apparent distress
  Head: Normocephalic; atraumatic.
  Eyes: PERRL
  Nose: The nose is normal in appearance without rhinorrhea
  Resp: Normal chest excursion with respiration; breath sounds clear and equal bilaterally; no wheezes, rhonchi, or rales

Card: Regular rhythm, without murmurs, rub or gallop.

Abd. The area appears morbidly obese. A moderate sized panniculus is present. The abdomen is non-tender to palpation and there is no palpable organomegaly or masses.

Ext: Carotid, radial, femoral and dorsalis pedis pulses are normal. Capillary refill is normal. Peripheral edema: pt right calf is 61 cm left calf is 61 cm, legs are without obvious edema, pt is morbidly obese, no redness or warmth to the lower extremity. Patient is positive for Homan's sign.

Skin: Normal for age and race; warm and dry; no apparent lesions

RESULTS:

ECG: Display of ECG

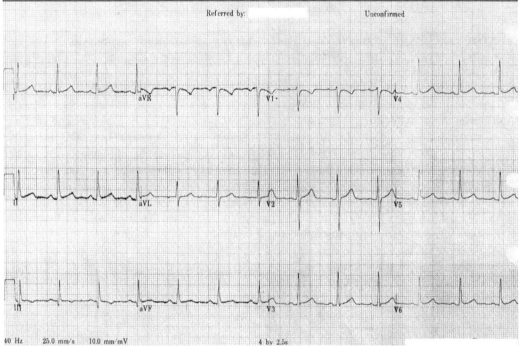

Time 10:52			Computer interpretation:
	Vent. rate	75 bpm	Normal sinus rhythm
Male	PR interval	170 ms	Normal ECG
	QRS duration	90 ms	
	QT/QTc	380/424 ms	
Technician:	P-R-T axes	60 48 26	
Test ind: R/O CARDIAC			

40 Hz   25.0 mm/s   10.0 mm/mV   4 by 2.5s

Venous Doppler (ordered at 11:39, results at 12:28): Negative for DVT per radiologist

DIAGNOSIS

1. Pain in limb, r/o DVT, 2. Obesity, 3. HTN

DISPOSITION - The patient was discharged to Home ambulatory and released from the ED at 14:53.

Gregory L. Henry comments:

"When in doubt, believe your instincts and not just one test"

The chief complaint and history in this case are clear. The patient has had worsening pain in the right calf and the onset of shortness of breath; this is a very difficult history to ignore in light of his previous DVTs. A pulse ox is often equivocal; at least 15% of people with PEs have a normal pulse ox on initial presentation. Tachycardia does not have to be present with smaller PEs. The fact that the patient's physical exam is strongly suggestive of DVT, along with his history, puts him into a high-risk category. It is inadequate to have one Doppler study of the leg and decide that no DVT exists. In fact there is some data suggesting that as a clot matures and breaks off, the leg study may be negative as the lung study becomes positive. General evaluation of the patient gathered the correct normal data, but did not pursue deeply enough that on a Wells criteria basis, this person has to be at least intermediate probability for PE.

If it looks like a duck and squawks like a duck, it is a duck. When in doubt, believe your instincts and not just one test. This patient has a previous history of DVTs, which is an independent risk factor for future DVTs. Secondly he has put "tender leg" and "shortness of breath" in the same sentence. It takes a very unusual physician who does not become upset with that combination.

Documentation in this case is appropriate.

The principal concern in this case is the decision making. This physician has the feeling that one Doppler study can erase a considerable number of positive features. In a case such as this, it would be perfectly appropriate to start the patient on heparin, send him for a helical CT of the chest, and await results. There is little evidence to suggest that VQ scans help. The intermediate scan is essentially useless. This patient needs a test that is a decision maker, because subjecting the patient to 6 months of Coumadin is not a benign process. If there were positive findings on the CT scan of the chest, the diagnosis is made and the patient can be managed as new onset pulmonary embolus. If the CT scan is equivocal, then the patient may need to be admitted, placed on heparin, and receive an angiogram of the chest, which would definitively rule in or out a pulmonary embolus. The wisest approach is to treat this patient as if he had a DVT until proven otherwise.

- Thoroughness of Documentation: 8 out of 10.

- Thoroughness of Patient Evaluation: 7 out of 10.

- Risk of Serious Illness Being Missed: High risk.

- Risk Management Legal Rating: High risk.

PRIMARY CARE VISIT—1 DAY LATER

Seen by his primary physician and was sent for a V/Q. Results showed multiple mismatched wedge-shaped perfusion defects. This includes at least two moderate large subsegmental defects in the right lung base and 1 to 2 moderate to large subsegmental defects in the left lower lobe. There is a small subsegmental mismatched defect in the left upper lobe anteriorly. There is moderate subsegmental mismatched defect in the right upper lobe. A patient's recent chest x-ray demonstrates no corresponding infiltrates.

IMPRESSION: High probability for pulmonary embolus. Report called to the referring physician's office immediately following the examination. He was referred to the ED.

34 YEAR OLD MALE WITH LEG PAIN

—Second ED Visit: Same Day as PCP Visit—

CHIEF COMPLAINT (at 14:37): Leg pain and shortness of breath

VITAL SIGNS							
Time	Temp	Pulse	Resp	Syst	Diast	Pulse	Ox
15:22	96.5		96	20	142	80	98%

HISTORY OF PRESENT ILLNESS (at 16:07): Pt states RLE, posterior pain/aching for 1 week, no swelling. Had mild intermittent shortness of breath with exertion only for 1wk. No chest pain at that time. Last night about 6pm after he had returned home from the ED, he noted significant increase in SOB and mild right anterior chest tightness lasting for about 4 hours. Had difficultly singing at church last night. Feels fine today but still with exertional shortness of breath, but no chest pain or tightness. Still has mild RLE pain, no edema. Called his PCP who ordered CXR and V/Q scan, after scan pt was told to come to ER. Pt was seen here yesterday for R/O DVT. Venous doppler was negative and he was sent home yesterday afternoon. Pt also states clear runny nose with mild epistaxis and noted hemoptysis with cough 5 days ago but none since. Pt states he was admitted twice about 4-5 years ago for cellulitis and probable DVT of his RLE. Was on Heparin and home on Coumadin for a period of time afterwards.

PAST MEDICAL HISTORY/TRIAGE:
Medications: Ziac
Allergies: No known allergies.
PMH: HTN, DVT
PSH: None

EXAM (documented at 17:47):
General: Well-appearing; Morbidly Obese, in no acute respiratory distress

Head: Normocephalic; atraumatic

Eyes: PERRL; EOM intact; sclera anicteric,

ENT: TM's normal; normal nose; no rhinorrhea; normal pharynx with no tonsillar hype ___

Neck: Supple; non-tender; no cervical lymphadenopathy;

Card: The heart has a regular rate and rhythm; normal S1, S2; no S3 or S4; no murmurs, rubs, or gallops. The pulses are equal bilaterally and there is brisk capillary refill. There is no peripheral edema of the extremities.

Resp: Normal chest excursion with respiration; breath sounds clear and equal bilaterally; no wheezes, rhonchi, or rales

Ext: Normal ROM in all four extremities; non-tender to palpation; distal pulses are normal, Negative Homan's sign or cords. No peripheral edema.

Skin: Normal for age and race; warm; dry; good turgor; no rash noted

ORDERS (at 16:56):
Heparin sodium 10,000 units IVP then 1,200 units/hr

RESULTS:

Test	Flag	Value	Units	Ref. Range
WBC	H	11.3	K/uL	4.6-10.2
HGB		13.2	G/DL	12.0-16.0
PLT		158	K/uL	142-424

PT/INR and PTT - WNL
ABG (at 17:16): pH 7.42, PCO2 41, PO2 74, O2 SAT 96%

DIAGNOSIS (at 16:54):
1. PE and infarction
2. Unspecified essential hypertension

DISPOSITION: Admitted to the hospital and transferred to the floor at 19:07.

HOSPITAL COURSE PER PULMONOLOGIST:

DISCHARGE DIAGNOSIS AND DISCUSSION PER PULMONOLOGIST:
1. **Pulmonary embolus.** We will plan for heparin at this time, as well as concomitant Coumadin. The amount of time that he will be on anticoagulation is unclear at this point. I would think he would need at least a year, if not a lifetime of Coumadin, depending on whether or not he is able to lose weight and adopt a more active lifestyle. We will check a 2D echo at some point to be sure that he does not have significant pulmonary hypertension or RV overload since some of this may have been chronic.
2. **History of hypertension.**
3. **Sleep apnea.**
4. **Morbid obesity.**

Disposition: The patient will be discharged to home and I will see him again in 2 weeks. The timing of anticoagulation will be dependent on how long he has his risk factors including his obesity. I will keep him on Coumadin for probably a year, if not longer. We will plan a V/Q scan in 3 weeks.

FINAL DIAGNOSIS: Pulmonary embolism

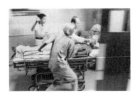

DIAGNOSIS AND MANAGEMENT OF PULMONARY EMBOLISM

Jeffrey A. Kline, MD

I. SUMMARY OF CASE

The patient prudently returned to his primary care physician, who astutely ordered an appropriate test for a patient with shortness of breath and calf pain. The ventilation perfusion lung scan was diagnostic for the presence of pulmonary vascular occlusion, most consistent with thrombotic embolism. After this outpatient test, the patient returned to the emergency department and was appropriately treated.

Clearly this clinical diad should raise the question of extremity venous thrombosis together with pulmonary embolsim (PE) in the mind of most, if not all, board certified emergency physicians. Accordingly, the burden is on the emergency physician to rule out both DVT and PE with appropriate testing.

II. DEFINITION AND DISCUSSION OF "SHORTNESS OF BREATH"

This patient described a classic story for PE, which is essentially breathlessness without obvious cause. Before moving to objective testing, I would like to comment on several points documented in the history and physical exam. I believe that one of emergency physicians' biggest mistakes is to dismiss unexplained dyspnea when the physician thinks the patient has "no risk factors for PE." The finding of unexplained dyspnea remains one of the strongest independent predictors of the presence of PE in ambulatory patients.[1] By unexplained, I mean the absence of prior lung disease, such as COPD or asthma, especially in a non-smoker with a clear chest radiograph.

As a digression, dyspnea itself can be difficult to define. One medicolegal and technical definition is "the pathological sensation of breathlessness." The perception of "shortness of breath" can vary between ages and with ethnicity. In the experience of our research team, we often find that older men are reluctant to admit shortness of breath, even when it is obvious that they are panting while in semi-Fowler's position! Often it is helpful to ask a family member if the patient has he had difficulty breathing with exertion. Often, family members will say, "That's the reason we brought him in, because he gets so short of breath when we go to the mall." I'm not sure why patients are reluctant to admit their shortness of breath. Maybe it's fear of admitting that they are getting older. PE often causes such a vague sensation to patients that they can't differentiate whether their symptoms are concerning or not.

III. EVALUATION OF CALF PAIN AND SHORTNESS OF BREATH

It seems that we were taught in medical school and residency that PE is an abrupt, dramatic event. Well, guess what? That teaching came from the cases that our teachers were able to diagnose. Our goal is to recognize the insidious (and common) syndrome of the cumulative, dyspnic embolism, which is the effect of progressive occlusion of the vasculature over weeks.[1,2] This syndrome is common, in my experience representing the presentation of 55% of all PEs diagnosed in the ED. This syndrome is sneaky because less than half of the patients will tell you chest pain exists, and very few will describe the symptom onset as abrupt.[3] More often than not, PE is a slow process of successive, segmental-sized embolism of the lungs, wherein each embolic event was barely noticed by the patient. Much like multi-infarct dementia, this is a cumulative process that pushes the patient's V/Q mismatch to the point where the patient can't tolerate the resultant fatigue and exertional dyspnea any more, and is brought to the emergency department by family.

Patients with PE frequently describe exertional shortness of breath, probably owing to inducible pulmonary hypertension.[4] One difference between heart failure and PE is that PE does not reliably cause orthopnea, whereas left ventricular failure almost always causes worsening shortness of breath in the recumbent position. Depending on the orientation of the clot(s) in the lung vasculature, about 30% of patients with PE complain of platypnea, stating that lying down feels better than sitting up.[5] Some patients feel better sitting up, but have better pulse ox readings lying down (thus manifesting orthodeoxia).

The definition of pleuritic chest pain warrants delineation. The definition that has stood the test of peer review is "pain between the clavicles and the costal margin that is worse with deep breathing or cough." Does this mean that substernal pain that gets worse with deep breathing or cough is pleuritic? I personally think so, unless the substernal pain is constant. I should caution that segmental lung infarctions sometimes refer distally. I personally have seen patients with pulmonary infarctions presenting with right upper quadrant pain that faked everyone into thinking the cause was biliary, and I have seen an apical lung infarction present with shoulder pain.

Our patient had a history of hemoptysis. In general, hemoptysis with PE occurs approximately 2 days after onset of pleuritic chest pain. This is about the time frame required for the lung ischemia to cause an inflammatory response, destroying the alveolar-capillary membrane junction and leading to erythrocyte exudation to the alveolar compartment. In contrast, patients with pneumonia more often develop hemoptysis almost coincident with symptom onset.

Our patient made it more difficult for us because he did not complain of hemoptysis on his first visit (I find this commonly). The second physician was able to elicit the history that hemoptysis had occurred 5 days previous. In addition, he had no pleuritic chest pain, and I would submit that this is unusual. I will bet that with further questioning, he would recall a twinge of peripheral chest pain. Often hemoptysis as a result of PE manifests as a small amount of streaking of blood in otherwise clear sputum. What probably happened is that this patient embolized a week or even longer ago, and developed a mild pulmonary infarction which resulted in hemoptysis. If he is like patients I have seen in the past, he might not even remember having thoracic pain. He might have ascribed it to a cold that caused epistaxis and thought that the hemoptysis was related to a nose bleed. In this particular case, I am reasonably certain that the hemoptysis came from the lung, rather than the nose, based on the results of the V/Q scan. In real practice, when I am not being a Monday morning quarterback (and I do not have the V/Q scan results), I believe that hemoptysis has to be taken seriously; virtually every author who collects databases on ambulatory patients evaluated for PE finds hemoptysis to be a strong predictor of PE. [3,6-8]

Regarding the physical examination of our patient, one descriptive phrase is very important. That is the simple observation as to whether the patient has asymmetrical calves or not. The second physician notes "no peripheral edema," but sometimes the swelling from DVT occurs more from venous engorgement than transudation of fluid into the subcutaneous space. Accordingly, when you are evaluating a patient with possible PE or DVT, the best single physical exam technique is to put your hands under the patient's heels, lift up the legs, and visually compare the calves. If they do not look symmetrical, then you have found unilateral leg swelling, which increases the probability of either DVT or PE 3 or 4 fold. [3,9]

IV. RISK OF PE WITH A NEGATIVE VENOUS DOPPLER

Regrettably, even well-trained physicians believe a negative bilateral lower extremity venous Doppler-ultrasound is reasonable evidence disproving the presence of PE. It is probably true that most PEs, even in ambulatory patients, originate in the leg veins, but ambulatory patients are far less likely than hospitalized or post-op patients to have a discoverable DVT. [10] One potential explanation for this phenomenon is that ambulatory patients, by definition, walk more than hospitalized patients, and therefore may have more muscular contractions that could dislodge a clot. Many experts in the study of thromboembolism overemphasize the connection between DVT and PE; I think their goal is to emphasize the importance of DVT prophylaxis in hospitalized patients, but the message ends up as "Every patient with PE has a DVT somewhere." Unfortunately this then gets transmuted into the belief that a patient with symptoms of PE and a normal pulse oximetry reading and venous doppler will be just fine.

Some doctors think implicitly that "even if he has a clot in his lungs, it is minor and will not hurt him, and since there is no DVT, he will not re-embolize and will not worsen." This concept makes no sense from either a clinical or biological standpoint. Simply put, clots in the legs don't kill people; clots in the lungs do. We know from serial studies of post-op orthopedic surgery patients, and from data pursuing the so-called "economy class syndrome" from long-distance air travel, that patients can develop a new DVT and embolize some or all of the new clot over a course of only 6 hours.

So, what is the quantitative value of one negative bilateral leg venous Doppler ultrasound in an ambulatory emergency department patient with symptoms of PE? The answer is the best case likelihood ratio is about 0.5. [11] The worst case likelihood ratio is near unity, suggesting no diagnostic utility. So a negative venous Doppler ultrasound of both legs will cut the probability of PE by about one-half. If your initial pretest probability of PE is approximately 2%, then a negative Doppler will reduce the posttest probability to approximately 1%, which might be acceptable. (Note to evidence based medicine (EBM) aficionados: I purposely ignored the conversion of probability to odds and back again). This patient's pretest probability was far higher than 2%.

V. RISK OF PE WITH D-DIMER TESTING

The immunoturbidimetric or ELISA D-dimer has a sensitivity of about 95% and a specificity at about 50% (LR- = 0.1) in emergency department patients. Note that the sensitivity and specificity of the qualitative D-dimers is more like 85% and 65%, respectively.[14]

What if the venous Doppler ultrasound had been used together with a D-dimer test? In general, a negative venous Doppler ultrasound used in conjunction with a negative quantitative D-dimer assay (either immunoturbidimetric, or ELISA, measuring a D-dimer concentration <500 nanograms/mL) rules out PE and DVT with defensible certainty. Although I cannot point to any specific study of the combination of a venous doppler and a quantitative D-dimer, if we chain the likelihood ratios (LRs) of the 2 tests together (LR(-) = 0.1 for the D-dimer <500 ng/mL and LR(-) =0.5 for the negative doppler), then both tests negative almost certainly produce an LR(-) < 0.1.[12,13] If we could say the patient's pretest probability was below 15%, this test combination would produce a posttest probability below 1%.

Whether or not a negative ultrasound plus a negative D-dimer would rule out PE in a patient like this remains a matter of debate, as his pretest probability was approximately 15% (see below), but I believe they would provide a reasonably defensible level of care.[14]

The latest controversy brewing in the research community is whether a negative quantitative D-dimer can be used independently of pretest probability. From an evidence-based standpoint, the answer is "no." A negative D-dimer can only rule out PE in patients with a low, or maybe moderate, pretest probability of disease. However, a number of prominent researchers believe that a negative D-dimer is just as good in high pretest probability patients. Their main reasoning for this position is that high pretest probability patients should also have an elevated D-dimer, mainly because of their high clot burden. [28]

VI. RISK PE WITH NORMAL VITAL SIGNS AND PULSE OX OF 99%

I mentioned "pretest probability" in the previous section on diagnostic tests and, to some degree, I put the cart before the horse. If we wish to use evidence based quantitative medicine, we have to determine a way to produce a quantitative pretest probability and then link it to a likelihood ratio to produce a quantitative posttest probability. While published diagnostic accuracy studies and meta-analyses do a pretty good job of telling us the likelihood ratio negative of diagnostic tests, there is less evidence to give us a very good quantitative pretest probability assessment. Scoring systems such as those promulgated by myself, Wells or Perrier tend to give estimates of pretest probability, lumped into low, moderate, or high categories. While these lumps do have some clinical utility in helping us to decide which diagnostic test to order, these scoring systems have very little utility in producing a specific posttest probability of PE, and essentially no utility in deciding when no test is the best test.

VII. CALCULATING PRETEST AND POSTTEST PROBABILITY OF PE

What we would really like to know about this patient is the following: the percentage probability of the outcome of PE for a 35 year old male with dyspnea, recent hemoptysis, a history of deep venous thrombosis, normal vital signs, a pulse ox of 99% on room air, and no unilateral leg swelling, and is the percentage probability low enough to rule out PE without testing. In other words, it would be helpful to have a database of several dozen or more patients just like this man, and know how many of these patients, matched for age, risk and vital signs, went on to have a PE. This invokes the concept of attribute matching. Such a system is commercially available (see www.pretestconsult.com) and represents an innovative way of using a computer program to mine a large database of patients who were evaluated for possible PE in emergency departments across the US. The screenshot below shows how the system works.

In the image, the attributes for this particular patient are: age 35–50 with dyspnea, no pleuritic chest pain, presence of hemoptysis, pulse ox >95%, heart rate <100, positive history of DVT, no unilateral leg swelling, and no recent surgery or immobilization. We find that out of a database of 5,200 patients, 26 had an identical profile to this patient and 4 of these patients had a PE within a 90-day follow up period. This gives a pretest probability of 4/26 or 15.4%, which is far too high of a pretest probability to allow the doctor to safely forgo additional testing for PE. A test with a likelihood ratio negative of 0.5, such as a negative venous doppler, would only reduce the posttest probability to approximately 7%, which is still too high to rule out PE.[15] By clicking a button, this Pretest Consult system automatically computes the posttest probability in view of results of commonly performed tests, such as a CT angiography, a D-dimer or V/Q scan, using best-evidence likelihood ratio data. The system also allows the pretest probability query to be stored as a medical record. The drawback to this system is that it is not free.

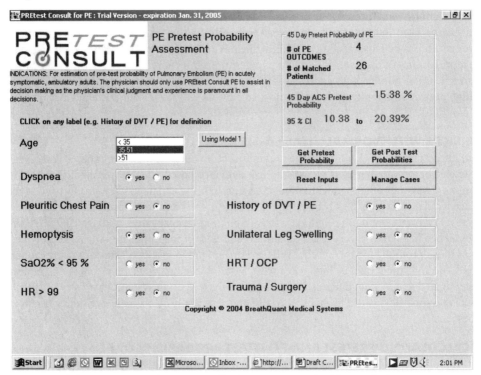

Copyright © 2004 BreathQuant Medical Systems. Used with permission.
Dr. Kline is a partner in Pretest Consult LLC

Occasionally we will approach a patient with normal vital signs and pulse ox who has symptoms suggestive of PE, no hemoptysis, and no prior PE/DVT. In this low risk type of patient, it's difficult to decide if D-dimer or any type of imaging test is necessary. To assist in this decision, Kline et al developed the PE rule out criteria (the PERC Rule). [16] This rule states that if a patient is aged <50, has a heart rate <100, pulse oximetry >94%, no prior DVT or PE, no estrogen use, no recent surgery or trauma requiring hospitalization or endotracheal intubation, no hemoptysis, and no unilateral leg swelling, then the pretest probability is <2% and the patient does not need evaluation at all for PE. The 2% number comes from a complex computation that is described in reference 14. Of note, our patient had 2 criteria that flunked the PERC Rule, including hemoptysis and prior DVT. The PERC rule has been validated in 2 separate databases outside of the U.S. and it's free of charge. Its disadvantage is that it may be hard to remember, it does not give you a discrete pretest probability estimate, and you cannot compute post-test probabilities when a patient "flunks" the rule.

VIII. HOW GOOD IS THE CT SCAN COMPARED TO THE V/Q SCAN?

It is worth commenting on the sensitivity and specificity of ventilation perfusion scan versus a helical chest CT to rule out PE. In this particular case, the V/Q scan showed multiple wedge shaped mismatched perfusion defects. This is diagnostic of pulmonary vascular occlusion and is a "no-brainer" for the radiologist and the doctor. V/Q scan reading remains as much as an art form as a science; the test is very good at the extremes, as in when it is obviously positive (in the present case), or when there is absolutely homogenous distribution of the perfusion label, showing a normal V/Q scan result. In emergency department patients, V/Q scans are normal or diagnostic positive in approximately 50% of cases, leaving the emergency department physician on the hook half the time. Most of the other 50% of "non-diagnostic V/Q scans" are low probability. The standard zeitgeist in most practices is that a low probability V/Q scan, together with a low clinical suspicion, rules out PE.

This brings us back to the discussion of pretest probability. The likelihood ratio negative for a low probability V/Q scan is approximately 0.3. [17] To reduce the posttest probability of PE below 1%–an accepted threshold to rule out most fatal diseases–the pretest probability has to be <4% as baseline. [15] A quantitative argument can be made that a low probability V/Q scan and a low-risk Wells score, or a low-risk Geneva score, will reliably produce a posttest probability <1% (note the acceptable posttest probability to rule out PE is lower than the acceptable pretest probability to exclude PE without diagnostic testing, or "testing threshold"). A better way of quantitatively making this decision is to perform attribute matching, obtain an exact percentage pretest probability, and then have the device compute an exact posttest probability. The device that was described earlier does all of this automatically for the physician.

The nice thing about the CT scan is that it gives us the performance of a binary output: positive or negative. The bad news is this binary appearance is an illusion because about 15% of CT scans should be read as indeterminate because of inadequate technique. Moreover, we don't know the real truth of the sensitivity and specificity of CT scans; the best answer will come from the results of "PIOPED II" due out later in 2005. This is a multicenter study funded by the NIH that will compare CT scanning to the best possible gold standard, as well as clinical follow up. Most rigorous meta analyses currently suggest that single-channel CT scan of the chest has approximately 85% sensitivity and 90% specificity. [18-20] The details matter because the multi-channel detectors (16 channel and up), the technique of injection (use of a timing run to ensure vascular opacification), and the skill of the reader, all make a big difference. A CT scan with adequate opacification of the pulmonary vasculature, performed with a GE light speed or Siemens SOMATOM™ Sensation 64 CT scanner, read by a board certified radiologist with fellowship training in body imaging, will have the best possible sensitivity and specificity of any test that we can order for PE. On the other hand, a CT scan performed without adequate timing, with a large bolus of contrast sitting in the right atrium without good pulmonary vascular opacification, and the patient exhibiting motion artifact on the images, has almost no diagnostic utility. It is important for the emergency physician to ask, especially when there is high pretest probability, whether the CT scan was done with good technique and if there is confidence in the interpreting radiologist.

IX. CT VENOGRAPHY
Lastly, it is worth mentioning the issue of CT venography. CT venography can pick up additional clots that would not be picked up with CT angiography alone. In the emergency department setting, for every 100 patients scanned for PE, CT venography will pick up about 2 cases of DVT that otherwise would require additional testing.[21] Because CT venography is done with the same bolus of contrast and simply requires some cuts taken from the knees up to the acetabulum, it does make logistical sense to do this test. The main problem with CT venography is that it has relatively low interobserver agreement when a DVT is observed without a PE. It is my opinion that CT venography, when the veins are well opacified, rules out DVT in a patient with suspected PE. However, I don't believe that a patient without evidence of PE on CT scan, and with evidence of DVT on CT venography, should be committed to Coumadin treatment without a follow up venous ultrasound to confirm the presence of clot.

X. MANAGEMENT OF PE
This patient had some nose bleed and hemoptysis 5 days ago. I would consider this a relative contraindication to thrombolysis, but not a contraindication to anticoagulation. He was started on unfractionated Heparin which is a perfectly reasonable treatment for PE. In 2004, a Cochrane meta analysis of randomized controlled trials demonstrated superiority of low molecular weight Heparin over unfractionated Heparin for the treatment of deep vein thrombosis. By "superiority," this means in terms of recurrence of thromboembolism (PE or DVT), overall mortality, and hemorrhagic complications (Van Dongen CJJ, Cochrane database).

The evidence is less clear as to whether low molecular weight Heparin is a better treatment for PE. The best-evidence answer is that low molecular weight Heparin is not inferior to unfractionated Heparin, and I believe it will eventually be shown to be superior in terms of reduction of clot size and recurrence of PE.[22] Unfortunately, low molecular weight Heparin is relatively difficult to reverse and has a long half life. Whereas protamine will rapidly reverse the augmenting effect of unfractionated Heparin on antithrombin, protamine doesn't reverse the inhibitory effect of short-chain Heparins on factor Xa. In our patient with a history of nosebleed and hemoptysis, that would prompt me to lean toward using unfractionated Heparin rather than fractionated Heparin.

XI. FINAL DISCUSSION OF CASE
Concerning whether the patient would benefit from thrombolytic treatment for PE, based on the evidence presented, I would say no. Patients with PE and a persistent pulse oximetry reading below 95%, an elevated troponin measurement (troponin I above 1 ng/mL or T above 0.1 ng/mL), a brain

natriuretic peptide concentration above 100 pg/ML, or patients with signs of pulmonary hypertension on electrocardiogram [23-27] are at high risk of death and should strongly be considered for thrombolytic therapy. Patients with a dilated or hypokinetic right ventricle on echocardiography should also be considered strongly for thrombolytic therapy. I don't believe that this patient would meet any of these criteria and think he would do just fine with Heparin anti-coagulation followed by Warfarin.

TEACHING POINTS ABOUT CASE 9:

- A negative lower extremity Doppler does not rule out a diagnosis of PE.
- Unexplained dyspnea remains one of the strongest independent predictors of the presence of PE in ambulatory patients.
- All concerning symptoms documented in the chart (such as shortness of breath in this case) should be addressed during the patient visit and discussed in the progress note.
- Previous history of thrombotic disease is a strong predictor of subsequent disease.

Author's notes: Thank you for the chance to opine on this case. I can back up any statement I made, either through my own research databases or through published work. Any reader who has a question or comment should not hesitate to email me at jkline@carolinas.org.

REFERENCES

1. Susec O, Boudrow D, Kline J. The clinical features of acute pulmonary embolism in ambulatory patients. Acad Emerg Med 1997; 4:891-7.
2. Stein PD, Henry JW. Clinical characteristics of patients with acute pulmonary embolism stratified according to their presenting syndromes. Chest 1997; 112:974-9.
3. Kline JA, Nelson RD, Jackson RE, et al. Criteria for the safe use of D-dimer testing in emergency department patients with suspected pulmonary embolism: A multicenter United States study. Ann Em Med 2002; 39:144-52.
4. Sharma GV, Folland ED, McIntyre KM, et al. Long-term benefit of thrombolytic therapy in patients with pulmonary embolism. Vascular Medicine 2000; 5:91-5.
5. Sharma GV, McIntyre KM, Sharm S, et al. Clinical and hemodynamic correlates in pulmonary embolism. Clin Chest Med 1984; 5:421-37.
6. Wells PS, Anderson DR, Rodger M, et al. Derivation of a simple clinical model to categorize patients probability of pulmonary embolism: Increasing the models utility with the SimpliRED D-dimer. Thromb Haemost 2000; 83:416-20.
7. Wicki J, Perneger T, Junod A, et al. Assessing clinical probability of pulmonary embolism in the emergency ward: A simple score. Arch Inter Med 2001; 161:92-97.
8. Miniati M, Monti S, Bottai M. A structured clinical model for predicting the probability of pulmonary embolism.[comment]. Amer J Med 2003; 114:173-9.
9. Wells PS, Anderson DR, Rodger M, et al. Derivation of a simple clinical model to categorize patients probability of pulmonary embolism: Increasing the models utility with the SimpliRED D-dimer. Thromb Haemost 2000; 83:416-20.
10. Daniel KR, Jackson RE, Kline JA. Utility of the lower extremity venous ultrasound in the diagnosis and exclusion of pulmonary embolism in outpatients. Ann Emerg Med 2000; 35:547.
11. Daniel KR, Jackson RE, Kline JA. Utility of the lower extremity venous ultrasound in the diagnosis and exclusion of pulmonary embolism in outpatients. Ann Emerg Med 2000; 35:547.

12. Brown MD, Lau J, Nelson RD, et al. Turbidimetric D-Dimer in the diagnosis of pulmonary embolism: A meta-analysis. Clinical Chemistry 2003; 49:1846-53.

13. Brown MD, Rowe BH, Reeves MJ, et al. The accuracy of the enzyme-linked immuno-absorbent assay D-dimer test in the diagnosis of pulmonary embolism: A meta-analysis. Ann Em Med 2002; 40:133-44.

14. Kline JA, Webb WB, Jones AE, et al. Impact of a rapid rule-out protocol for pulmonary embolism on the rate of screening, missed cases, and pulmonary vascular imaging in an urban U.S. emergency department. Ann Emerg Med. 2004; 44:490-502.

15. Kline JA, Wells PS. Methodology for a rapid protocol to rule out pulmonary embolism in the emergency department. Ann Emerg Med 2003; 42:266-275.

16. Kline JA, Mitchell AM, Kabrhel C, et al. Clinical criteria to prevent unnecessary diagnostic testing in emergency department patients with suspected pulmonary embolism. J Thrombosis Haemostasis 2004; 2:1247-1255.

17. PIOPED Investigators. Value of the ventilation/perfusion scan in acute pulmonary embolism. JAMA 1990; 263:2753-9.

18. Safriel Y, Zinn H. CT pulmonary angiography in the detection of pulmonary emboli: a meta-analysis of sensitivities and specificities. Clinical Imaging 2002; 26:101-5.

19. van Beek EJ, Brouwers EM, Song B, et al. Lung scintigraphy and helical computed tomography for the diagnosis of pulmonary embolism: a meta-analysis. Clinical & Applied Thrombosis/Hemostasis 2001; 7:87-92.

20. Kline JA, Johns KL, Coluciello SA, et al. New diagnostic tests for pulmonary embolism. Ann Emerg Med 2000; 35:168-80.

21. Richman PB, Wood J, Kasper DM, et al. Contribution of indirect computed tomography venography to computed tomography angiography of the chest for the diagnosis of thromboembolic disease in two United States emergency departments. J Thrombosis Haemostasis 2003; 1:652-7.

22. Dolovich LR, Ginsberg JS, Douketis JD, et al. A meta-analysis comparing low-molecular-weight heparins with unfractionated heparin in the treatment of venous thromboembolism: examining some unanswered questions regarding location of treatment, product type, and dosing frequency. Arch Intern Med 2000; 160:181-8.

23. Kline JA, Hernandez J, Newgard CD, et al. Use of pulse oximetry to predict in-hospital complications in normotensive patients with pulmonary embolism. Am J Med 2003; 115:203-8.

24. Konstantinides S, Geibel A, Olschewski M, et al. Importance of cardiac troponins I and T in risk stratification of patients with acute pulmonary embolism. Circulation 2002; 106:1263-8.

25. Daniel KR, Courtney DM, Kline JA. Assessment of cardiac stress from massive pulmonary embolism with 12-lead electrocardiography. Chest 2001; 120:474-81.

26. Kucher N, Printzen G, Goldhaber SZ. Prognostic role of brain natriuretic peptide in acute pulmonary embolism. Circulation 2003; 107:2545-7.

27. ten Wolde M, Tulevski II, Mulder JW, et al. Brain natriuretic peptide as a predictor of adverse outcome in patients with pulmonary embolism. Circulation 2003; 107:2082-4.

28. Samuel Z. Goldhaber, personal communication, May, 2003, Boston, MA.

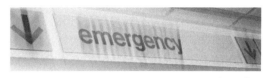

CASE 10

50 YEAR OLD MALE WITH GALLBLADDER INFLAMMATION

Commentary:
Gregory L. Henry, MD, FACEP

CEO, Medical Practice Risk Assessment, Inc., Ann Arbor, Michigan
Clinical Professor, Department of Emergency Medicine
    University of Michigan Medical School, Ann Arbor, Michigan
Past President, American College of Emergency Physicians (ACEP)

Discussion:
Jud E. Hollander, MD, FACEP

Professor of Medicine, University of Pennsylvania
    Philadelphia, Pennsylvania
Past member, Society of Academic Emergency Medicine (SAEM)
    Board of Directors
Past Chair of Scientific Review Committee ACEP
Past Chair of SAEM Program Committee
Deputy Editor, Annals of Emergency Medicine
Reviewer for JAMA, NEJM, JACC, Academic Emergency Medicine,
    American Journal of Emergency Medicine
ACEP Award for Outstanding Contribution in Research, 2001

Esther H. Chen, MD

Assistant Professor, Department of Emergency Medicine
    University of Pennsylvania, School of Medicine

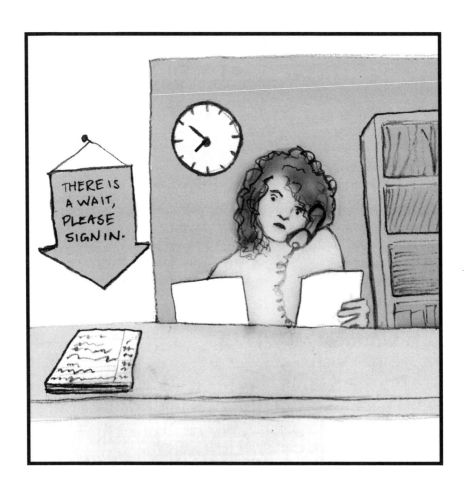

50 YEAR OLD MALE WITH GALLBLADDER INFLAMMATION

—Initial Visit*—

*Authors' Note: The history, exam and notes are the actual documentation of the physicians and providers, including abbreviations (and spelling errors)

CHIEF COMPLAINT (at 19:51): Gallbladder inflammation

```
VITAL SIGNS
Time      Temp      Pulse     Resp     Syst     Diast    Pulse Ox
20:25     96.4      162       16       112      54       94%
```

HISTORY OF PRESENT ILLNESS (at 20:32): The patient is a 50-year-old man with a past history of myocardial infarction 5 years ago who presents today with complaints of right upper quadrant abdominal discomfort which began this morning. He feels like his gallbladder is inflamed. He feels a discomfort and it feels swollen. He does have some lightheadedness when he stands. There are no other symptoms. He had a negative cardiac stress test 3 years ago. No complaints of chest tightness, discomfort, pain, or pressure. No diaphoresis, shortness of breath, pain in the lower extremities, peripheral edema, cough, fevers, or orthopnea. No chest discomfort with exertion. The patient does have a very healthy lifestyle, exercises every day, and does eat very healthy foods. He took his home medications today, including aspirin, prior to arrival.

PAST MEDICAL HISTORY/TRIAGE:
Medications: Toprol, Aspirin
Allergies: No known allergies.
PMH: CAD, MI
FamHx: Adopted
SocHx: Nonsmoker

EXAM (at 20:34):
HEENT: His throat is normal. Pupils equal, round, and reactive to light.
Lungs: On anterior exam are clear with good breath sounds.
Heart: Regular and tachycardic. No murmur.
Abdomen: Soft and nontender. No pulsatile abdominal mass.
Extremities: Lower extremities without edema. Nontender. Peripheral pulse is 2+ and equal in the lower extremities.
Skin: Warm and dry with no rash or diaphoresis.

ORDERS: IV, O2, Cardiac Monitor, EKG, CXR, CBC, Chem7, CK-MB, Troponin

	Vent. rate	164 bpm
Male	PR interval	264 ms
	QRS duration	150 ms
	QT/QTc	338/558 ms
	P-R-T axes -134 -103 26	

Computer interpretation:
*** SUSPECT ARM LEAD REVERSAL, INTERPRETATION ASSUMES NO REVERSAL
UNUSUAL P AXIS, POSSIBLE ECTOPIC ATRIAL TACHCARDIA WITH FUSION COMPLEXES
NON-SPECIFIC INTRA-VENTRICULAR CONDUCTION BLOCK
RIGHT VENTRICULAR HYPERTROPHY
INFERIOR INFARCTION OF INDETERMINATE AGE
ANTEROLATERAL INFARCT, POSSIBLY ACUTE
** ** ** ** * ACUTE MI * ** ** ** **
ABNORMAL ECG

Technician:
Test ind: RAPID HEART RATE

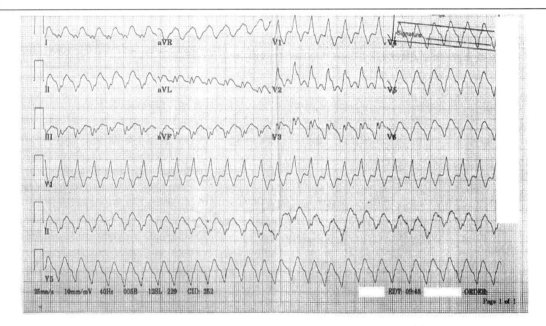

EMERGENCY DEPARTMENT COURSE:

19:51 – Pt arrived in triage with chief complaint of "gallbladder inflammation"

20:25 – Triaged with vital signs listed above

20:41 – Initial ECG. The ED physician discussed the initial ECG with a second ED doctor and it was agreed that this was ventricular tachycardia.

20:47 – He received Lidocaine 100 mg IV, which caused him to become transiently dizzy. There was no change in rhythm.

20:52 – He received Adenosine 6 mg IV x 2 then 12 mg IV, which did absolutely nothing.

21:14 – He then received Procainamide drip 20 mg per minute, which did not really improve his rhythm at all. Cardiology was called and a copy of the ECG and rhythm strip was faxed to the cardiologist who agreed that this was ventricular tachycardia. He asked us to continue the Procainamide and we did that.

21:44 – Pt. denied having any chest pain.

22:00 – He did have an episode of hypotension with a BP of 88/60 and a recheck was 93/65. Cardiology was paged again and he asked that the patient to be given Lopressor 5 mg IV every 5 minutes x 3 and the Procainamide be stopped, which we did. We thought this might cause his heart to slow down and allow his heart to fill better and empty better. The patient did have decrease in his heart rate to the 130s and then to 120s. After the Lopressor, first dose, 5 mg was given, the patients pressure did decrease to a systolic pressure of 67. He was placed in Trendelenburg. He was given IV fluids with a rapid infusion through 2 IVs and also had Dopamine started at 5 mcg/kg per minute.

22:24 – A second ECG was done which showed an acute anterolateral myocardial infarction. (see below) A heart alert was called (Mobile ICU automatically put 'on the road' to the hospital, pharmacist to the ED) and Cardiology was again notified. They recommended against thrombolytic, but did recommend ReoPro and Heparin and emergent transfer to a sister hospital which was able to perform invasive catheterization. The patient's pressure did minimally improve to 77/52.

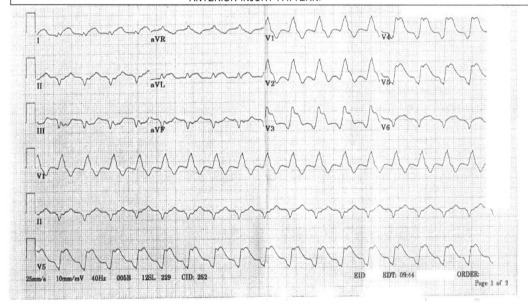

	Vent. rate 107 bpm	**Computer interpretation:**
	PR interval * ms	*** POOR DATA QUALITY, INTERPRETATION MAY BE ADVERSELY AFFECTED
Male	QRS duration 172 ms	SINUS RHYTHM WITH
	QT/QTc 374/499 ms	ACCELERATED JUNCTIONAL RHYTHM
	P-R-T axes 78 -97 52	WITH A COMPETING JUNCTIONAL PACEMAKER
		NON-SPECIFIC INTRA-VENTICULAR CONDUCTION BLOCK
		RIGHT VENTRICULAR HYPERTROPHY
Technician:		LATERAL INFARCT OF INDETERMINATE AGE
Test ind: CP		INFERIOR INFARCTION OF INDETERMINATE AGE
		ANTERIOR INJURY PATTERN.

RESULTS:

Test	Flag	Value	Units	Ref. range
WBC	H	19.5	K/uL	4.6-10.2
HGB		15.8	G/DL	13.5-17.5
PLT		273	K/uL	142-424

(continued on next page)

Test	Flag	Value	Units	Ref. range
NA		142	MMOL/L	135-144
K		3.8	MMOL/L	3.5-5.1
CL		101	MMOL/L	98-107
CO2		25	MMOL/L	22-29
BUN		9	MG/DL	7-18
CREAT		1.1	MG/DL	0.6-1.3

Test	Flag	Value	Units	Ref. range
CK	H	2,269		
CKMB	H	284	NG/ML	0.0-5.0
TROPI	H	24.4	NG/ML	.00-.27
REL INDEX	H	12.5		

—Continuation of CASE 10—

22:42 - The mobile intensive care unit team arrives, and the patient emergently transferred for emergency cardiac catheterization. Cardiology again notified.

23:13 - The patient arrests in the parking lot of the receiving hospital. Attempts at resuscitation are unsuccessful.

FINAL DIAGNOSIS: Acute anterolateral myocardial infarction with wide complex tachycardia and hypotension.

Gregory L. Henry comments:

"Transport of critically ill patients has inherent d⌐ patient in a hospital that cannot prov⌐

Patients tell you many things that need interpretation. A patiᵕ blood pressure, and low pulse ox does not generally equate to gaᵢᵤ the patient has an extensive history with this disease entity, the diagnosis ᵢᵤ the physicians in this case avoided the trap of falling into the patient's line of tᵣᵢᵢᵤ

A chief complaint is only that; a complaint presented by the patient. The chief complaint may be taken by an emergency medicine clerk, LPN, or emergency tech, and may not actually indicate the kind of medical evaluation that a nursing or physician appraisal might produce. The chief complaint is often vague and not borne out by the final diagnostic impression. The intelligent emergency physician knows to reserve judgment until further information is gathered.

The evaluation of this patient seems perfectly appropriate. It should be noted that the patient had no abdominal tenderness. It would be wise to comment specifically on the right upper quadrant since the patient had come in with a complaint of gallbladder disease, but essentially no one with an inflamed gallbladder has a normal abdominal examination. It appears that orders and evaluation took place in a most expeditious manner.

My compliments for the documentation recorded in this case. The key to proper nursing charting is to document the times of all therapies given, procedures performed, and response to such interventions. The shorter the initial nursing evaluation, the better. Lawsuits are often determined on a minute-to-minute evaluation of what was happening to a patient. This chart nicely summarizes the actions taken.

The emergency physicians in this case were not diverted by the initial EKG; whether this represents a broad, junctional rhythm or a true ventricular tachycardia is difficult to assess. The key point is that an abnormal cardiac rhythm in such a patient, particularly with his history of myocardial disease, should be considered a manifestation of cardiac ischemia—the rhythm is almost inconsequential. It must be determined if a coronary artery lesion exists and can be resolved to improve vascularity to the heart.

The patient did have some improvement with medications given and the second EKG did show the injury pattern and the junctional rhythm. The problem at this point is transfer for cardiac catheterization. Transport of critically ill patients has inherent dangers, but so does keeping a patient in a hospital that cannot provide the necessary intervention. Although this patient did die in transfer, I believe it was a noble effort and one that I would want done for my own family. The only real salvation for this patient was immediate catheterization and restoration of blood flow to the cardiac conduction system. Although criticism occasionally is heard about transferring patients, there is no question that this patient needed high quality and sophisticated cardiac intervention.

er of patients with involvement of the cardiac conduction system from acute
ae. This is an unfortunate but inevitable truth in emergency medicine.

- Thoroughness of documentation: 9 out of 10.

- Thoroughness of Patient Evaluation: 10 out of 10.

- Risk of Serious Illness Being Missed: Low risk.

- Risk Management Legal Rating: Medium risk.

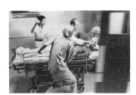

EVALUATION OF ACUTE CORONARY SYNDROME AND MANAGEMENT OF CARDIAC ARRHYTHMIAS

Jud E. Hollander, MD
Esther H. Chen, MD

I. PRESENTATIONS OF ACUTE CORONARY SYNDROME

The classic presentation of acute coronary syndrome (ACS): substernal chest pressure associated with diaphoresis, dyspnea, and nausea, is still taught in major medical textbooks, yet those of us in practice have since learned that few people ever present classically. Misdiagnosis occurs most often when pain is absent (e.g., in diabetic, female, or elderly patients),[1] or when a subxiphoid location of pain is attributed to indigestion or some other gastrointestinal process. Both may result in significant delay to seeking medical care[2] and a poorer prognosis. Astute clinicians must be aware of these atypical presentations and use their clinical judgment along with other objective data (i.e., physical exam, ECG, cardiac markers) to appropriately risk stratify patients for possible ACS.

As illustrated in this case, this patient presented with right upper quadrant discomfort, thinking his gallbladder was inflamed. Patients will often diagnose themselves using medical knowledge they acquire from the internet, television, or magazines, which may or may not be accurate. Do not be led astray by your misinformed patient. In this case, the absence of gastrointestinal symptoms and objective abdominal exam findings makes a biliary problem much less likely. Gallbladder inflammation causing a pulse of 162 would be expected to result in an impressive abdominal exam! With ultrasound now available in many emergency departments, a "quick look" at the gallbladder will quickly put this organ to rest.

II. EVALUATION OF ACUTE CORONARY SYNDROME WITH STRESS TESTING

Once biliary disease is excluded, ACS moves up in our differential diagnosis. The role of the emergency physician in patients with suspected ACS is to identify and effectively manage those patients at risk for adverse events. However, risk stratification of acute chest pain patients proves to be very difficult, despite consensus guidelines and risk stratification tools.[3,4] The guidelines seem to be most useful for patients with classical, not atypical, presentations. The pretest probability of ACS in our patient is at least intermediate, and his risk for cardiac ischemic events, using the TIMI risk score,[5] would be about 13%. Do not be misled by his history of a negative stress test; it does not exclude ACS. Radionucleotide imaging has a sensitivity and specificity for detecting coronary artery disease of 70–94% and 43–97%, respectively.[6] Moreover, noninvasive imaging will more easily detect significant plaques (>70% stenosis) because of its obstructive effects on blood flow, although these plaques are not likely to rupture and cause a cardiac event. Less significant plaques (< 70% stenosis) are actually more likely to rupture and cause an ischemic event, but are also easily missed by stress testing.[7] Therefore, even if our patient had a negative stress test last week, he could still have a coronary event from a missed "insignificant plaque" that suddenly ruptured.

III. ADVERSE EVENTS ASSOCIATED WITH ACUTE CORONARY SYNDROME

Adverse events associated with ACS are well established, including but not limited to death, heart failure, and life-threatening dysrhythmias. Evidence suggests that ACS patients in the early phase of their disease (≤ 72 hours) should be monitored in telemetry or intensive care units so that a malignant dysrhythmia may be treated with anti-arrhythmic medications or defibrillation.[8] There is less convincing data for mandatory monitoring of all admitted chest pain patients and growing evidence supporting the safety of managing low risk patients (normal initial ECG and cardiac biomarkers) in unmonitored beds.[9] The risk of life-threatening cardiac arrhythmias in these patients is so low that continuous monitoring makes very little difference in their management.

IV. MANAGEMENT OF ARRHYTHMIAS

Although ventricular fibrillation (VF) and ventricular tachycardia (VT) are the most serious arrhythmias, other cardiac arrhythmias including supraventricular arrhythmias (atrial fibrillation and flutter), bradyarrhythmias (variable heart blocks), and accelerated idioventricular and junctional rhythms, may develop in patients with ST-elevation myocardial infarction (STEMI).[4] Treatment of cardiac arrhythmias in the setting of ACS generally follows ACLS guidelines. Any dysrhythmia that causes hemodynamic instability requires electrical intervention, either cardioversion or defibrillation, depending on the degree of cardiovascular compromise. Atrial fibrillation or flutter in patients with ongoing ischemia, but without hemodynamic compromise, should receive β-adrenergic blockade for rate control and anti-coagulant therapy. In contrast, no treatment (particularly prophylactic lidocaine) is recommended for premature ventricular beats or couplets, non-sustained VT, and accelerated idioventricular or junctional rhythms. These rhythms are no longer considered to be ventricular warning arrhythmias resulting in VF.[4]

Treatment for VT and VF is slightly more complicated. ACS patients with either VT or VF have a 5-fold to 15-fold higher 6-month mortality rate, especially in patients with STEMI.[10] Our patient's initial ECG revealed sustained VT, so prompt treatment was indicated. Cardioversion (starting energy 100J) or defibrillation is recommended for patients with hemodynamic instability or clinical evidence of pulmonary edema. Sustained monomorphic VT without angina, hypotension, or pulmonary edema may be treated with an amiodarone infusion or cardioversion (starting energy 50J). There is also some data supporting the use of a procainamide bolus and infusion in these patients. This was attempted in our patient, but was stopped when hypotension worsened. Finally, in patients with refractory polymorphic VT, there is sufficient evidence to justify attempts to reduce the myocardial ischemia (e.g., β-adrenergic blockade, intra-aortic balloon pump, and emergency percutaneous intervention) and to normalize potassium and magnesium levels.[4]

V. DIFFERENTIATING VENTRICULAR TACHYCARDIA FROM SVT WITH ABERRANCY

Recognizing a wide complex tachycardia on ECG may seem straightforward, but distinguishing VT from SVT with aberrancy, or monomorphic from polymorphic VT, may be confusing. Pathophysiologically, VT occurs during active ischemia or from previous scar tissue, through either a re-entry phenomenon or triggered automaticity.[11] Monomorphic VT exhibits a regular beat-to-beat QRS morphology as compared to polymorphic VT where there are numerous QRS morphologies (Figure 1), with variable R-R interval.[11] Monomorphic VT is more common, especially in patients with ACS.

Figure 1. Polymorphic and Monomorphic Ventricular Tachycardia
A. Monomorphic VT.   B. Polymorphic VT.   C. Torsades de pointes.

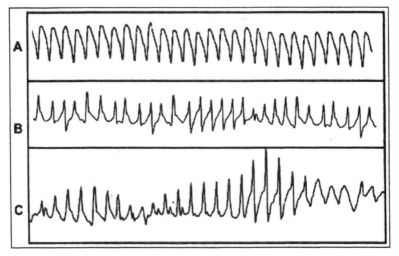

Source: Hudson KB, Brady WJ, Chan TC, et al. Electrocardiographic manifestations: ventricular tachycardia. J Emerg Med 2003; 25:303-14. Used with permission.

It is important to distinguish VT from SVT with aberrancy, because misidentification may have serious clinical implications. Figure 2 shows an algorithmic approach to the ECG interpretation of wide complex tachycardias. If all these rule make your head swim, the good news is that 80% of wide complex tachycardias are VT,[11] so in the setting of ACS, treat them as VT until proven otherwise.

Using the Brugada algorithm,[12] we can interpret the patient's initial ECG as monomorphic VT, probably due to ACS. The subsequent ECG eventually demonstrates the anterolateral STEMI. According to the American College of Cardiology guidelines described above, patients with this rhythm may be treated medically with amiodarone or procainamide, or electrically with cardioversion. Our patient was treated initially treated with lidocaine, which only made him slightly dizzy, but didn't change his rhythm. This was followed by adenosine, which also made no difference in his rhythm, but further confirmed that the rhythm was VT. However, when procainamide produced similar results and the patient became hypotensive, the next appropriate step should have been cardioversion, not lopressor.

Figure 2. Brugada criteria for Distinguishing VT from SVT wi

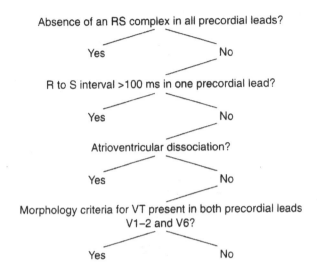

Absence of an RS complex in all precordial leads?

Yes   No

R to S interval >100 ms in one precordial lead?

Yes   No

Atrioventricular dissociation?

Yes   No

Morphology criteria for VT present in both precordial leads
V1–2 and V6?

Yes   No

Source: Brugada P, Brugada J, Mont L, et al. A new approach to the differential diagnosis of a regular tachycardia with a wide QRS complex. Circulation 1991; 83:1649-59. Copyright 1991, American Heart Association. Used with permission.

VI. EMERGENT CARDIOLOGY CONSULTATIONS

At this moment, the physicians were faced with a patient who seemed to be refractory to initial intervention, so they appropriately consulted their cardiologist for guidance. Dealing with consultants can be frustrating for emergency physicians. Often, consultation is for a specific question that needs to be answered, as occurred in this case (i.e., consulting a cardiologist to assist you in reading a difficult ECG) or to arrange an intervention that emergently needs to occur (i.e., emergency revascularization for a patient with STEMI). Crucial information to convey during the conversation is the acuity of the patient, a brief summary of initial interventions, and the reason for the consultation. Consultants who recognize the urgency of a critically ill patient will likely help you manage the patient at the bedside. However, if your institution's consultant is unhelpful, using a regional referral center's consultants may be more appropriate, especially if a higher level of care is anticipated.

VII. CARDIOGENIC SHOCK

Unfortunately, sometimes we do all the right things for the patient, but have a bad outcome. This patient eventually developed cardiogenic shock from his anterolateral STEMI, and expired despite the aggressive management. Cardiogenic shock is well recognized as a complication of ACS and a major cause of death in these patients, with an in-hospital mortality rate of 60–70%.[13]

Pharmacologic treatment begins with IV dopamine or other vasopressors, and dobutamine, for its inotropic effects, if the systemic vascular resistance is high. Because shock is related to the ongoing cardiac ischemia, emergency revascularization may actually improve cardiac function and

.nodynamics. Moreover, intra-aortic balloon pumps in conjunction with revascularization may further improve patient outcomes.[13]

VIII. TRANSFER OF UNSTABLE PATIENTS

Unfortunately, in this case our patient had his STEMI in a hospital without emergency revascularization capabilities, and died during transfer to a facility with those capabilities. Transferring unstable patients is always associated with very high risks, but the patient probably would have suffered the same outcome without definitive therapy. Ultimately, the physicians made a noble effort to give this patient the best chance for survival.

TEACHING POINTS ABOUT CASE 10:

- Any ACS patient may present with atypical symptoms, although this is more common in elderly, female, and diabetic patients.
- A wide-complex tachycardia seen on the ECG of a patient with potential ACS should be treated as ventricular tachycardia until proven otherwise.
- A recent negative stress test does not exclude the diagnosis of ACS.
- Cardiogenic shock is the most common cause of death in patients with ACS. Definitive treatment remains emergent revascularization.
- Though a patient may like to believe that their symptoms are from a benign etiology, if they were 100% sure, they wouldn not be in your ED. Waiting 34 minutes for a bed is not appropriate for patients with a pulse of 162, even if it is just from gallbladder inflammation!

REFERENCES

1. Coronado BE, Pope JH, Griffith JL, et al. Clinical features, triage, and outcome of patients presenting to the ED with suspected acute coronary syndromes but without pain: a multicenter study. Am J Emerg Med. 2004; 22(7):568-74.
2. Goldberg RJ, Steg PG, Sadiq I, et al. Extent of, and factors associated with, delay to hospital presentation in patients with acute coronary disease (the GRACE registry). Am J Cardiol 2002; 89:791-796.
3. Braunwald E, Antman EM, Beasley JW, et al. ACC/AHA 2002 guideline update for the management of patients with unstable angina and non-ST-segment elevation myocardial infarction—summary article: a report of the American College of Cardiology/American Heart Association task force on practice guidelines (Committee on the Management of Patients With Unstable Angina). J Am Coll Cardiol 2002; 40:1366-74.
4. Antman EM, Anbe DT, Armstrong PW, et al. ACC/AHA guidelines for the management of patients with ST-elevation myocardial infarction—executive summary. A report of the American College of Cardiology/American Heart Association Task Force on Practice Guidelines (Writing Committee to revise the 1999 guidelines for the management of patients with acute myocardial infarction). J Am Coll Cardiol 2004; 44:671-719.
5. Antman EM, Cohen M, Bernink PJ, et al. The TIMI risk score for unstable angina/non-ST elevation MI: A method for prognostication and therapeutic decision making. JAMA 2000; 284:835-42.
6. Lee TH, Boucher CA. Clinical practice. Noninvasive tests in patients with stable coronary artery disease. N Engl J Med 2001; 344(24):1840-5.

7. Gibbons RJ, Abrams J, Chatterjee K, et al. ACC/AHA 2002 guideline update for the management of patients with chronic stable angina—summary article: a report of the American College of Cardiology/American Heart Association Task Force on practice guidelines (Committee on the Management of Patients With Chronic Stable Angina). J Am Coll Cardiol 2003; 41:159-68.

8. Drew BJ, Califf RM, Funk M, et al. Practice standards for electrocardiographic monitoring in hospital settings: an American Heart Association scientific statement from the Councils on Cardiovascular Nursing, Clinical Cardiology, and Cardiovascular Disease in the Young: endorsed by the International Society of Computerized Electrocardiology and the American Association of Critical-Care Nurses. Circulation 2004; 110:2721-46.

9. Hollander JE, Sites FD, Pollack CV, Jr., et al. Lack of utility of telemetry monitoring for identification of cardiac death and life-threatening ventricular dysrhythmias in low-risk patients with chest pain. Ann Emerg Med 2004; 43:71-6.

10. Al-Khatib SM, Granger CB, Huang Y, et al. Sustained ventricular arrhythmias among patients with acute coronary syndromes with no ST-segment elevation: incidence, predictors, and outcomes. Circulation 2002; 106:309-12.

11. Hudson KB, Brady WJ, Chan TC, et al. Electrocardiographic manifestations: ventricular tachycardia. J Emerg Med 2003; 25:303-14.

12. Brugada P, Brugada J, Mont L, et al. A new approach to the differential diagnosis of a regular tachycardia with a wide QRS complex. Circulation 1991; 83:1649-59.

13. Hasdai D, Topol EJ, Califf RM, et al. Cardiogenic shock complicating acute coronary syndromes. Lancet 2000; 356(9231):749-56.

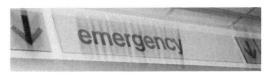

CASE 11

37 YEAR OLD MALE WITH HEADACHE

Commentary:
Gregory L. Henry, MD, FACEP

CEO, Medical Practice Risk Assessment, Inc., Ann Arbor, Michigan

Clinical Professor, Department of Emergency Medicine
   University of Michigan Medical School, Ann Arbor, Michigan

Past President, American College of Emergency Physicians (ACEP)

Discussion:
Michael Para, MD

Pomerene Professor of Infectious Diseases

Associate Dean of Clinical Research

The Ohio State University College of Medicine
   Columbus, Ohio

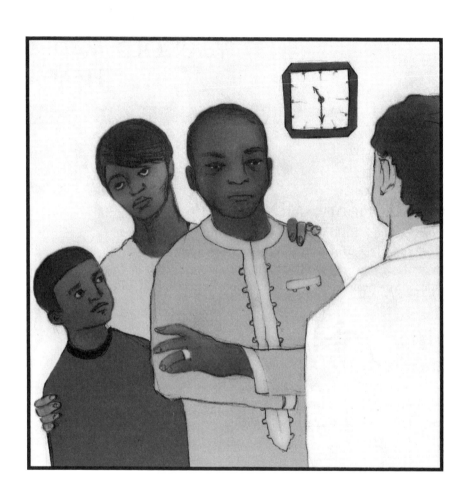

37 YEAR OLD MALE WITH HEADACHE

—Initial Visit*—

*Authors' Note: The history, exam and notes are the actual documentation of the physicians and providers, including abbreviations (and spelling errors)

CHIEF COMPLAINT (at 11:22): Headache

VITAL SIGNS					
Time	Temp	Pulse	Resp	Syst	Diast
23:30	98.9	104	18	112	68

HISTORY OF PRESENT ILLNESS (at 11:54): Pt. is a 37 year old male who presented with complaint of 20 year history of headaches which occur about once per month. The patient was returning from church the day previously and had a constant pain in the frontal region associated with nausea and one episode of vomiting and was similar to past headaches, but lasted longer. No complaints of rhinorrhea, cough, sore throat, earache, dizziness, neck pain, rash, numbness, slurred speech or facial droop, chest pain, SOB, or abdominal pain.

PAST MEDICAL HISTORY/TRIAGE:
  PMH: Negative
  PSH: Negative
  Medications: None
  SH: Works for Buckeye steel

PHYSICAL EXAM (AT 12:00):
  General: Alert and oriented X3, well-nourished, in no apparent distress
  Head: Normocephalic; atraumatic.
  Eyes: PERRL, EOMI
  Nose: The nose is normal in appearance without rhinorrhea
  Respir.: Breath sounds clear and equal bilaterally; no wheezes, rhonchi, or rales
  Cardiac: Regular tachycardic rhythm, without murmurs, rub or gallop
  Abd.: Non-distended; non-tender, soft, without rigidity, rebound or guarding
  Skin: Normal for age and race; warm and dry; no apparent lesions
  Neck: No jugular venous distention, no lymphadenopathy, supple without nucal rigidity.
  Neuro: Patient is alert and oriented times three. Cranial nerves III-XII are intact. Sensory and motor functions are intact. Strength is 5/5 for flexion and extension in all 4 extremities. Patellar DTRs are equal and intact. Finger to nose testing is equal and normal bilaterally.

DIAGNOSIS (AT 13:11): Acute cephalgia, recurrent

PLAN: Rx for vicodin and phenergan, work excuse, instructions for HA, follow up family practice clinic

Gregory L. Henry comments:

"The real question is, "Why is this headache different? What brought him in today?"

When approaching a patient with a headache, the history must be directed. The emergency physician must feel comfortable with the evaluation of intercerebral bleeding, infection, and chemical irritations such as carbon monoxide, since it is easy to be led astray by historical red herrings. The signal-to-noise ratio in emergency medicine is high; we are receiving multiple inputs that may obscure a diagnosis.

The patient reports headaches for the past 20 years, occurring about once a month. The real question is, "Why is this headache different? What brought him in today?" He certainly has not been visiting an emergency department every month for 20 years! The difference in this headache as opposed to others should be elucidated.

The onset of a headache is important to document. In the largest series ever done on subarachnoid hemorrhage, the only historical feature that could be directly related to subarachnoid hemorrhage was the acuity of onset. When a headache goes from nonexistent to maximum intensity within a few minutes, the possibility of vascular rupture needs to be considered. When a patient has a loss of consciousness with a headache, the patient should not be discharged; the outcomes are severe enough, the patient need to be aggressively evaluated.

The evaluation of this patient seems perfectly appropriate. It is interesting to note, under the eye examination, that extra-ocular movements and pupil size and reactivity are documented, but examination of the fundi is not. It is rare that abnormal extra ocular movements and altered pupils are noted in patients with normal mental status. The important questions during the evaluation of headaches have to do with the underlying brain. The second cranial nerve is not a true cranial nerve, but an extension of the diencephalon of the brain; the only place on the body where the brain can be visualized is therefore the fundus of the eye. Fundoscopic examination, although most likely normal in this case, should be performed in every headache patient. The rest of the neurologic examination and the neck exam all appear perfectly appropriate and are well done.

The disposition on this case is also appropriate. With a normal examination, no specific laboratory testing is required. The response to pain medication in the department can be noted, but does not rule out a more serious underlying condition.

Documentation on the history, except for its weaknesses in the onset and location of the headache, is acceptable. The documentation of the physical exam, with the exception of the absence of a funduscopic exam, is also acceptable.

Documentation is weaker in the area of instructions. Whenever it says follow-up with family practice clinic, the obvious question is "when?" All discharge instructions need to be two things: 1) time-specific, and 2) action-specific. Exactly when is the patient supposed to follow-up, and why? This rather obvious shortcoming is a deficiency in a large number of medical/legal actions against emergency physicians.

- Thoroughness of Documentation: 7 out of 10.

- Thoroughness of Patient Evaluation: 9 out of 10.

- Risk of Serious Illness Being Missed: Medium risk.

- Risk Management Legal Rating: Medium Risk.

37 YEAR OLD MALE WITH HEADACHE

—Second Visit: 3 Days Later—

CHIEF COMPLAINT (at 08:44): Headache

```
VITAL SIGNS
Time      Temp     Pulse    Resp    Syst    Diast
08:47     98.6      80       16      112      58
```

HISTORY OF PRESENT ILLNESS (at 09:09): Pt. returns with frontal headache present for 4 days. Seen by his primary care physician 2 days ago (one day after first ED visit) and diagnosed with sinusitis and prescribed zithromax. Pain is constant and worse with bending over. Complains of emesis and decreased appetite. Denies trauma, photophobia, fever, chills or cough. No relief from vicodin prescribed 3 days ago.

PAST MEDICAL HISTORY/TRIAGE:
  Medications: Zithromax, Vicodin, Phenergan

PHYSICAL EXAM (at 09:17): (summary) No change from initial exam, except nasal mucosa edematous and erythematous and he is tender to palpation over the frontal and maxillary sinuses

RADIOLOGY (results received at 10:49):
  Brain CT: 1. No acute intracranial findings. 2. A small air-fluid level or mucoperiosteal thickening is seen within the right maxillary sinus antrym. Is there clinical evidence for sinusitis?

ED COURSE (at 11:28): Given imitrex before the CT without relief. Given Demerol and phenergan IM with marked improvement.

DIAGNOSIS: Cephalgia and sinusitis

PLAN (at 11:35): Rx for entex, he should continue the vicodin and zithromax

---

—Third Visit: 2 Days Later—

CHIEF COMPLAINT (at 06:15): Headache

VITAL SIGNS					
Time	Temp	Pulse	Resp	Syst	Diast
06:23	97.4	84	20	110	60

HISTORY OF PRESENT ILLNESS (at 06:57): Pt. was seen 2 times previously and was having rhinorrhea and facial pressure on the right side and nausea. Saw family doctor yesterday (second visit to family doctor) and received additional pain medication. No relief from the vicodin and motrin, one day left of the zithromax. Does complain of vomiting X 1 yesterday and facial pressure on the right side. No cp, SOB, visual changes, earaches, stiff neck, numbness, weakness of extremities. He has never had anything like this before.

MEDICATIONS: Zithromax, Entex, Vicodin, Motrin, Phenergan

PHYSICAL EXAM (at 07:02): (summary)
No change from initial exam except it was noted that he was in mild discomfort. Extensive exam is normal.

ED COURSE (at 07:44): Demerol and phenergan IM

DIAGNOSIS: Acute cephalgia secondary to sinusitis

PLAN (at 08:03): Antibiotic changed to Augmentin, instructions for sinusitis, continue vicodin and phenergan as instructed, follow up PCP 5-7 days

—Fourth Visit: Same Day, 10 Hours Later—

CHIEF COMPLAINT (at 16:33): Headache

```
VITAL SIGNS
Time     Temp    Pulse   Resp    Syst    Diast
16:40    99.0    76      16      116     74
```

HISTORY OF PRESENT ILLNESS (at 16:49): 37 year old African American male from Guinea who has been in the US for 6 years with headache for one week which is getting worse. States had fevers at home. States is worst headache of his life. No visual changes, vomiting, neck pain, photophobia, neck stiffness.

Medications: Augmentin, Entex, Vicodin, Motrin, Phenergan

PHYSICAL EXAM: (summary) Afebrile, VSS
Exam normal except somewhat tender on bilateral frontal sinuses

ED COURSE AND MEDICAL DECISION MAKING (at 19:59): Pt. was from Guinea and did not have risk factors for HIV, but there is a large HIV population there and I was concerned about atypical infection, without a high suspicion. Was also concerned about an abscess based on poor clinical response to antibiotics for sinusitis. CT head with IV contrast showed perhaps some minimal mucoperiosteal thickening in the right maxillary sinus which was demonstrated on previous CT. Pt. received benadryl and compazine for pain without help, then morphine with a little improvement. LP was performed (results below). I spoke with the pathologist who felt this was secondary to the traumatic tap.

CSF RESULTS: Blood tinged initially then clear and colorless without xanthochromia. RBC 11 in tube 3 (there were 250 in tube one), WBC 5 (1 poly, 4 lymph) which were irregularly shaped.

DIAGNOSIS:
1. Sinusitis
2. Complicated cephalgia

PLAN (at 22:07): Change vicodin to percocet. With his history being from Guinea, will add cryptococcal antigen to his CSF, but I do not feel this is likely, but I thought it might be worthwhile investigating. Discharged to home.

After the initial visit, he returned for multiple other visits. One of my rules is on a second visit the patient needs to be thoroughly re-examined. Most cases of second visits are due to either instructions not understood, or disease entity not properly diagnosed. A return to the emergency department is rarely the patient's fault. A third visit is a bigger medical/legal risk, and equals admission until proven otherwise. If a patient comes back three times, something is definitely wrong. We may not know what the problem is, but there should be other minds brought in to investigate the problem. This was particularly true with this patient; with a change in headache pattern that has gone on for 20 years, this seems to be a very unusual case.

37 YEAR OLD MAN WITH HEADACHE

—Fifth Visit: Early Morning (A Few Hours Later)—

CHIEF COMPLAINT (at 01:58): Called to return with positive LP results

```
VITAL SIGNS
Time      Temp     Pulse    Resp    Syst    Diast
02:01     97.4     96       16      130     72
```

HISTORY OF PRESENT ILLNESS (at 02:33): Lab had called the ED with positive cryptococcal stain by India ink. Pt. states headache is completely resolved after the LP. No more nausea and vomiting. Weight loss of 35 poounds over the last 8 months. Married for the last 6 years, his wife lives in New Jersey. No history of IV drug use or sex with men or prostitutes. No history of HIV test.

MEDICATIONS: Augmentin, Entex, Vicodin, Motrin, Phenergan

PHYSICAL EXAM: (summary)
Exam normal, no oral thrush or oral hairy leukoplakia. No adenopathy

RESULTS (at 03:03):

```
Test  Flag  Value   Units    Ref. Range
WBC         4.4     K/uL     4.6-10.2
HGB    L    11.0    G/DL     13.5-17.5
PLT         295     K/uL     142-424

HIV, CD4 and viral load pending.
```

DIAGNOSIS: Cryptcoccal meningitis

PLAN (AT 03:22): Started on Amphotericin B, admitted to infectious disease specialist.

HOSPITAL COURSE:
Was found to have AIDS and was successfully started on antiretroviral therapy.

FINAL DIAGNOSIS: Cryptococcal meningitis, AIDS

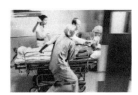

DIAGNOSIS OF HIV, EVALUATION OF HEADACHES IN PATIENTS WITH HIV/AIDS, & CRYPTOCOCCAL MENINGITIS

Michael Para, MD

I. INTRODUCTION
The history on the fourth visit now mentions that the patient is African. This fact, at this point in his evaluation, expands the possible etiologies for his headache. The complaint of fever supports the diagnosis of an infectious etiology. Though he has been in the US for 6 years, it would be helpful to know when he last visited Africa in order to rule out a recently acquired zoonotic infection. With HIV infection present in approximately 10% of all sub-Saharan Africans and up to 40% of adults in some African countries, HIV infection must be moved into the differential diagnosis of persistent headache and fever. This is what occurred in this case; the physician tested the CSF for Cryptococcus and the result came back positive.

Opportunistic infections such as cryptococcus or toxoplasmosis typically occur in the later stages of HIV infection when the CD4 count is under 200. Since the CD4 cell count falls 60–100 cells per year of HIV infection, it may take years after the initial viral infection for patients to present with an opportunistic infection (OI). This patient's picture would be typical of someone 6–10 years after HIV infection presenting with an OI.

II. DIAGNOSING HIV DISEASE—HISTORY AND PHYSICAL
ED physicians should consider the possibility of HIV infection when the patient has a history of HIV-positive sexual contacts, potential exposure from injection drugs, or multiple unknown sex partners. White, gay men no longer represent the majority of new HIV infections in the US; over a third of recently infected individuals acquired HIV via heterosexual contact and 46% by homosexual contact. Over half of new infections are diagnosed in African-Americans, and 27% are in women. Direct questioning about prior HIV testing is appropriate. It may have been performed because of exposures, for blood donations, or insurance applications.

What else might have clued the ED physicians to a diagnosis of HIV infection? AIDS patients presenting with major opportunistic infections typically give a history of repeated minor mucocutaneous infections such as thrush, recurrent herpes simplex, or shingles. Weight loss, night sweats and anorexia are commonly present in late stage HIV. Organ system specific complaints usually relate to the particular opportunistic infection e.g., progressive dyspnea with PCP.

Physical exam clues to HIV diagnosis also depend on the CD4 count. Examination of the skin of HIV-infected individuals with CD4 counts < 200 commonly shows seborrheic dermatitis especially over the malar eminences, zoster scars, genital or perianal herpes simplex virus (HSV), and tinea. Oral lesions are also common and include thrush, oral hairy leukoplakia (pathognomonic for HIV) and linear gingivitis. Generalized lymphadenopathy, with strings of 1–2 cm nodes in the posterior cervical chain, are typically found. A funduscopic exam may reveal cotton wool spots. Papilledema can be seen with cryptococcus, toxoplasmosis, or CNS lymphoma.

III. DIAGNOSING HIV DISEASE—LABORATORY STUDIES

In November 2002, reliable, rapid testing for HIV antibodies became available, making the diagnosis of HIV in the ED quick and simple.[1] In fact, the CDC has a campaign to encourage ED physicians to obtain HIV testing of 'at risk' and potentially HIV-infected persons. The new OraQuick Rapid HIV-1 Antibody Test (OraSure Technologies Inc., Bethlehem, Pennsylvania US) can be performed using either a fingerstick blood sample, a tube of blood, or salivary secretions. The results are available in 20–30 minutes. Sensitivity and specificity are excellent and compare favorably with the routine EIA. Furthermore, these rapid assays are CLIA-waived and can be performed in the ED. Studies have shown that ED personnel can perform the test reliably with minimal training.[2] As with positive EIA tests for HIV, all positives rapid assay tests need to be confirmed with a Western blot or other confirmatory assay.

Routine laboratory studies commonly show abnormalities and can support suspicions of undiagnosed HIV infection. Leukopenia with lymphopenia is the rule; its absence argues against HIV. A normochromic, normocytic anemia is common but not universal. Thrombocytopenia is seen in 10% of patients. Patients are commonly co-infected with hepatitis, resulting in abnormal LFTs.

IV. EVALUATION OF HEADACHES IN PATIENTS WITH HIV

In this patient, the chronicity of the headache argues against acute bacterial meningitis. In patients with AIDS, the differential diagnosis of headache includes CNS mass lesions, and a spinal tap should be withheld until a head CT scan is performed, confirming there is not a midline shift. The lack of mass lesion in the brain parenchyma in our patient's contrast enhanced CT makes B-cell lymphoma and toxoplasmosis less likely. Sinus infection can cause headaches in HIV infected patients, but this has been treated without resolution. While cryptococcus would be the most common cause of subacute meningitis in an AIDS patient in the US, other opportunistic infections of the central nervous system that could present as headache include cytomegalovirus (CMV), herpes simplex virus (HSV), herpes zoster (VZV), progressive multifocal leukoencephalopathy (PML), tuberculosis (TB), Mycobacterium avium complex (MAC), syphilis, listeria, histoplasmosis, and coccidioides. A CSF examination and cultures of the CSF are needed to help sort out these possibilities.

V. CRYPTOCOCCAL MENINGITIS—SYMPTOMS AND DIAGNOSIS

Cryptococcus is a ubiquitous organism with a portal of entry via the lungs. It spreads to the CNS hematogenously. With a diagnosis of cryptococcal meningitis, blood cultures and CXR are indicated to more fully evaluate its dissemination.

The most common symptoms of cryptococcal meningitis in HIV patients are chronic headache, fever, and malaise.[3] Physical signs suggestive of chronic HIV infection are not noted in our patient's record. However, the lack of nuchal rigidity is typical in cryptococcal disease; less than half of patients have a stiff neck. Other physical findings in late stage HIV usually reflect the extent of underlying cell-mediated immunodeficiency. The mucocutaneous signs/symptoms noted above would be expected in an AIDS patient presenting with a major OI. Fever occurred late in this patient, which is usually the case. Temperatures normally do not exceed 39° C, and are absent in a quarter of patients.[4]

In AIDS patients with cryptococcal meningitis, the CT scan is normal in most patients, but hydrocephalus and gyral enhancement can be found in some. Cortical atrophy is seen in a third of patients.

An LP was performed on our patient, but no opening pressure was noted. This would have been helpful and may have suggested the diagnosis as opening pressures are elevated (>200 mm of water) in three-fourths of patients with cryptococcal meningitis and AIDS. In fact, the increased intracranial pressure not infrequently causes cranial nerve palsies and visual impairment and is the main determinant of outcome.[4]

The large polysaccharide capsule of cryptococcus shields the fungus from the host response, so it causes minimal inflammation in the CSF, especially in patients with AIDS. The CSF protein may be slightly elevated and glucose depressed, but the CSF may be entirely normal throughout the course of cryptococcal meningitis. Making the diagnosis more confusing, HIV infection alone can cause mild CSF lymphocytic pleocytosis and increased protein.

While the cell counts and chemistries of the CSF may appear entirely normal in cryptococcal meningitis in AIDS patients, the organism load is very high. The India ink examination is positive in over 80% of the cases.[4] Cryptococcal polysaccharide is also present in high concentration and can be detected using the EIA or latex agglutination assays. These tests are more than 90% sensitive and specific in both the CSF and the serum. In fact, since the cryptococcal antigen is positive in the serum in almost all cases of cryptococcal meningitis, this assay can be used to screen AIDS patients with headache for cryptococcal disease.[5] A positive serum test does not always equate with meningitis since it can be seen with extraneural cryptococcal infection alone.

As expected, the LP relieved our patient's intracranial hypertension, and his headache, nausea, and vomiting were improved. A repeat spinal tap will be required to assess the severity of the intracranial hypertension. A large volume of spinal fluid may need to be removed to control the headache. Daily taps may be necessary to keep the pressure down and relieve cranial nerve palsies and visual impairment.[6]

VI. CRYPTOCOCCAL MENINGITIS—TREATMENT

Amphotericin remains the initial therapy for cryptococcal meningitis. Higher doses (0.7 mg/kg/day) seem to be most effective. Liposomal preparations have similar efficacy but less toxicity.[7] The addition of flucytosine at 100 mg/kg/d helps sterilize the CSF earlier, but is associated with increased bone marrow toxicity in AIDS patients. After approximately two weeks of therapy, if there is clinical and CSF improvement, the patient can be switched to fluconazole at 400 mg/d. The short term prognosis is predicted by the patient's mental status at presentation and by the burden of yeast present in the CSF. Decreased levels of consciousness and a cryptococcal antigen titer >1:1028 or a CSF WBC < 20 are all bad signs. The long term prognosis and duration of therapy depends on the immune response to antiretroviral therapy.

VII. SUMMARY OF CASE

This patient's initial visit seemed uncomplicated, and the evaluation and management were reasonable. During the subsequent visits, it seems that the history and physical exam were changing to fit his previous diagnosis of sinusitis without concerted efforts to look for other causes of headache. Red flags included his fever and the fact that he was of African descent (first mentioned by his doctor on his fourth visit). Pain worse when bending over (mentioned on the third visit) suggested the possibility of increased intracranial pressure, though this can also occur with sinusitis.

The onset of this patient's cryptococcal meningitis was insidious, as was his AIDS. It was only through repeat visits and good thinking that the diagnosis was found. There are some clues on history and physical exam, such as fatigue, fevers, lymphadenopathy, oral thrush and seborrheic dermatitis, which may be suggestive of immunosuppression due to HIV/AIDS, but from examining the charts, it is difficult to say if these processes were occurring in our patient. The correct diagnosis was eventually made and the patient was appropriately treated, but his outcome could have been far different…

TEACHING POINTS ABOUT CASE 11:
- Frequent returns to the ED are concerning and demand extreme vigilance.
- Cryptococcal meningitis may be present with normal CSF glucose, protein, and cell count. The opening pressure is > 200 mm Hg in 75% of patients.
- HIV can be diagnosed in the ED with the OraQuick Rapid HIV-1 Antibody Test. This test is CLIA-waived and can be quickly performed in the ED.
- Follow-up instructions should be time- and action-specific.

REFERENCES

1. Centers for Disease Control and Prevention. Notice to readers: approval of a new rapid test for HIV antibody. Morb Mortal Wkly Rep 2002; 51:1051.
2. Kendrick SR, Kroc KA, Couture E, et al. Comparison of point-of-care rapid HIV testing in three clinical venues. AIDS 2004 18:2208-10.
3. Powderly WG. Cryptococcosis. In: AIDS Therapy. Dolin R, Masur H, Saag M, eds. New York, NY: Churchill Livingstone, 1999:400-11.
4. Van der Horst C, Saag M, Cloud G, et al. Treatment of cryptococcal meningitis associated with the acquired immunodeficiency syndrome. National Institute of Allergy and Infectious Diseases Mycoses Study Group and AIDS Clinical Trials Group. N Engl J Med 1997; 337:15-21.

5. Powderly WG, Cloud GA, Dismukes WE, et al. Measurement of cryptococcal antigen in serum and cerebrospinal fluid: value in the management of AIDS-associated cryptococcal meningitis. Clin Infect Dis 1994; 18:789-92.
6. Graybill JR, Sobel J, Saag M, et al. Diagnosis and management of increased intracranial pressure in patients with AIDS and cryptococcal meningitis. Clin Infect Dis 2000; 30:47-54.
7. Leenders AC, Reiss P, Portegies P, et al. Liposomal amphotericin B (AmBisome) compared with amphotericin B both followed by oral fluconazole in the treatment of AIDS-associated cryptococcal meningitis. AIDS 1997; 11:1463-71.

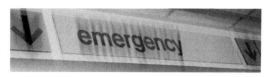

CASE12

42 YEAR OLD FEMALE WITH HEADACHE

Commentary:
Gregory L. Henry, MD, FACEP

CEO, Medical Practice Risk Assessment, Inc., Ann Arbor, Michigan
Clinical Professor, Department of Emergency Medicine
   University of Michigan Medical School, Ann Arbor, Michigan
Past President, American College of Emergency Physicians (ACEP)

Discussion:
Stephen Karas, Jr., MD, FACEP

Clinical Professor at UCSD in Emergency Medicine, San Diego, California
Member, ACEP Clinical Policy Committee, 1991–2000
Author of ACEP publications: *Guidelines for Cost Containment in Emergency Medicine*
   and *Cost Effective Diagnostic Testing in Emergency Medicine*

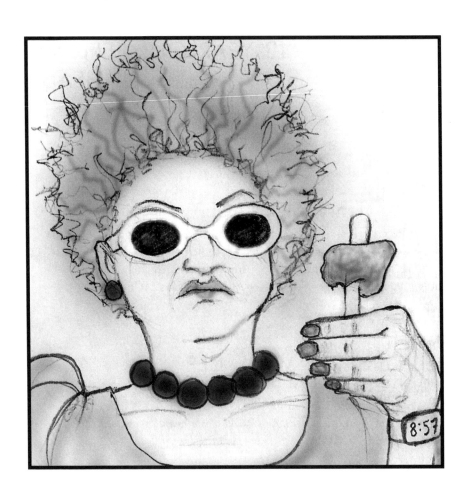

42 YEAR OLD FEMALE WITH HEADACHE

—Initial Visit*—

*Authors' Note: The history, exam and notes are the actual documentation of the physicians and providers, including abbreviations (and spelling errors)

CHIEF COMPLAINT (at 05:02): Headache

VITAL SIGNS						
Time	Temp	Pulse	Resp	Syst	Diast	Pain
05:11	97.7	104	20	122	82	10

HISTORY OF PRESENT ILLNESS (at 05:39): She is a 42 year old woman with a headache which began 5 hours ago. Similar episodes of cephalgia for approx 1 yr. Location: right temporal region that radiates to the right occipital region. Quality: "real bad ache." c/o Phonophobia and photophobic. c/o vomiting earlier. Denies paresthesias or focal weakness of the upper or lower extremities. Took Excedrin - no relief. Denies fever or chills, diarrhea or cough. This is not a new onset headache or a change in her normal headache pattern. Neck and back are tightening up. Has had a recent thorough neurological work-up which was negative for identifiable pathology. She states that her mother died recently and that she has recently been laid off from her job, and that the neurologist has attributed her headaches to stress. She has a normal MRA circle of Willis 8 days ago.

PAST MEDICAL HISTORY/TRIAGE:
  Medications: None
  Allergies: No known allergies.
  PMH: None
  PSH: None

EXAM (at 05:45):
  General: Well-nourished; A&O X 3
  Head: Normocephalic; atraumatic.
  Eyes: PERRL, wearing sun glasses
  Resp: Normal chest excursion with respiration; breath sounds clear and equal bilaterally; no wheezes, rhonchi, or rales
  Card: Regular rhythm, without murmurs, rub or gallop
  Abd: Non-distended; non-tender, without rigidity, rebound or guarding
  Skin: Normal for age and race; warm and dry; no apparent lesions
  Vascular: 2+ pulses bilaterally, no mottling or cyanosis of the extremities. Brisk capillary refill
  Neck: The neck appears normal and is non-tender to palpation. ROM is normal. Pt. is able to touch chin to knee.

Neuro: Alert and oriented to person, place and time. Cranial nerves II-XII intact. Motor strength and sensation intact.

ORDERS (at 05:59): Compazine 2.5mg IM, Toradol 60 mg IM, Decadron 10 mg IM, Demerol 75 mg IM

PROGRESS NOTES (at 07:04): Patient is feeling much better. Patient is ready to go home.

DIAGNOSIS:
Headache

DISPOSITION (at 07:29):
Pt. called cab for ride home. Security advised of pt.'s car in parking lot. Excused from work for 1 day

42 YEAR OLD FEMALE WITH HEADACHE

—Second Visit: 1 Day Later—

CHIEF COMPLAINT (at 06:09): Migraine

```
VITAL SIGNS
Time      Temp    Pulse   Resp   Syst   Diast   Pain
06:24     97.5    110     16     130    76
07:46             80      20     130    80      5
```

HISTORY OF PRESENT ILLNESS (at 06:28): Plagued with headaches for 2-3 weeks, seen last night for status migraine and treated with IM Toradol, Compazine, Demerol, and Decadron. Discharged home and slept for 3 hours until 18:00 last night. Headache worsened at this point and has been unresponsive to Excedrin and relaxation techniques. Pain remains in the same location as before with associated paracervical spasm. No focal neurologic symptoms. No fever/chills or head injury.

PAST MEDICAL HISTORY/TRIAGE:
  Medications: None
  Allergies: No known allergies.
  PMH: None
  PSH: None

EXAM (at 06:36):
  General: The patient is well-appearing and well-developed. The patient is in apparent moderate distress due to pain. She appears to have objective photophobia and is holding an ice pack to the head. She is freely engaged in conversation and feels it is important to relate multiple details

of her PMH despite being assured by myself that this was information that I had reviewed from her records and was aware of it. This seems to be inconsistent with most migraneurs I see whose pain often limits their ability to relate any details.

Eyes: Conjunctiva: O.U. normal.

Sinuses: There is no tenderness to palpation of the frontal and maxillary sinuses. There is no rhinorrhea.

Muscles/meninges: Bilaterally the paracervical muscles are moderately painful with palpation. There is muscle spasm present. There is limited ROM. There is pain with rotation.

Neuro: Alert and oriented to person, place and time. Speech is normal. Cranial nerves II-XII grossly intact. Upper and lower extremity strength grossly normal. Biceps, patellar and Achilles reflexes normal bilaterally. Coordination and gait are normal.

ORDERS (at 06:46):
Compazine 10 mg IV, Benadryl 25 mg IV, Dilaudid 1 mg IV, **(at 08:05)** Dilaudid 1 mg IV

PROGRESS NOTES: Patient appears to be clearly poorly equipped to handle stress. As I presented my treatment plan she reacted dramatically insisting—drawing away, her crying stopped and she began making eye contact— that she couldn't have an IV started. She told me that she never had one started, never had blood drawn and was very fearful. I initially attempted to explain the benefits of using IV titration for her pain but this did not sway her. I was able to capture her attention by confronting this behavior and unfounded fear that she had. Old charts were reviewed.

SOCIAL WORK CONSULTATION (at 07:57): RN requested this staff to speak to pt about stressors and coping mechanism. Pt states "You are here because they think I am crazy but I am not." Pt tangential jumping from health problems, to stressors to stocks. Pt states in the past year she lost her parents and her job. States she is currently attending a grief group. pt very dramatic. Unable to finish conversation due to medical procedure. Will pass case to next shift social worker.

DIAGNOSIS: Headache

DISPOSITION (at 08:22): Discharged to home with prescription for Fioricet.

42 YEAR OLD WOMAN WITH HEADACHE

—Third Visit: 2 Days Later—

CHIEF COMPLAINT (at 03:19): Migraine

```
VITAL SIGNS
Time      Temp    Pulse    Resp    Syst    Diast    Pain
03:48     98.8     112      16      112      66       10
05:05              90       16      100      60       10
05:39              90       16      104      60       4
```

HISTORY OF PRESENT ILLNESS (at 04:02): The patient presents with a moderate occipital and non-radiating headache that began gradually today. The symptoms are constant. The pain began spontaneously. The patient describes the headache as sharp. It is associated with nausea, vomiting, and photophobia. The patient denies fever, ptosis, lacrimation, rhinorrhea, fainting, weakness, dizziness, extremity weakness, paresthesias, and hemiplegia. No modifying factors noted. Prior treatment includes prescription pain medication. This treatment was not effective. The patient has a prior history of tension headache

PAST MEDICAL HISTORY/TRIAGE:
  Medications: None
  Allergies: No known allergies.
  PMH: None
  PSH: None

EXAM (at 04:09):
  General: Well-appearing; well-nourished; A&O X 3, in no apparent distress
  Head: Normocephalic; atraumatic.
  Eyes: PERRL
  Nose: The nose is normal in appearance without rhinorrhea
  Skin: Normal for age and race; warm and dry; no apparent lesions .
  Neck: Supple without LN.
  Neuro/psych: Alert and oriented x3. Cranial nerves II-XII intact. Normal gait and normal mentation.

ORDERS (at 04:27):
Droperidol 5mg IVP
Toradol 30 mg IV
Demerol 50 mg IV
Ativan 1 mg IV

DIAGNOSIS:
Headache

DISPOSITION (at 06:01):
Disposition - Discharged: The patient was discharged to Home ambulatory accompanied by friend. The patient's diagnosis, condition, and treatment were explained to patient or parent/guardian. The patient/responsible party expressed understanding. A discharge plan has been developed. Aftercare instructions were given to the patient. Follow-up with your physician as scheduled

42 YEAR OLD FEMALE WITH HEADACHE

—Fourth Visit: 12 Days Later—

CHIEF COMPLAINT (at 08:13): Migraine

```
VITAL SIGNS
Time      Temp    Pulse   Resp    Syst    Diast   Pain
08:36     98.3    104     18      120     70      10
10:14             72      20      108     70      7
```

HISTORY OF PRESENT ILLNESS (at 08:49): The patient presents with a severe frontal headache that began gradually 12 hour(s) ago. The symptoms are constant.. The discomfort is currently and 9/10. The pain began while working. The patient describes the headache as sharp. Patient complains of photophobia, nausea, vomiting and denies fever, paresthesias, weakness of the extremities, skin rash, rhinorrhea. The pain improved with lying down in a dark room. Prior treatment includes aspirin. This treatment was minimally effective. The patient has a prior history of tension headache. Patient has had identical headache in the past. Patient is under the care of a neurologist. Patient has had a negative head CT in the past. She sees a psychiatrist and has also seen her primary care physician for these symptoms. She had a negative MRI and MRA and was told these were stress headaches. No suicidal thoughts or plan. Is in the process of setting things up to see a counselor. She denies drug use and lives alone.

PAST MEDICAL HISTORY/TRIAGE:
Medications: None
Allergies: No known allergies.
PMH: None
PSH: None

EXAM (at 08:57):
General: Well-appearing; A&O X 3, in no apparent distress, very animated affect, holding a melted green popsicle to her head (it is in a plastic bag), asking for a shot of Ativan and Demerol
Head: Normocephalic; atraumatic.
Eyes: PERRL
Resp: Normal

Card: Regular rhythm, without murmurs, rub or gallop

Abd: Non-distended; non-tender, without rigidity, rebound or guarding

Skin: Normal for age and race; warm and dry; no apparent lesions

Neck: No jugular venous distention, no lymphadenopathy, supple without nuchal rigidity.

Neuro: Patient is alert and oriented times three. Cranial nerves III-XII are intact. Sensory and motor functions are intact. Strength is 5/5 for flexion and extension in all 4 extremities. Patellar DTRs are equal and intact. Finger to nose testing is equal and normal bilaterally.

ORDERS (at 09:04):

Demerol 100 mg IM

Phenergan 25 mg IM

Droperidol 5 mg IM

PROGRESS NOTE:

At 09:05 I spoke with her primary care physician who last saw her on 11 days ago and he wanted her to see a counselor but she did not and he did think this was related to the grief of losing her mother 4 months ago. He would like to see her in the office this week. He thought that pain meds were really a "band aid" for a deeper underlying problem, but that we should treat her pain today and have her follow up.

SOCIAL WORK CONSULTATION (at 10:09):

Pt is a 42 yo divorced female presenting to ER for Migraine. This is pt's fourth visit in past month. Pt presents anxious and tearful and dramatic, saying she feels stupid for coming to ER for headache when it is only stress related. When SW initially met with pt she stated, "your here because you think I am a psychopath." Pt has been under a lot of stress recently, losing her mother 4 months ago and losing her job in the past two months. Pt denies any support system. Pt has been referred to a psychologist from her PCP, which she has not contacted. SW offered to assist with getting appt for psychologist but pt refused. Pt reports she is planning to call for an appt this week. Pt reports she has recently started attending a grief support group that meets once a week. Pt appears to have flight of ideas and attention span is short. Pt denies any mental health hx or previous suicide attempts. Pt denies any current suicidal ideations. Pt denies hx of or current use of drugs or alcohol. Pt denies any needs to this SW.

DIAGNOSIS:

Headache

DISPOSITION (at 10:55):

The patient left prior to completing examination.

42 YEAR OLD FEMALE WITH HEADACHE

—Fifth Visit: 8 Days Later—

CHIEF COMPLAINT (at 08:01): Migraine

```
VITAL SIGNS
Time      Temp    Pulse    Resp    Syst    Diast    Pain
08:33     96.8     78       18      128      78       8
10:27              84       16      80       50       6
```

HISTORY OF PRESENT ILLNESS (at 08:51) : 43 year old white female presents here with frontal generalized migraine starting last week. Pt states this has been getting worst for the last few days associated w/ photophobia but no fevers, chills or vomiting. Pt states this HA is like others and is tearful and stressed out. Pt has no neck stiffness and describes this as throbbing. Pt had previous evaluation by neurologist with MRI and CT all neg. Pt more tearful concerning the death of her close mother and disagreements w/ her sister. Pt states also laid off of a good job and has no good support system. Pt feelings more stressful and tearful but no homicidal or suicidal ideation. Pt has seen a counselor. Pt also mentioned divorce and w/o any children

PAST MEDICAL HISTORY/TRIAGE:
  Medications: None
  Allergies: No known allergies.
  PMH: None
  PSH: None

EXAM (at 08:54):
  General: The patient is well-appearing and is thin. The patient is in moderate distress due to anxiety disheveled. Mood is inappropriate. Manner is appropriate.
  Ears: Auricles and external auditory canals are normal. Both tympanic membranes are normal.
  Cardiac: Cardiac rhythm: regular Murmur: None noted. No gallop rhythms are present.
  Resp: Respiratory rate and effort appear normal. The lungs are clear to auscultation bilaterally. No retractions noted.
  GI: Abdomen appears normal. Bowel sounds are normal. Abdomen soft and nontender. There is no pain on palpation. There is no organomegaly. No scars. No masses.
  Skin: Normal exam. Warm and dry, no rash or lesions noted.
  Neuro/psych: Alert and oriented x3. Cranial nerves II-XII intact. Normal gait and normal mentation.

ORDERS (at 09:11): Toradol 30 mg IV, Reglan 10 mg IV, Ativan 1 mg IV, 0.9NS 1 liter bolus

SOCIAL WORK CONSULTATION (at 10:10): Patient has had number of visits to ER in past two months for headache which patient reports is stress related. Patient was seen by the social worker last visit and referred to outpatient counseling. This social worker will meet with patient to determine patient's current mental health status. This social worker met with patient in treatment room. Patient is alert, O x 3, patient is dressed in distressed, worn clothing and her hair is uncombed and disheveled. Patient's speech is coherent; slurred; her responses are tangential and patient has flight of ideas. Patient's mood is sad and patient is crying and histrionic in affect. Patient 's Hx is difficult to clarify due to tangential nature of her responses. Patient denies any mental health Hx. Patient reports she did follow up with her PCP and he referred her to a psychologist, with whom patient reports she has made an appointment. Patient denies any suicidal or homicidal ideation or gestures in past of any attempt to harm herself. She is able to complete tasks at work and her difficulty staying focused today is due to her HA. Recommendation: Patient to continue working with her PCP and consequent referrals for outpatient counseling and treatment for HA and depression.

DIAGNOSIS: Migraine and neurotic depression

DISPOSITION (at 11:13): Discharged ambulatory to home.

Gregory L. Henry comments:

"There is nothing more disconcerting to the emergency physician than the positive sunglass sign"

This is the quintessential emergency department patient. Multiple visits, multiple times, for a disease entity that exists ... or does not exist! These are the patients who try men's souls. The overall approach should be one of "killing the patient with kindness." EMTALA and most supporting state laws require that each person be seen each time they present to an emergency department. My compliments to these physicians, as there was a respectable examination performed with each visit. There is nothing more disconcerting to the emergency physician than the positive sunglass sign. It is important to remember that multiple visits and detestable personalities in no way protect patients from disease, and they deserve a proper evaluation each time.

The chief complaint and history are well done. The fact that the patient has not had a change in her headache pattern, and that she has been worked up by neurology in the recent past (including a normal MRI/MRA study), is extremely helpful. It would be unlikely that performance of a CT scan, lumbar puncture, or anything else would be of value in working up this patient. The lack of the thunderclap onset, as well as this headache's repetitive pattern, should give some solace and comfort to the emergency physician.

On physical examination I recommend performing a fundoscopic exam, but otherwise the evaluation performed is satisfactory. She did receive excellent results from her pain medication, was advised to follow up with her physician, and was excused from work for the day. Subsequent ED visits showed excellence in history taking and physical examination. Each time the patient presented, a proper evaluation was performed.

The documentation in this case is also quite excellent. Not only do we see a physician evaluation, but social work consultation was also utilized. A multi-disciplined approach to these patients is important.

Recurrent pain patients are among the most frustrating ED cases. The emergency department is not the location to handle most of these problems. Recurrent pain patients usually have deep underlying psychological problems; primarily depression. Management by the patient's neurologist or a specific pain center is essential.

An excellent stance for the emergency department to take is to slowly build a corral around such patients and their symptoms. Each time the patient presents, a thorough evaluation must be performed. Also, a letter should be sent from the director of the department, with copies to the chart, encouraging the patient to follow up with a chronic pain clinic—the ED can even help in arranging the appointment. As the patient becomes more and more noncompliant with these follow up exams, the emergency department can feel comfortable in giving less and less narcotics. If there is a simple answer to this question, I do not know it; getting mad at the patient only increases the tension and does nothing to lessen return visits.

- Thoroughness of Documentation: 9 out of 10.

- Thoroughness of Patient Evaluation: 10 out of 10.

- Risk of Serious Illness Being Missed: Low risk.

- Risk Management Legal Rating: Low risk.

42 YEAR OLD FEMALE WITH HEADACHE

—Sixth Visit: 8 Days Later—

CHIEF COMPLAINT (at 06:17): Migraine

VITAL SIGNS						
Time	Temp	Pulse	Resp	Syst	Diast	Pain
06:36	97.8	86	16	108	62	8

HISTORY OF PRESENT ILLNESS (at 06:42): The patient presents with a severe frontal occipital headache that began gradually 7 hour(s) ago. The symptoms are constant. The symptoms have worsened in the last 2 hour(s). The discomfort is currently 9/10. The pain began while at rest. The patient describes the headache as sharp. Patient complains of photophobia and nausea. She denies fever, rash, paresthesias, confusion, aura, rhinorrhea, neck stiffness, diaphoresis, dizziness, vomiting. Prior treatment includes prescription pain medication. This treatment was not effective. The patient has a prior history of a tension headache. Patient has had identical headache in the past. Patient has had a negative head CT in the past. Patient is under the care of a neurologist. She has seen her primary care physician and a neurologist recently and she had a negative MRI and MRA and was told these were stress headaches.

PAST MEDICAL HISTORY/TRIAGE:
Medications: None
Allergies: No known allergies.
PMH: None
PSH: None

EXAM (at 06:57):
Constitutional: Well-appearing; well-nourished; A&O X 3, in no apparent distress, wearing dark glasses. She does have an odor of alcohol and is disheveled
Head: Normocephalic; atraumatic.
Eyes: PERRL
Nose: The nose is normal in appearance without rhinorrhea
Resp: Normal chest excursion with respiration; breath sounds clear and equal bilaterally; no wheezes, rhonchi, or rales
Card: Regular rhythm, without murmurs, rub or gallop
Abd: Non-distended; non-tender; without rigidity, rebound or guarding
Skin: Normal for age and race; warm and dry; no apparent lesions
Neurological: Patient is alert and oriented times three. Cranial nerves III-XII are intact. Sensory and motor functions are intact. Strength is 5/5 for flexion and extension in all 4 extremities. Patellar DTRs are equal and intact. Finger to nose testing is equal and normal bilaterally. No papilledema.

ORDERS (at 07:01): Toradol 60 mg IM, CBC, Chem-7, TSH and urine and serum Tox screen

PROGRESS NOTES (at 07:45):
When I suggested checking lab work and urine, she stated it has already been done but it was not done in the ED as I have checked all of our old records. I did confront her with this and she stated that she actually had it done in the distant past by her primary care physician. She then did get up and say that she did not want to stay for her Toradol shot and did not want her blood or urine checked and she wanted to go home. I am very concerned about her frequent ED visits and have encouraged her to follow up with her doctor, her neurologist and her counselor. I am very uncomfortable with continuing to give her narcotics, especially as she did have an odor of alcohol today and it was noted she had an odor of alcohol at the last visit and she does need intensive outpatient evaluation. I am also concerned that she mentioned at a previous visit that she did not want her neurologist contacted, and today told me that she has an appointment with him

FINAL DIAGNOSIS (at 08:22): Headache, Probable drug seeking behavior

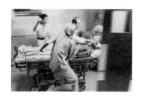

EVALUATION AND MANAGEMENT OF FREQUENT HEADACHE PATIENTS AND POTENTIAL DRUG-SEEKING BEHAVIOR

Stephen Karas, Jr., MD, FACEP

I. INTRODUCTION—EVALUATION OF RECURRENT HEADACHES

Despite presenting to the emergency department 6 times over 31 days with complaints of headache, this patient remained without a diagnosis or a clear plan to prevent their reoccurrence.

When a patient presents to the emergency department with recurrent headaches, the history should include (as it did in this case) if this headache was similar to previous headaches. In addition, it must be determined if the patient was adequately evaluated in the past, and if the results are consistent with a benign or primary headache like migraine, tension, or cluster headaches. At each visit, a careful history and physical should be performed to ensure that more serious causes, such as subarachnoid hemorrhage, cerebral venous thrombosis (CVT), temporal arteritis, or dissection of the vertebral artery have been excluded.[1,2,3] In this case, through multiple careful reviews and adequate history and physical exam, it was determined that the patient did not have a serious cause of her headache, and she was treated appropriately.[4,5,6] The general ED workup for adults with headaches is covered more completely elsewhere is this book.

II. DIAGNOSIS OF POTENTIAL DRUG SEEKING BEHAVIOR AND ITS EVALUATION AND MANAGEMENT IN THE ED

When the patient arrived for her sixth visit her care had unraveled. She seems to be in worse condition than she was at the time of her first visit. Recognition of drug-seeking behavior is very difficult; in this case it took six visits. This patient's headache is confounded by co-morbid conditions including depression. Drug-seeking behavior and psychiatric illness often coexist and are called "a dual diagnosis."[7] They both need to be recognized and treated to have any chance of helping the patient. This can be initiated from the ED but must be followed up outside the ED by a caring physician—these cases require a lot of attention.

Initially, the patient must be informed that the headache is likely being triggered by depression or anxiety and that it will not help to continue to seek care for her headaches unless she can seek help first for her underlying psychiatric disorder.[8] In our facility we have a psych liaison that evaluates all psychiatric related cases and comes up with recommendations for follow up. They often recommend initiation of medications to address anxiety, depression or psychosis until follow up can be arranged. Medications may include antidepressants, anticonvulsants, muscle relaxants, 5-HT1 agonists, ergots, and anti-anxiety agents.[9] This often will ablate triggering of the headache. A referral to a neurologist will facilitate alternative treatment to modulate severity and prevent recurrences.

In addition, the drug-seeking behavior must be addressed. This patient came in 6 times in 1 month requiring pain medication. During these initial visits, her immediate pain needs were addressed by medication.[4,5,6] She appeared to get the best relief from narcotics, which were correctly used as a rescue drug. However, continued use of narcotics can lead to addiction and failure to ablate the pain. This will eventually require increasing dosages and more frequent administration. There were hints that she was drug seeking when recommendations by the emergency physician and the primary MD were not followed; she also knew that tests were not indicated because they would not point to any medical cause, and could reveal her drug-seeking behavior.

Leaving against medical advice before a treatment plan could be addressed, not following through with the recommendations, recurrent visits, and lack of a medical etiology of the pain are all clues that the patient is drug-seeking. Other information which may be helpful can be found in medical records of recent visits, from nearby hospitals, or from the patient's primary physician. Often a pattern will become evident.

She should be advised to follow up with her primary care physician, and may need to follow up with a neurologist, psychiatrist or pain center. A treatment plan should be devised, and the ED should consider very carefully whether to give her narcotics in the future. The QA director or group director should review the patient's previous pattern of visits for pain control, and any communications with her outside physician to see if there is a problem with drug-seeking behavior. If there is a problem, then a letter can be sent to the patient. (addendum 1, below) Subsequently, the name is added to the habitual patient file.[10] This approach has worked well for us, and we have not been involved in any medical or legal problems.

III. ADDITIONAL RESOURCES

Many facilities have health educators funded by the federal government who try to interview all teen and adult patients to assess their drug or alcohol dependency and suggest appropriate follow up. Their opinions are given to the physician and then their findings can be supported by the physician intervention. This reinforces the recommendation for follow up.

IV. SUMMARY

In summary, dealing with the chronic benign primary headache patient is difficult. A multidisciplinary approach works best, but sometimes patients, including the patient in this case, are not amenable to this approach.

TEACHING POINTS FROM CASE 12:
- With each visit, perform a complete history, physical exam, and review of past history and previous workups to eliminate a serious cause of headache.
- Initially treat pain with rescue medications such as narcotics.
- Seek underlying triggers or conditions, such as anxiety or depression, that may exacerbate the headaches and consider initiating prophylactic pharmacological treatment of chronic headaches.
- Utilize available resources including a psychiatry liaison, social worker, health educator, neurologist, primary MD, psychiatrist and pain management specialist.
- If it is determined that drug-seeking behavior is present, consider sending the patient a letter concerning use of narcotics in the emergency department.

Addendum 1.

Dear xxxx,

Our records indicate that you have been treated in our Emergency Department multiple times over the past few months for problems related to chronic pain. The majority of these visits involve your request for, and subsequent administration of, narcotic pain medication. Our medical group has become concerned regarding your frequent need for pain management, and we are no longer comfortable providing you with this type of care.

Chronic pain management is a specialized field of medicine, which requires a level of expertise that an Emergency Department simply cannot provide. Multiple repeat visits for narcotic pain medicine are not the answer, and will not control your problem in the long run. For this reason, we strongly encourage you to develop a relationship with a physician who specializes in this area (i.e., a pain management specialist) so that you can receive optimum care for your chronic pain.

With this in mind, our Emergency Department (physicians and nurses) will be glad to evaluate and treat you at any time for any new <u>emergency</u> medical condition. However, we will no longer treat you with <u>narcotic</u> pain medication of any kind for any condition related to chronic pain (i.e., migraines, back pain, etc.). Should you at any time develop a new emergency medical condition for which pain medication is required, this will be evaluated on a case-by-case basis.

We hope you realize that, in our best judgment, this is truly what is best for you and your medical condition.

Sincerely,

Director, Emergency Department

REFERENCES

1. Godwin SA, Villa J. Acute headache in the ED: evidence-based evaluation and treatment options. Emerg Med Prac 2001; 3:1-36.
2. American College of Emergency Physicians. Clinical policy for the initial approach to adolescents and adults presenting to the emergency department with a chief complaint of headache. Ann Emerg Med 1996; 27:821-44.
3. American College of Emergency Physicians. Clinical policy: critical issues in the evaluation and management of patients presenting to the emergency department with acute headache. Ann Emerg Med 2002; 39:108-22.
4. Wilsey B. Pain Management in the ED. Am J Emerg Med 2004; 22: 51-7.
5. Vinson DR. Variations among emergency departments in the treatment of benign headache. Ann Emerg Med - 01-JAN-2003; 41(1): 90-7.
6. Vinson DR. Treating Headache in the Emergency Department: Avoiding the Migraine-Meperidine Trap. - Ann Emerg Med - 2003 Jul; 42(1); 161-162..
7. Regier DA, Farmer ME, Rae DS, et al. Comorbidity of mental disorders with alcohol and other drug abuse-results from the Epidemiologic Catchment Area (ECA) study. JAMA 1990; 264:2511-8.

8. Jacobson SA. Psychiatric perspectives on headache and facial pain. Otolaryngol Clin North Am - 01-DEC-2003; 36(6): 1187-200.
9. Redillas C, Solomon S. Prophylactic pharmacological treatment of chronic daily headache. Headache. 2000 Feb(2):83-102.
10. Geiderman, JM. Keeping lists and naming names: habitual patient files for suspected nontherapeutic drug-seeking patients. Ann Emerg Med. 2003;42:873-881.

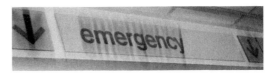

CASE 13
71 YEAR OLD FEMALE WITH
BIPOLAR DISEASE & SHOULDER PAIN

Commentary:
Gregory L. Henry, MD, FACEP

CEO, Medical Practice Risk Assessment, Inc., Ann Arbor, Michigan
Clinical Professor, Department of Emergency Medicine
   University of Michigan Medical School, Ann Arbor, Michigan
Past President, American College of Emergency Physicians (ACEP)

Discussion:
Stephen F. Pariser, MD

Professor of Clinical Psychiatry
Professor of Clinical Obstetrics and Gynecology
The Ohio State University College of Medicine
Columbus, Ohio

Douglas A. Rund, MD, FACEP

Professor and Chair
   Department of Emergency Medicine
Associate Dean, College of Medicine and Public Health
President, Ohio State University Physicians
   The Ohio State University College of Medicine
   Columbus, OH
Past President, American Board of Emergency Medicine
Editor-in-Chief, Textbook *Essentials in Emergency Medicine, 2nd Edition*

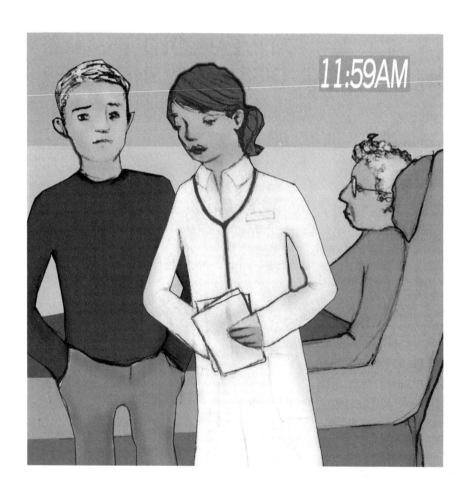

71 YEAR OLD FEMALE WITH
BIPOLAR DISEASE & SHOULDER PAIN

—Initial Visit*—

*Authors' Note: The history, exam and notes are the actual documentation of the physicians and providers, including abbreviations (and spelling errors)

CHIEF COMPLAINT (at 08:39): Arm pain

VITAL SIGNS

Time	Temp(F)	Rt.	Pulse	Resp	Syst	Diast	O2 sat	O2%
08:43	96.8	Tym.	81	20	204	81	97	RA
11:59			68	18	140	70		

HISTORY OF PRESENT ILLNESS (at 09:58): She complains of left periscapular or posterior shoulder pain which is intermittent and a "pulling, sharp and stabbing" quality. She denies injury or trauma other than lifting her great-grandson recently. The pain is worse when she gets up in the morning and she feels that she injured her right elbow getting out of bed because of compensating for her left periscapular region. She has taken no medication for pain. The pain has become progressively worse over the last 3-4 days. The pain is worse if she lays a certain way. She denies history of similar pain in the past. She has had malaise for the last few months. She has had an occasional nonproductive cough and clear rhinorrhea which is chronic. No fever, unexplained weight change, SOB, n/v/d, abd. pain, urinary frequency, HA, rash.

PAST MEDICAL HISTORY/TRIAGE:
Allergies: Penicillin
Meds: Premarin, Lithium, Multivitamins
Past medical history: GERD, Diverticulitis, Manic-Depression, Irritable Bowel
Past surgical history: Hysterectomy, Cholecystectomy

EXAM (at 10:03)
General: Alert and appropriately conversant.
Head: Normocephalic; atraumatic.
Eyes: No scleral icterus.
Nose: The nose is normal in appearance without rhinorrhea.
Resp: Normal chest excursion with respiration; breath sounds clear and equal bilaterally; no wheezes, no rhonchi, or rales.
Card: Regular rhythm, without rub or gallop.
Abd.: Non-distended; non-tender, soft, without rigidity, rebound or guarding. Bowel sounds are present. There is no CVA tenderness.
Skin: Normal for age and race; warm and dry; no apparent acute lesions.

Neuro: Cranial nerves II-XII intact. Motor and sensory exam of the upper and lower extremities are grossly intact with no cerebellar deficits.

Shoulder: The left periscapular region and approx 4th left paraspinal region is focally tender to palpation. The left shoulders appear normal and is mildly tender to palpation. ROM is normal but provokes pain about the aforementioned area.

ORDERS: Toradol 30mg IVP

RESULTS (at 10:45):

Test	Flag	Value	Units	Ref. Range
WBC	H	11.4	K/uL	4.6-10.2
HGB		13.8	G/DL	12.0-16.0
PLT		330	K/uL	142-424

Test	Flag	Value	Units	Ref. Range
NA		139	MMOL/L	135-144
K		4.1	MMOL/L	3.5-5.1
CLH		108	MMOL/L	98-107
AGAP		12.1	MMOL/L	6.0-18.0
CO2		23	MMOL/L	22-29
BUN		13	MG/DL	7-18
CREAT		0.9	MG/DL	0.6-1.3

Test	Flag	Value	Units	Ref. Range
CKMB		0.0	NG/ML	0.0-5.0
TROP I		.05	NG/ML	.00-.27
LITHIUM	L	.44	MMOL/L	.50-1.50

Urinalysis – WNL

RADIOLOGY:
  PA and lateral chest: Normal PA and lateral chest.
  Left shoulder, four views: Normal left shoulder.

DIAGNOSIS
  1. Shoulder sprain
  2. Syncope - near
  3. Bipolar affective disorder
  4. Leukocytosis

DISPOSITION (at 13:02): Discharged home with prescription for ibuprofen and aftercare instructions for shoulder sprain and instructions to follow up with her family doctor in 4 days.

Gregory L. Henry comments:

"We cannot, and should not, be in the business of solving all problems, and pursuing all workups"

The emergency department cannot be all things to all people. Evaluation of non-traumatic pain during an emergency department visit is difficult; we cannot, and should not, be in the business of solving all problems, and pursuing all workups. To workup every case as if it were a new internal medicine visit, would be incredibly cost- and time-inefficient for the system. This patient did present with shoulder pain, and the emergency physician's principal job is to determine if the pain is musculoskeletal in origin and whether some intervention would be required in the ED. The key to such a case is follow-up; the primary care physician can order additional studies as necessary.

The chief complaint in this case is unrelated to a specific trauma. The activities of daily living really do not count; the patient does not relay a fall or major accident, so bone or joint irritation unrelated to direct trauma need to be considered but not worked up in the emergency department. The patient's initial chart indicates no systemic symptoms such as weight loss.

The evaluation from an emergency medicine standpoint was reasonable; adequate history was taken, and the patient's history of bipolar disease and medication history was considered.

The physical examination, including evaluation of the shoulder, seems reasonable. Initial blood studies were done, but whether these studies were necessary is questionable. One of the diagnoses was "near syncope," a complaint not found in the history. Cardiac enzymes were ordered; one wonders what disease entity is being sought. If this is a screen for cardiac disease, it is an inadequate screen. If just a general acquisition of laboratory data, it is probably unnecessary. Additional x-rays did not shed light on this problem.

- **Thoroughness of Documentation:** 8 out of 10.

- **Thoroughness of Patient Evaluation:** 8 out of 10.

- **Risk of Serious Illness Being Missed:** Low risk.

- **Risk Management Legal Rating:** Low risk.

71 YEAR OLD FEMALE WITH
BIPOLAR DISEASE & SHOULDER PAIN

—Second Visit: 1 Month Later—

CHIEF COMPLAINT (at 07:35): Arm pain

VITAL SIGNS								O2		Pain
Time	Temp(F)	Rt.	Pulse	Resp	Syst	Diast	Pos.	sat	O2%	scale
08:00	98.4	Oral	88	20	122	70	L			
09:54			88	20	159	77	S	97	RA	4
11:16			78	16	128	74	S			2

HISTORY OF PRESENT ILLNESS (at 08:22): 71 y/o female transported by EMS c/o right arm pain x two wks. States past hx of mmc. States she was seen in this ER for similar symptoms as today but in the opposite arm. Denies any trauma or strain to right arm or shoulder. States she got a cortisone shot in the left shoulder 3 weeks ago and this is when the current pain started. Pt states her lithium levels have been low and she has been taking an extra pill at night to increase her levels. Admits to chronic diarrhea secondary to IBS and diverticulosis. States she vomited several times last night and admits she has lost some weight because she has "not been eating well." States pain is sharp and is intermittent. Pt states she is concerned she has cancer because she has a family hx of liver cancer. Denies fever. Denies fever, malaise, ear or throat pain, chest pain, SOB, edema, cough, abd. pain, HA.

PAST MEDICAL HISTORY/TRIAGE:
   Allergies: Penicillin, sulfa
   Current meds: Premarin, Lithium, Pepcid, Amitriptyline, and Triam/hctz
   Past medical history: GERD, Diverticulitis, Manic-Depression, Irritable Bowel. Bipolar was diagnosed 23 years ago and she did see her PCP 4 days ago and lithium dose was increased.
   Past surgical history: Hysterectomy, Cholecystectomy

EXAM (at 09:12)
   General: Sitting comfortably in the cart, well-nourished, well appearing, in no apparent distress
   Head: Normocephalic; atraumatic.
   Eyes: PERRL
   Nose: The nose is normal in appearance without rhinorrhea
   Resp: Normal chest excursion with respiration; breath sounds clear and equal bilaterally; no wheezes, rhonchi, or rales
   Card: Regular rhythm, without murmurs, rub
   Abd.: Non-distended; non-tender, soft, without rigidity, rebound or guarding
   Skin: Normal for age and race; warm and dry; no apparent lesions

Ext: No obvious deformity noted in right UE. No bruising noted. FROM of shoulder and elbow noted. No pain with palpation of shoulder or elbow. (+) pain with palpation of humerus. Sensation is grossly intact, 2+ pulses noted.

Neck: No jugular venous distention, Minimal lymphadenopathy, supple without nucal rigidity.

ORDERS: Toradol 30mg IV, phenergan 6.25mg IVP, phenergan 6.25mg IVP

RESULTS (at 09:53):

Test	Flag	Value	Units	Ref. Range
WBC	H	21.4	K/uL	4.6-10.2
HGB		14.1	G/DL	12.0-16.0
PLT	H	579	K/uL	142-424

Test	Flag	Value	Units	Ref. Range
NA	L	134	MMOL/L	135-144
K		4.2	MMOL/L	3.5-5.1
CL		99	MMOL/L	98-107
CO2	L	20	MMOL/L	22-29
BUN		18	MG/DL	7-18
CREAT		1.2	MG/DL	0.6-1.3

Test	Flag	Value	Units	Ref. Range
LITHIUM		1.35	MMOL/L	.50-1.50
ION CAL		1.34	MMOL/L	1.15-1.37
MG		2.2	MG/DL	1.8-2.4
PHOS		3.5	MG/DL	2.5-4.9

Nursing and social worker notes (at 10:10): The patient's sister explained the patient has manic depression and refuses to take her lithium. Sister states she vomits it up and believes she has cancer and is dying from it. Sister states her mother died of cancer so she believes that she has cancer. She has had OCD-type behaviors for many years stemming from fear of developing liver cancer; will not any food that may cause cancer; she has not eaten fruit for 10 years as she heard it ferments in the stomach, drinks mostly Ensure as she heard substances in water can cause cancer, many vitamin supplements. Patient is lethargic and spends most of her time in bed, she does have crying spells. Was very energetic until last month.

RADIOLOGY (at 12:53):

Right shoulder: Suspicious erosive process of the bone is noted in the proximal humerus about the neck region. Remaining bones of the shoulder appear unremarkable. Further evaluation with bone scan is recommended.

CT chest: The lung bases demonstrate several small, noncalcified indeterminate lung nodules, the largest of which was 9 mm in size at the left lung base. These are nonspecific and they are concerning for pulmonary metastases.

CT chest: Multiple hepatic lesions in the liver, predominantly in the right lobe, the largest of which measures about 7 cm in size in the posterior inferior aspect of the right lobe. The spleen, pancreas, kidneys, and adrenal glands are unremarkable.

DIAGNOSIS:
1. Leukocytosis
2. Nausea and vomiting
3. Cancer - liver, primary or secondary
4. Possible bone CA

DISPOSITION (at 13:44): Admitted to medical bed

HOSPITAL COURSE:

Discharge summary: Was seen by an oncologist, hospitalist and palliative care specialist. She was noted to have a flat affect and did not even shake her head when asked questions. A bone scan was done showing multiple skeletal lesions, highly suggestive of metastatic disease. CT of the brain shows 3 enhancing masses suspicious for metastatic disease. CT of the neck shows nodules in the thyroid, and a 12-mm nodule in the right supraclavicular region, which is not definitely pathologic, but is suspicious. Mild enlargement of the right lobe of the thyroid. CT of the chest shows multiple lung masses, including 1 large mass within the right upper lobe, extending to the right hilum. There is also mediastinal adenopathy. CT of the abdomen and pelvis showed multiple hepatic lesions as well as a 6.3 cm cystic lesion of her left pelvis. It was later learned that she had lost 20-25 pounds in the last year and 6-7 pounds in the last month. She has had 2-3 months of intermittent nausea, diarrhea, abdominal cramps, and decreased appetite. It was learned that she did have a CT done 1 ½ years prior to this admission which showed a 5X6 cm cystic mass in the left side of the pelvis. It was nonspecific and was thought to be secondary to the ovary. It was unknown if she had an oophorectomy with her hysterectomy.

Follow up: It was thought the primary source was gastrointestinal. Biopsy showed adenocarcinoma. Pt. was subsequently referred for hospice/palliative care.

FINAL DIAGNOSIS: Adenocarcinoma of the GI tract with metastases to the brain, bone, lungs, liver and pelvis.

Additonal comments by Gregory L. Henry:

Missing this diagnosis for a month did not affect the outcome of this case as she unfortunately had wide spread metastatic carcinoma. All the king's horses and all the king's men were not going to change the outcome. If it is now expected that emergency physicians workup everyone for every disease, then we cannot practice rapid evaluation and movement of patients—the essence of emergency medicine. We would become unscheduled internal medicine, which does not serve the public interest, the vast majority of our patients, or the rest of the medical community.

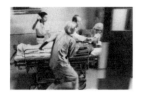

EVALUATION OF PATIENTS WITH KNOWN PSYCHIATRIC ILLNESS, DISCUSSION OF BIPOLAR MOOD DISORDER, AND LITHIUM TREATMENT

Stephen F. Pariser, MD
Douglas A. Rund, MD, FACEP

I. SUMMARY OF CASE

The ultimate diagnosis was adenocarcinoma with bone metastases, which presumably caused the presenting symptoms of right shoulder pain. She had known psychiatric illness and, during the second visit, the patient's sister and social worker described numerous symptoms which they attributed to the bipolar mood disorder, including abnormal eating patterns, weight loss, and lethargy. Her history was difficult to elicit; she had a flat affect and did not even shake her head when asked questions.

II. LIFE-THREATENING CONDITIONS WHICH MAY CAUSE PSYCHOSIS

A patient with known psychiatric illness displaying symptoms and signs of the illness can present a challenging problem. Teasing out the medical components from the psychiatric components is a common expectation for emergency physicians and is sometimes discussed in our literature as "medical clearance of the psychiatric patient;"[1] patients who appear to be showing manifestations of psychiatric illness should not be routinely sent to a psychiatric unit or psychiatrist for care until medical illness has been reasonably excluded. The literature in this area regularly notes that life-threatening illnesses can present with psychosis or altered mood or behavior. The list of potentially life-threatening illnesses includes hypoxia, hypotension, head trauma, sepsis, hypoglycemia, CNS infection (meningitis, encephalitis) post-ictal state, hypothermia, exogenous corticosteroids, CVA, or HIV-related conditions. In addition, intoxication or withdrawal from substances such as alcohol, amphetamines, cocaine, LSD, PCP, and aromatic hydrocarbons can cause psychosis.

III. HISTORY AND PHYSICAL EXAM OF PATIENTS WITH ABNORMAL THOUGHT OR BEHAVIOR

The emergency evaluation of all patients presenting with abnormal thought or behavior should include history obtained from relatives, police, EMS, bystanders, and friends. If no accompanying source of history is available, then check medical records and call the number listed on the patient's driver's license. Physical exam should include vital signs (including pulse ox), exam of the head (signs of trauma); eyes—pupils (extra-ocular movements, nystagmus); mouth (trauma, vomiting, signs of ingestion); and neck (suppleness). Based on patient symptoms, additional examination can also include chest (observation, palpation for trauma, breath sounds); abdomen (palpation); back (observe for traumas); extremities (effects of restraints, needle tracks, trauma); neurological (gross motor movement bilaterally, general level of consciousness). Laboratory studies for such purposes are discussed in several recent publications on this topic.[2,3]

IV. BIPOLAR MOOD DISORDER

This patient (or family) indicated that the patient has bipolar mood disorder. In this case, the patient's bipolar diagnosis appears to be incidental to her chief complaint and emergency presentation. The history of manic depressive illness, now referred to as bipolar disorder, was apparently elicited during the process of obtaining the past medical history and as a result of information gathered from her sister. The clinical features of bipolar mood disorder are shown in Table 1. Nothing in the patient's acute presentation in the emergency department suggests depression, mania, or mood cyclicity. However, the patient's sister's description of the patient's obsessional concerns or delusions about developing cancer are perhaps compatible with bipolar or unipolar depression with psychosis. Psychotic symptoms are common in bipolar patients, especially during manic episodes. Bipolar depression can also present with psychotic features.

Table 1. Bipolar Mood Disorder

1. The essential feature of bipolar mood disorder is a clinical course that is characterized by the occurrence of at least one or more manic episodes; such patients have often experienced at least one major depressive episode.
2. Criteria for manic episode
   a. Elevated, expansive or irritable mood lasting more than one week (or requiring hospitalization).
   b. Three or more of the following symptoms:
      i. Grandiosity
      ii. Decreased need for sleep
      iii. Pressure to keep talking
      iv. Racing thoughts
      v. Distractibility
      vi. Increased goal-directed activity
      vii. Increased involvement in pleasurable, but risky behavior
   c. Episodes interfere with social and occupational functioning.
   d. Disorder not due to a medical cause, including substance use or withdrawal.

Adapted from the American Psychiatric Association, Diagnostic and Statistical Manual, 4th ed., 2000.

We have no specific information that would formally support a diagnosis of obsessive compulsive disorder (OCD) at this point, although a more thorough evaluation might suggest that the patient does have comorbid OCD. We do not have a time frame, but the documentation of the patient's history (tearfulness, lethargy and more time in bed) may suggest a worsening of her bipolar disorder, or may reflect the depressive symptoms that can be seen in patients with many types of neoplasm.

V. LITHIUM CARBONATE

Given the diagnosis of metastatic adenocarcinoma, the patient's age, and the finding of poor treatment compliance, the patient's refusal to take lithium is not at all surprising. Because of declining GFR (lithium is renally excreted), lithium must be used very carefully in older adults. Serum levels, electrolytes, ECGs, thyroid function, and urine must all be monitored frequently. Because of these concerns and given the other treatment options for bipolar patients, lithium is not an ideal agent in the elderly.

Lithium carbonate can cause side effects, even when patients have subtherapeutic lithium levels. Of course, delusional ideation related to this patient's concerns about cancer can also play an important role in the patient's decision not to take lithium. Commonly encountered lithium side effects include nausea, fatigue, intention tremor, cognitive slowing, frequent urination and hyponatremia (frequently linked to lithium induced nephrogenic diabetes insipidus), weight gain, and hypothyroidism (based on laboratory assessment and clinical evaluation). Chronic lithium use can also cause renal insufficiency, which may subsequently raise serum lithium levels.

Symptoms attributed to side effects of lithium may actually be from lithium toxicity. Prescription and over-the-counter medications can significantly raise lithium levels, increasing the risk of side effects and lithium toxicity. Our patient was taking a combination of triamterene/hydrochlorathiazide. Examples of prescription medications that can raise serum lithium levels include nonsteroidal anti-inflammatory drugs (NSAIDs), diuretics, calcium channel blockers and ACE inhibitors.

VI. OTHER MEDICATIONS USED TO TREAT BIPOLAR DISORDER

Other agents that are FDA approved for the treatment of bipolar disorder include divalproex sodium, the atypical antipsychotics (olanzapine, risperidone, quetiapine, ziprasidone and aripiprazole) and the anticonvulsant lamotrigine (approved for maintenance phase treatment and commonly prescribed for patients with bipolar depression). All of the drugs approved for the treatment of mania or maintenance phase bipolar disorder require attention to potential side effects including the increased risk of developing the metabolic syndrome, hyperlipidemia, weight gain or diabetes (or worsening of diabetes).

Tricyclic antidepressants (this patient was taking amitripyline) can also cause problems, inducing cycling. Amitriptyline is a poor choice for bipolar depression in this patient because of her lethargy and age. Amitriptyline has anticholinergic effects and can cause cardiac arrhythmias. Serum levels and ECG monitoring should be ordered in patients who take tricyclic antidepressants. This is especially true in the elderly; most geropsychiatrists are reluctant to prescribe tricyclics to the elderly.

Once an accurate diagnosis of bipolar disorder is made, it is a lifetime diagnosis with high likelihood of mania, hypomania, depression, and mixed episodes throughout the patient's lifespan. For this reason, lifetime maintenance treatment is commonly recommended for patients with bipolar disorder in order to avoid relapse, hospitalization, comorbidity, and even suicide.

VII. FINAL THOUGHTS

The final issue for discussion from a psychiatric perspective is the link between depression and cancer.[4,5] Higher levels of IL-6 have been reported in cancer patients and may contribute to depressive symptoms.[6]

Bipolar or unipolar depression in a cancer patient, even a patient with terminal cancer, should be treated. Treatment may consist of medical management and/or psychotherapy. Appropriate treatment may reduce the impact of pain and greatly enhance the quality of life, even for patients as they approach the end of life.

TEACHING POINTS ABOUT CASE 13:
- Patients with psychiatric illness may also have organic illness.
- Input from family and friends is often instrumental in making a diagnosis, but may be misleading.
- Lithium and amitriptyline are not the best psychiatric medications in the elderly.

REFERENCES
1. Korn CS, Currier, GW, Henderson, SO. Medical clearance of psychiatric patients without medical complaints in the Emergency Department. J Emerg Med 2000; 18:173-6.
2. Broderick KB, Lerner EB, McCourt JD, et al. Emergency physician practices and requirements regarding the medical screening examination of psychiatric patients. Acad Emerg Med 2002; 9:88-92.
3. Zun LS, Hernandez R, Thompson R, et al. Comparision of EP's and psychiatrists' laboratory assessment of psychiatric patients. Am J Emerg Med 2004; 22:175-80.
4. Fras I, Litin EM, Bartholomew LG. Mental symptoms as an aid in the early diagnosis of carcinoma of the pancreas. Gastroenterology 1968; 55: 191-8.
5. Massie M J. Prevalence of depression in patients with cancer. J Natl Cancer Inst Monogr 2004 (32): 57-71.
6. Musselman DL, Miller AH, Porter MR, et al. Higher than normal plasma interleukin-6 concentrations in cancer patients with depression: preliminary findings. Am J Psychiatry 2001; 158:1252-7.

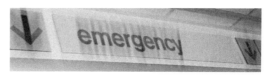

CASE14
55 YEAR OLD MALE WITH LUQ ABDOMINAL PAIN S/P MVA

Commentary:
Gregory L. Henry, MD, FACEP

CEO, Medical Practice Risk Assessment, Inc., Ann Arbor, Michigan
Clinical Professor, Department of Emergency Medicine
    University of Michigan Medical School, Ann Arbor, Michigan
Past President, American College of Emergency Physicians (ACEP)

Discussion:
Tom Lukens, MD, PhD, FACEP

Operations Director, Emergency Department, MetroHealth Medical Center
Associate Professor, Case Western University School of Medicine
    Cleveland, Ohio
Member, ACEP Clinical Policies Committee
Member, ACEP Clinical Policy Subcommittee on Blunt Abdominal Trauma

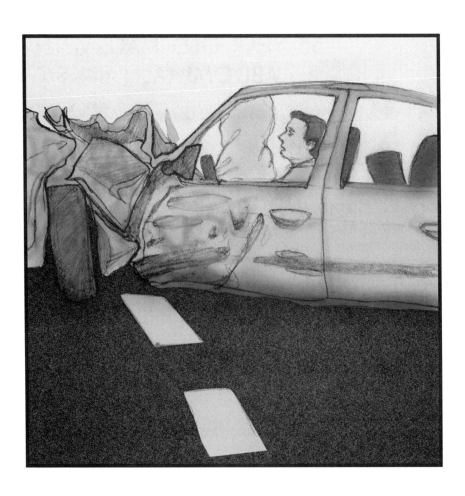

55 YEAR OLD MALE WITH LUQ ABDOMINAL PAIN S/P MVA

—Initial Visit*—

*Authors' Note: The history, exam and notes are the actual documentation of the physicians and providers, including abbreviations (and spelling errors)

CHIEF COMPLAINT: MVA

VITAL SIGNS							
Time	Temp(F)	Rt.	Pulse	Resp	Syst	Diast	Pos.
16:41	96.9	Oral	76	18	98	68	L

HISTORY OF PRESENT ILLNESS (documented by the physician assistant **at 16:52**): This patient is a 55 y/o male who presents with L ant and post chest pain, LUQ abd pain s/p MVC at 15:30. The pt was restrained driver going approx 5 mph when he was hit R passenger front side from oncoming vehicle. Air bags were deployed. No head/neck trauma. The pt reports constant throbbing, aching, pressure sensation chest and abd. aggravated with movement, no alleviating factors. No meds taken prior to arrival. The pt c/o shortness of breath since the injury. Apparently, pt refused treatment originally, when sudden onset of L post chest / back pain occurred. Does have nausea and vomiting. No h/o pericarditis, pulmonary or lung abnl, DM. No paresthesia/incontinence. No h/o PE, TE, DVT, no hormones, no recent surgery. Denies calf pain, palp, peripheral edema, fever, visual changes, cough, diarrhea, hematuria, HA, mental status changes, chest pain, neck stiffness.

PAST MEDICAL HISTORY/TRIAGE:
Allergies: No known drug allergies.
Medications: None
PMH: Staphylococcal pneumonia 10 yrs ago.
Social history: Nonsmoker
Nurse triage notes: Pt. was restrained driver involved in MVA this afternoon where he was T boned on drivers side of his vehicle. Denies hitting his head or loc. He had initially refused transport at the scene, however had severe low back pain and " nearly passed out according to the police officer that took him home".

EXAM (at 16:56):
General: Well-appearing; well-nourished; A&O X3, no apparent distress, no evidence of shock; appears to be in pain.
Head: Normocephalic; atraumatic. No battle sign, raccoon eyes or evidence of CSF drainage
Eyes: PERRL, EOMI
Ears: No hemotypanus or TM rupture

Neck: The patient denies any neck pain. The patient does not appear to be intoxicated or have a distracting injury. As such, they appear to be a candidate to have their cervical spines clinically cleared. With the head and neck in the neutral position I carefully loosened the hard collar. Palpating the posterior elements of the cervical spine I found no tenderness, step-off or crepitance. I then loosened the forehead taping to allow the patient to display ROM as pain allows. The patient displayed a full range of motion. This patient meets all criteria established in the NEXUS study for bedside cervical spine clearance. At this point spinal precautions were discontinued. The exam reveals no tracheal deviation, JVD, seat belt signs or hematoma. No midline spinal tenderness throughout

Nose: The nose is normal in appearance without rhinnorrhea

Mouth: Normal with intact dentition

Resp: Normal chest excursion with respiration, no paradoxical motion, subcutaneous emphysema, seatbelt signs. The breath sounds are clear and equal bilaterally; no wheezes, rhonchi, or rales

Cardiovascular: Regular rhythm, without murmurs, rub or gallop

Chest: Tenderness to palpation left side of the chest

Abdomen: No distention, ecchymosis, seatbelt signs. The abdomen is normal in appearance with bs in all 4 quadrants; There is mod pain with palpation LUQ and abd. is firm; No rigidity, rebound, but there is slight guarding. No HSM.

Back: No CVAT

Pelvis: No laxity or tenderness with palpation or compression; femoral pulses = and intact bilat.

Extremities: Good ROM without tenderness, deformity. Pulses 2+ in 4 extremities

Neuro: Patient is alert and oriented to person, place, and time. Cranial nervies III-XII are intact. Sensory and motor functions are intact. Strength is 5/5 for flexion and extension in all 4 extemities. Patellar DTR's are equal and intact. Finger to nose testing is equal and normal bilaterally. No evidence of incontinence.

ORDERS at 17:07: CBC, electrolytes, BUN/creatinine. CT abdomen/pelvis with IV contrast

Physician progress Note at 17:28: He has LUQ abd. pain, no ecchymosis, no other abd. pain. Pelvis stable. Will get CT to r/o splenic injury

—Continuation of ED visit follows Gregory L. Henry comments—

Gregory L. Henry comments:

"I am a huge advocate of emergency medicine, but trauma bleeding of the abdomen is a surgical disease, and requires surgical intervention"

One maxim must be followed when a trauma patient presents to the emergency room—too little, too late is no good. The emergency physician should know what backup, personnel, and radiographic techniques are available. If there is inadequate backup, immediate transfer is required. Having reviewed this case, I can say that I want this emergency physician in the department if I ever need emergency care. Getting from point A to point B is important.

In an awake, alert patient, the clinical clearing of the C-spine is perfectly appropriate and excellent in this case. Moving on as quickly as possible to obtain studies and stabilize the patient is absolutely essential. Laboratory studies are only a baseline; no one makes decisions based on a patient's initial hemoglobin. The overall condition of the patient is what counts.

The chief complaint is anatomic. A splenic rupture must be considered in a patient with left upper quadrant pain following a t-bone car collision. With a history of presyncope and lower than expected blood pressure, internal bleeding must be suspected. The lack of tachycardia should not dissuade the physician from considering blood in the abdomen causing reflex bradycardia. Tachycardia may occur only late in the course of such bleeding.

The history, physical examination, and the studies all seem appropriate. The documentation, including the reference to the NEXUS criteria for C-spine clearance, all seemed exemplary.

—Continuation of ED Visit—

```
VITAL SIGNS
Time   Temp(F)  Rt.  Pulse  Resp  Syst  Diast  Pos.  O2 Sat  O2%
18:09                 80     18    92    60     L
18:49                 84     18    81    61     L     100     RA
19:13                 90     18    68    48     L     100     4L NC
```

ED COURSE: He was taken for CT at 18:11 and returned to the ED at 18:32. At 18:49, just prior to receiving the results of the CAT scan the patient did become hypotensive with BP of 81/61. At that point I did make the decision that he would need to go to a trauma hospital and I did speak with the surgeon on call at 19:05, who told me that he does not do trauma at our hospital and asked that the pt. be sent to a trauma center (where he is an attending). We did contact our transportation team and did arrange transport, however just after this his blood pressure decreased to the seventies. He did seem too unstable to transport. At 19:06 blood was cross matched for 2 units and coagulation studies were ordered. He was placed on a cardiac monitor. One of our general surgeons happened to be walking through the emergency Department, and I asked him if he would be kind enough to take this patient to surgery, even though he was not on call. He agreed and the patient was immediately taken up to the operating room. Prior to this time he did have a second IV line. He has IV fluids running wide open, and we did type and screen and type and cross matched two units of packed red blood cells. When he left the emergency Department his blood pressure was in the sixties but he was conversant. He was weak and pale, but alert and oriented. This was all discussed with his wife who is in agreement and does understand the severity of the situation.

RESULTS at 18:20

Test	Flag	Value	Units	Ref. Range
WBC	H	19.3	K/uL	4.6-10.2
HGB	L	13.1	G/DL	13.5-17.5
PLT		247	K/uL	142-424

Test	Flag	Value	Units	Ref. Range
NA		137	MMOL/L	135-144
K		3.5	MMOL/L	3.5-5.1
CL		104	MMOL/L	98-107
AGAP		10.5	MMOL/L	6.0-18.0
CO2		26	MMOL/L	22-29
BUN		18	MG/DL	7-18
CREAT		1.2	MG/DL	0.6-1.3

RADIOLOGY: CT ABDOMEN/PELVIS: Splenic laceration with a large amount of intra-abdominal hemorrhage. Additional fluid is seen around the liver capsule and dissecting along the paracolic gutters bilaterally. Additional fluid is seen within the small bowel mesentery and these fluid collections are continuous with a large pelvic fluid collection. The findings suggest a significant amount of blood loss due to the splenic injury.

CXR: Fractured ribs numbers 7 and 8. Otherwise no active disease in the chest.

DIAGNOSIS: 1. Acute splenic fracture S/P MVA, 2. Hypotension, 3. Left 7th and 8th rib fractures

HOSPITAL COURSE:

SURGEON NOTES: He was brought to the operating room for exploratory laparotomy and was found to have several liters of fresh blood in his abdomen. This was copiously irrigated and the bleeding was found to be isolated to the spleen. A splenectomy was performed. Upon completion of the splenectomy, there was found to be a large retroperitoneal hematoma on the right. The retroperitoneum at this juncture was opened and the retroperitoneum was explored up to the right kidney including the vena cava. There was found to be no active bleeding and it was presumed that this was blood that dissected down from the splenic rupture. The patient left the hospital in good condition.

FINAL DIAGNOSIS: Acute traumatic splenic rupture.

Additional Gregory L. Henry comments:

The real fun started in this case while the patient was at CT scanning. Blood pressures were taken periodically, which was important, but I would suggest they should have been done more frequently.

It was clear that the patient's blood pressure was going down as he returned from the CT scan, and the emergency physician immediately sought surgical consultation. It is important to realize when a disease process requires a specialist. I am a huge advocate of emergency medicine, but traumatic bleeding in the abdomen is a surgical disease, and requires surgical intervention. It is fortuitous that the emergency physician was able to find a general surgeon at his own hospital willing to take the patient to the operating room. Depending on the length of transport time, this could have been a very sticky situation; if the physician was unable to locate a surgeon at his hospital, the patient needs immediate transport which may require extra IV lines and continuous infusion of O negative blood.

It is interesting that the ruptured spleen was managed with splenectomy. This is an intra-operative surgical choice—some physicians are treating ruptured spleens with closure and not splenectomy depending on the condition of the spleen. Also, it is a surgical maxim that one enters the retroperitoneal space at his/her own peril; fortunately for this case, the bleeding was only secondary to the spleen injury and no untoward affect resulted from the entrance into the retroperitoneum.

- **Thoroughness of Documentation:** 10 out of 10.

- **Thoroughness of Patient Evaluation:** 10 out of 10.

- **Risk of Serious Illness Being Missed:** Low risk.

- **Risk Management Legal Rating:** Low risk.

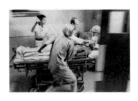

EVALUATION OF PATIENTS WITH BLUNT ABDOMINAL TRAUMA

Tom Lukens, MD, PhD, FACEP

I. OVERVIEW

Evaluation of the patient with blunt chest and abdominal trauma can be challenging, as injuries can range from minor contusions to life-threatening multi-system damage. Many conditions, such as bowel lacerations, manifest over time, sometimes leading to catastrophic results if not anticipated. In this country, victims of trauma are often taken to the nearest emergency department. Studies indicate that morbidity and mortality is decreased when patients are cared for in verified trauma centers, particularly the most severely injured and geriatric patients.[1,2,3]

II. SUMMARY OF CASE—HISTORY

In this case, a 55 year old male restrained driver was t-boned on the front passenger's side. Air bags were deployed. The patient was ambulatory at the scene and evidently refused transport to the hospital. A telling piece of history is obtained by the triage nurse—the patient "nearly passed out" while being transported home, possibly the first indication of hemodynamic instability from blood loss.

The sudden onset of left posterior chest and back pain prompted the patient to come to the hospital. The mechanism of injury suggests that the patient was thrown against his door, hitting his left chest and abdomen to produce the ensuing pain. Injuries to the left lung and/or spleen can be anticipated in this situation. He arrived at the hospital a little over an hour after the accident.

In the ED, the patient reported left sided chest, back, and LUQ abdominal pain that was aggravated by movement—typical of musculoskeletal injury but by no means specific for it. The shortness of breath may have been related to splinting or, more worrisome, a primary lung injury such as contusion or pneumothorax. Nausea and vomiting are also elicited in the history but both are non-specific findings and don't portend the possible severity of the patient's injuries.

III. EXAMINATION OF THE TRAUMA PATIENT

The ED physician's assessment proceeded with a complete physical examination. An orderly method of initial evaluation, as recommended by the Advanced Trauma Life Support (ATLS) system with primary attention to ABCs, does improve outcomes.[4] Routine labs were ordered and an abdominal CT was appropriately arranged. However, the patient waited approximately 1 hour to get the CT scan, and "crashed" soon after the test was done, becoming hypotensive. Had the diagnosis of spleen injury been made earlier while the patient was still stable, transport to a trauma center could have occurred rapidly. Of course, the decision to transfer always involves a risk benefit analysis, but once unstable, the transfer is definitely problematic. The fortuitous arrival of a general surgeon willing to immediately operate saved the day ... and the patient! An advantage of transfer directly to a trauma center is that CT and other capabilities are immediately available. A delay is sometimes found in smaller community hospitals as key personnel are not always available, and need to be "called in."

The concept of the "golden hour" for the trauma victim was formulated in the early 1970s by Dr. R. Adams Cowley, from his work at the Maryland Shock Trauma Center in Baltimore. Survival is increased if definitive treatment of a trauma patient begins within the first "golden hour" after the injury. It seems intuitive that the earlier care is begun, the better the outcome; this concept has spurred the development of trauma centers and trauma care systems without, interestingly, much scientific evidence to support it.[5] In this case, several hours passed before definitive care took place, potentially increasing morbidity.

In most ED's caring for trauma victims, vital signs are taken simultaneously with the patient evaluation. Our patient's blood pressure was lower than expected, particularly for someone in pain. A healthy 55 year old male would not usually run systolic pressures of 92 to 98; in retrospect, this should have been an initial cause for concern, prompting earlier contact with a trauma center to arrange a transfer. Perhaps the absence of tachycardia lulled the physician into a false sense of security, mistakenly reassuring him that major blood loss had not occurred. However, a normal heart rate, or even bradycardia, in the face of traumatic hemorrhage is actually common—present in over a quarter of hypotensive patients in one retrospective review.[6] The mechanism appears to be primarily mediated via an increase in cardiac vagal tone, a vasodepressor-cardio inhibitory mediated reflex. Blood in the peritoneum may also stimulate a parasympathetic reflex via the vagus nerve to blunt tachycardia.[7,8] Tachycardia is not the only response to acute hemorrhage and resulting hypovolemia. A failure to realize that a normal heart rate (or bradycardia) is consistent with acute hemorrhage is potentially hazardous.

Given the mechanism of injury, a cervical spine collar was appropriately placed on the patient prior to the ED evaluation. Clearance of the cervical spine was done using the NEXUS criteria: no posterior midline cervical tenderness in an alert patient with no evidence of intoxication, focal neurologic deficit, or distracting injury.[9] No other midline spinal tenderness was reported, and the spines were considered cleared. Importantly, the examination also demonstrated no evidence of a head injury.

The positive findings on examination were confined to the chest and abdomen. Chest wall tenderness was present, but clear and equal lung sounds with no palpable subcutaneous air were recorded, helping to rule out a pneumothorax, although it can be missed by clinical examination alone.[10] A chest radiograph was reported as showing two rib fractures and no other abnormalities. However, if suspicion still exists after viewing the chest radiograph, chest CT remains the gold standard for detection of pneumothorax and other injuries in the chest and lungs.[11,12] Recently, thoracic ultrasound has been demonstrated to be superior to chest radiographs for detection of traumatic pneumothorax.[12,13] This patient had a normal respiratory rate, without hypoxia and had no other findings on chest radiograph, so further assessment for chest injury was not indicated.

Indication of an abdominal injury was found during the physical examination with detection of LUQ tenderness, guarding, and firmness. Physical examination alone can be inaccurate in detecting abdominal injuries, especially in the face of the multiply injured patient, or if the patient has altered cognition.[14,15,16] Other modalities are available for further evaluation of patients with blunt abdominal trauma (BAT) including diagnostic peritoneal lavage (DPL), focused assessment with sonography for trauma (FAST), and computed tomography (CT) of the abdomen and pelvis.

IV. DIAGNOSIS OF BLUNT ABDOMINAL TRAUMA—DPL, CT, ULTRASOUND

DPL was introduced in the mid 1960s by Root et al[17] and it remains a rapid and very sensitive technique to determine if hemoperitoneum is present. It is superior to physical examination alone for predicting intra-abdominal hemorrhage.[18] Since its introduction, it has helped to decrease the number of trauma deaths[19]. As little as 20 ml of intraperitoneal blood can be detected with the technique. Disadvantages of DPL include the invasiveness of the procedure, failure to identify the bleeding site, and the inability to predict if an operation is necessary to correct the cause of the bleeding. The false positive rate of the procedure (nontherapeutic laparotomy after DPL) ranges from 13% to 50%.[20,21] False negative tests may occur, particularly when the DPL is done early in the course of evaluation of patients with bowel injuries that produce little bleeding.[22] Open or closed technique has equal accuracy.[23]

In the stable patient, abdominal CT has become the accepted standard in patients suspected of having an intra-abdominal injury. With the advent of helical and multidetector CTs, scanning is faster and more accurate than ever before. Solid organ injuries are easily identified and decisions concerning operative or non-operative management can be made. Sensitivities approaching 97% have been demonstrated. [24,25] One large multicenter prospective trial has shown that the negative predictive value of an abdominal CT in patients with blunt abdominal trauma is sufficiently high (99.6%) so as to permit safe discharge of patients after a negative abdominal CT.[26] An additional benefit of CT scanning in blunt abdominal trauma is the identification of retroperitoneal structures and clinically unsuspected injuries.[27]

Damage to the bowel and mesentery, which occurs in less than 5% of patients with BAT, can be difficult to diagnose and debate remains as to the utility of CT imaging in identifying these injuries. DPL is thought by some to be a more sensitive test for isolated bowel injuries.[28] Oral contrast typically has been given to patients undergoing CT to aid in identifying bowel loops, wall hematomas, hemorrhage, and the actual perforation site. Reported sensitivities for detecting bowel injuries ranged from 64% to 94%.[29,30,31] However, several recent studies, including two prospective trials, have concluded that, when using newer generation CT scanners to image patients not given oral contrast, sensitivity can approach 95% and specificity 99% for detecting bowel and mesenteric injuries.[32,33,34] Therefore, withholding oral contrast doesn't detract from the accuracy of CT in BAT. Diaphragm injuries, also uncommon in BAT and often clinically silent, are not easily detected with CT, being missed up to 43% of the time.[35] A high index of suspicion is needed if there is clinical concern for this injury.

A final criticism of CT in BAT is high expense and radiation exposure. Some have proposed that sonography become the primary diagnostic tool after physical examination, followed by laboratory testing and observation in the hospital. Unfortunately, there is not a combination of sonographic, non-CT radiographic and laboratory testing sufficiently sensitive to exclude intra-abdominal injury in BAT patients.[36] The approach of using clinical observation along with non CT investigations may actually be less cost-effective than obtaining a CT on all admitted BAT patients.[37]

Since the early 1990s, abdominal ultrasound has been gaining increasing acceptance in trauma centers and community hospitals for the rapid evaluation of BAT patients. Typically it is performed by emergency physicians and trauma surgeons, not radiologists. Focused assessment with sonography for trauma (FAST) is a rapidly performed, non-invasive test to determine if hemoperitoneum is present. It has largely supplanted DPL during the trauma evaluation. In one large prospective study, FAST was 100% sensitive and 100% specific in demonstrating hemoperitoneum in hypotensive patients with BAT.[38] Approximately 100-200 ml of free intraperitoneal fluid can be detected with a FAST examination,[39] making it somewhat less sensitive than DPL, although the difference may not be clinically noticeable.

FAST is particularly useful in the unstable patient because it rapidly identifies intra-abdominal bleeding usually resulting from organ damage. In one recent retrospective study, in patients hypotensive after BAT, a negative FAST essentially excluded a surgical injury. On the other hand, a positive ultrasound exam indicated surgical injury in only 64% of the patients.[40]

FAST isn't as effective in diagnosing solid organ defects or bowel injuries, nor is it useful in inspecting the retroperitoneal area. FAST does not normally identify the site of bleeding, only that bleeding is taking place. Using FAST to identifying all intra-abdominal injuries, including intestinal and solid organs injuries as well as hemoperitoneum, has a sensitivity of approximately 70%, which is not as sensitive as CT.[41] In the stable patient, ultrasound should not be considered to be a substitute for CT scanning, but rather an adjunct. If a FAST examination is used solely to evaluate the abdomen, then abdominal injuries will be under diagnosed.[42]

A simple algorithm for the evaluation of BAT in a stable patient as proposed by the EAST guidelines: [27]

1. Stable patients with reliable exam and no confounding injuries—observe and perform serial exams.
2. Stable patients with questionable exam and/or rib fractures, abdominal pain, abdominal wall contusion—CT (or FAST initially with CT in complementary role).
3. Unstable patient—FAST or DPL for the initial diagnostic test.

V. SUMMARY
Our patient had a splenic rupture with retroperitoneal hematoma, diagnosed at surgery. During the initial ED evaluation, a FAST examination would have probably demonstrated free intra-abdominal fluid, prompting earlier intervention and trauma center transfer. The patient's vital signs were an early clue to the internal bleeding that was occuring. CT scanning provides the most information short of an exploratory laparotomy in BAT patients, but when they are unstable, a CT is difficult to do and potentially unsafe. FAST is a rapid and easy-to-use modality in this situation, and provides critical information to aid in the management of the patient. Emergency physicians practicing in any type of hospital can master FAST, giving them an additional tool to evaluate trauma patients.

TEACHING POINTS ABOUT CASE 14:
- Maintain a high index of suspicion for splenic injury in trauma patients with LUQ pain and abnormal vital signs.
- Lack of tachycardia does not exclude acute blood loss.
- Accuracy, as well as timeliness, is important in managing ED patients.

REFERENCES

1. Piontek FA, Coscia R, Marselle CS, et al. Impact of American College of Surgeons verification on trauma outcomes. J Trauma 2003; 54:1041-6.
2. Abernathy JH, McGwin G Jr, Acker JE, et al. Impact of a voluntary trauma system on mortality, length of stay, and cost at a level I trauma center. Am Surg 2002; 68:182-92.
3. Meldon SW, Reilly M, Drew BL, et al Trauma in the very elderly: a community-based study of outcomes at trauma and nontrauma centers. J Trauma 2002; 52:79-84.
4. van Olden GD, Meeuwis JD, Bolhuis HW, et al. Clinical impact of advanced trauma life support. Am J Emerg Med 2004; 22:522-5.
5. Lerner EB, Moscati RM. The "golden hour": scientific fact or medical "urban legend?" Acad Emerg Med 2001; 8:758-60.
6. Demetriades D, Chan LS, Bhasin P, et al. Relative bradycardia in patients with traumatic hypotension. J Trauma 1998;45:534-9.
7. Thomas I, Dixon J. Bradycardia in acute hemorrhage. BMJ 2004; 328:541-3.
8. Snyder HS. Lack of a tachycardic response to hypotension with ruptured ectopic pregnancy. Am J Emerg Med 1990; 8:23-6.
9. Hoffman JR, Mower WR, Wolfson AB, et al. Validity of a set of clinical criteria to rule out injury to the cervical spine in patients with blunt trauma. National Emergency X-Radiography Utilization Study Group. N Engl J Med 2000;343:94-9.
10. Wall SD, Federle MP, Jeffrey RB, et al. CT diagnosis of unsuspected pneumothorax after blunt abdominal trauma. Am J Roentgenol 1983; 141:919-21.
11. Rowan KR, Kirkpatrick AW, Liu D, et al. Traumatic pneumothorax detection with thoracic US: correlation with chest radiography and CT—initial experience. Radiology 2002; 225:210-4.
12. Kirkpatrick AW, Sirois M, Laupland KB, et al. Hand-held thoracic sonography for detecting post-traumatic pnuemothoraces: the extended focused assessment with sonography for trauma (EFAST). J Trauma 2004; 57:288-95.
13. Dulchavsky SA, Schwarz KL, Kirkpatrick AW, et al. Prospective evaluation of thoracic ultrasound in the detection of pneumothorax. J Trauma 2001; 50:201-5.
14. Rodriguez A, DuPriest RW Jr., Shatney CH. Recognition of intra-abdominal injury in blunt trauma victims. A prospective study comparing physical examination with peritoneal lavage. Am Surg 1982;48:457-9.
15. Schurink GW, Bode PJ, van Luijt PA, et al. The value of physical examination in the diagnosis of patients with blunt abdominal trauma: a retrospective study. Injury 1997; 28:261-5.
16. Livingston DH, Lavery RF, Passannante MR, et al. Admission or observation is not necessary after a negative abdominal computed tomographic scan in patients with suspected blunt abdominal trauma: results of a prospective, multi-institutional trial. J Trauma 1998;44:273-83.
17. Root HD, Hauser CW, McKinley CR, et al. Diagnostic peritoneal lavage. Surgery 1965; 57:633-7.
18. Bivins BA, Sachatello CR, Daughtery ME, et al. Diagnostic peritoneal lavage is superior to clinical evaluation in blunt abdominal trauma. Am Surg 1978; 44: 637-41.
19. Nagy KK, Roberts RR, Joseph KT, et al. Experience with over 2,500 diagnostic peritoneal lavages. Injury 2000; 31:479-82.
20. Henneman PL, Marx JA, Moore EE, et al. Diagnostic peritoneal lavage: accuracy in predicting necessary laparotomy following blunt and penetrating trauma. J Trauma 1990; 30:1345-55.

21. Sozuer EM, Akyurek N, Kafali ME, et al. Diagnostic peritoneal lavage in blunt abdominal trauma victims. Eur J Emerg Med 1998; 5:231-4.
22. Kemmeter PR, Senagor AJ, Smith D. Dilemmas in the diagnosis of blunt enteric trauma. Am Surg 1998; 64:750-4.
23. Hodgson NF, Stewart TL, Girotti MJ. Open or closed diagnostic peritoneal lavage for abdominal trauma? A meta-analysis. J Trauma 2000; 48:1091-5.
24. Liu M, Lee CH, P'eng FK: Prospective comparison of diagnostic peritoneal lavage, computed tomographic scanning, and ultrasonography for the diagnosis of blunt abdominal trauma. J Trauma 1993; 35: 267-70.
25. Peitzman AB, Makaroun MS, Slasky BS, et al. Prospective study of computed tomography in initial management of blunt abdominal trauma. J Trauma 1986; 26:585- 92.
26. Livingston DH, Lavery RF, Passannante MR, et al. Admission or observation is not necessary after a negative abdominal computed tomographic scan in patients with suspected blunt abdominal trauma: results of a prospective, multi-institutional trial. J Trauma 1998; 44: 272-82.
27. Hoff WS, Holevar M, Nagy KK, et al. Practice management guidelines for the evaluation of blunt abdominal trauma: The East practice management guidelines work group. J Trauma 2002; 53:602-15.
28. Ceraldi, CM, Waxman K: Computerized tomography as an indicator of isolated mesenteric injury. A comparison with peritoneal lavage. Am Surg 1990; 56: 806-10.
29. Sherck J, Shatney C, Sensaki K, et al. The accuracy of computed tomography in the diagnosis of blunt small-bowel perforation. Am J Surg 1994; 168:670-5.
30. Butela ST, Federle MP, Chang PJ, et al. Performance of CT in detection of bowel injury. Am J Roentgenol 2001; 176:129-35.
31. Killeen KL, Shanmuganathan K, Poletti PA, et al. Helical computed tomography of bowel and mesenteric injuries. J Trauma. 2001;51:26-36.
32. Allen TL, Mueller MT, Bonk RT, et al. Computed tomographic scanning without oral contrast solution for blunt bowel and mesenteric injuries in abdominal trauma. J Trauma. 2004;56:314-322.
33. Stafford RE, McGonigal MD, Weigelt JA, et al. Oral contrast solution and computed tomography for blunt abdominal trauma. Arch Surg. 1999;134:622-627.
34. Stuhlfant JW, Soto JA, Lucey BC, et al. Blunt abdominal trauma: performance of CT without oral contrast material. Radiology. 2004;233:689-694.
35. Nchimi A, Szapiro D, Ghaye B, et al. Helical CT of blunt diaphragmatic rupture. Am J Roentgenol 2005; 184:24-30.
36. Poletti PA, Mirvis SE, Shanmuganathan K, et al. Blunt abdominal trauma patients: can organ injury be excluded without performing computed tomography? J Trauma 2004; 57:1072-81.
37. Navarette-Navarro P, Vazquez G, Bosch JM, et al. Computed tomography vs clinical and multidisciplinary procedures for early evaluation of severe abdomen and chest trauma: a cost analysis approach. Intensive Care Med 1996; 22:208-12.
38. Rozycki GS, Ballard RB, Feliciano DV, et al. Surgeon-performed ultrasound for theassessment of truncal injuries. Lessons learned from 1,540 patients. Ann Surg1998; 228:557-67.
39. Branney SW, Moore EE, Cantrill SV, et al. Ultrasound based key clinical pathway reduces the use of hospital resources for the evaluation of blunt abdominal trauma. J Trauma 1997; 42:1086-90.

40. Farahmand N, Sirlin CB, Brown MA, et al. Hypotensive patients with blunt abdominal trauma: performance of screening US. Radiology 2005; 235:436-43.
41. Tso P, Rodriguez A, Cooper C, et al. Sonography in blunt abdominal trauma: a preliminary progress report. J Trauma 1992; 33:39-43.
42. Miller MT, Pasquale MD, Bromberg WJ, et al. Not so fast. J Trauma 2003; 54:52-60.

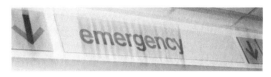

CASE15
45 YEAR OLD MALE WITH COUGH & SORE THROAT

Commentary:
Gregory L. Henry, MD, FACEP

CEO, Medical Practice Risk Assessment, Inc., Ann Arbor, Michigan
Clinical Professor, Department of Emergency Medicine
    University of Michigan Medical School, Ann Arbor, Michigan
Past President, American College of Emergency Physicians (ACEP)

Discussion:
Michael B. Weinstock, MD

Clinical Assistant Professor, Division of Emergency Medicine
    The Ohio State University, College of Medicine
    Columbus, Ohio
Attending ED physician, Director of Medical Education
    Mt. Carmel St. Ann's Emergency Department
    Westerville, Ohio

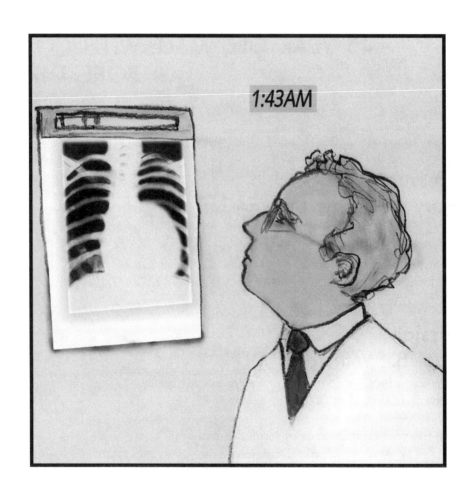

1:43AM

45 YEAR OLD MALE WITH COUGH & SORE THROAT

—Initial Visit*—

*Authors' Note: The history, exam and notes are the actual documentation of the physicians and providers, including abbreviations (and spelling errors)

CHIEF COMPLAINT (00:39): Sore throat

VITAL SIGNS								
Time	Temp(F)	Pulse	Resp	Syst	Diast	Pos.	O2 Sat	O2%
00:39	97.8	110	16	110	82	S	98	RA

HISTORY OF PRESENT ILLNESS (documented by physician assistant): 45 year old male c/o cough and throat pain x 1month. Admits to past hx of GERD. States he has been taking Zantac for a week. His PCP prescribed a cough medicine and an antibiotic, but the cough has not improved. Denies known fever. Admits to feeling hot and having intermittent chills. Denies n/v/d, abdominal pain, ear pain, chest pain, peripheral edema, calf muscle pain, shortness of breath, rhinorrhea. The history is provided by the patient. He refuses an interpreter.

PAST MEDICAL HISTORY/TRIAGE (at 00:26)
    Medication, common allergies: No known allergies.
    Current meds: Zoloft and Tramadol hcl and Zantac, and Lipitor
    Past medical/surgical history: Depression, Headache. No significant surgical history.

PHYSICAL EXAM (documented by physician assistant):
    General: Well-appearing; well-nourished; A&O X 3, in no apparent distress
    Head: Normocephalic; atraumatic
    Eyes: PERRL
    Nose: The nose is normal in appearance without rhinorrhea
    Neck: No JVD or distended neck veins
    Resp: Normal chest excursion with respiration; breath sounds clear and equal bilaterally; no wheezes, rhonchi, or rales
    Card: Regular rhythm, without murmurs, rub
    Abd: Non-distended; non-tender, soft, without rigidity, rebound or guarding
    Skin: Normal for age and race; warm and dry without diaphoresis ; no apparent lesions
    Extremities: No peripheral edema or calf muscle pain

RESULTS (01:43): PA and lateral CXR: The heart size is enlarged. The pulmonary vasculature is within normal limits. No acute infiltrates or evidence of CHF is seen. Impression: Cardiomegaly

PROGRESS NOTE (at 03:23) (documented by physician): I spoke with his PCP and discussed the case including getting a cardiac ECHO and to ensure follow up. I do not feel that he needs admission as there is no peripheral edema, crackles on exam, or pulmonary edema on CXR.

DIAGNOSIS: Cough, Gastritis

FOLLOW UP: Prescriptions for prilosec and hycodan. Follow up with primary physician in 3 days. Outpatient testing for cardiac ECHO ordered with results to be sent to PCP. Discharge time was 03:44

Gregory L. Henry comments:

"A sore throat is not a sore throat is not a sore throat"

A sore throat is not a sore throat is not a sore throat. This gentleman was not your typical sore throat patient. The fact that he is otherwise quite well should not dissuade one from thinking broadly on such a case.

The patient's sore throat is also tied up with a cough. The etiology may not be confined to the larynx and may involve the respiratory system. He has already been on antibiotics, and therefore has failed outpatient therapy. He denied most questions in the review of systems, including shortness of breath.

His evaluation is reasonable. It is not commented upon whether he has stridor or any tenderness over the larynx. When examining patients with a sore throat, the possibility of airway involvement should be explored. Stridor, difficulty swallowing, or significant discomfort with squeezing the larynx should raise the possibility of epiglottitis.

The documentation on this case is really quite good. It is important to note that since the patient is not a native speaker of English, an interpreter was offered and refused. It is neither the medical system nor the physician who is denying an important part of his care.

- Thoroughness of Documentation: 8 out of 10

- Thoroughness of Patient Evaluation: 8 out of 10

- Risk of Serious Illness Being Missed: Moderate risk

- Risk Management Legal Rating: Moderate risk

45 YEAR OLD MALE WITH COUGH & SORE THROAT

—Second Visit: 36 Hours Later—

CHIEF COMPLAINT (15:49): Difficulty breathing

```
VITAL SIGNS
Time    Temp(F)  Pulse  Resp  Syst  Diast  Pos.  O2 Sat  O2%
17:10    99              12    85    25     L     100     vent
17:18    94.1    106     24    75                 97      vent
17:38            106     38    59    25     L
18:16            98      12    72    0      L     100
18:46    94.6    99      12    81    58     L     100     vent
19:11            98      12    89    74     L     100     vent
```

HISTORY OF PRESENT ILLNESS (Time not recorded): Patient is a 45-year-old male who has no significant past medical history according to family. He is a smoker. The patient was seen in the emergency Department yesterday for a persistent cough for the last several days. He had already been placed on antibiotics per his primary care physician. His chest x-ray was clear with no infiltrates. He was noted to have cardiomegaly and was to have an outpatient cardiac echo done. The patient's son noted that he has not been eating and drinking for the last two days. He has had little in a way of urine output. His son believes that he may have had fevers although his temperature was not taken. He has had no vomiting. He has had increasing respiratory distress since last evening. He presented in marked respiratory distress, lethargic, unable to participate in it any extensive review of systems due to his critical condition.

PAST MEDICAL HISTORY/TRIAGE (15:50): Initially triaged to 'zone 3/urgent care area' of the ED
   Nursing assessment : The patient was brought to room by stretcher with EMS. Patient is awake and irritable with an affect that is anxious, responds to verbal stimuli, and responsive to painful stimuli. Patient speaks in brief phrases only. There is no nasal flaring. There are no retractions. Inspiration is severely labored with marked distress. There are crackles throughout the entire chest bilaterally. Capillary refill is greater than 5 seconds. The patient's color is pale and dusky. The skin is cool and dry. Skin turgor is poor.
   Allergies: No known allergies
   Current meds: Zoloft and Tramadol hcl and Zantac, and Lipitor and Hycodan
   Past medical/surgical history: Depression, Headache. No significant surgical history.

EXAM (Time not recorded):
   General: the patient is a slender middle-aged male who is lethargic and in severe respiratory distress.
   Head: Normocephalic; atraumatic.
   Eyes: EOMI, pupils are reactive.
   Nose: Normal nose; no rhinorrhea;

Throat: Normal pharynx with no tonsillar hypertrophy. Dry mucous membranes.

Neck: Supple; non-tender; no cervical lymphadenopathy.

Card: Regular rate and rhythm, no murmurs. No peripheral edema. The patient has marked bilateral JVD even when sitting upright.

Resp: Normal chest excursion; breath sounds clear and equal bilaterally; no wheezes, rhonchi, or rales.

Abd: Non-distended;soft, non-tender , without rigidity, rebound or guarding. Bowel sounds are positive.

Skin: Normal for age and race; warm and dry; no apparent lesions

Neuro: The patient is awake although lethargic. Cranial nerves are intact. He moves all extremities.

PROGRESS NOTES: The patient presented in severe respiratory distress.

- **At 15:49** he was triaged to zone 3.
- **At 16:00**, finger stick revealed a blood sugar of 20. Two IVs were established. The patient was given 1 amp of D50 at 16:14.
- ECG was done at 16:19 (see below).
- He went for CXR at 16:21 and returned at 16:27. He was given fluid wide open.
- **At 16:33** he was emergently moved to the main trauma room.
- **At 17:02** his condition had not improved, so he was given 3mg of IV versed and 100mg IV succinylcholine and intubated . A post intubation CXR was ordered (see below).
- He remained hypotensive and was placed on a dopamine drip at 17:08. This was titrated. The patient was acidotic with marked JVD and cardiomegaly on chest x-ray. He received 2 amps of sodium bicarb.
- He received IV fluids, with liters 3 and 4 hung at 17:42. Clinical suspicion was that of pericardial effusion with possible tamponade. I attempted twice to obtain a cardiac echo. The technician stated that this would require a cardiologist to approve this procedure. I had spoken with the intensivist, who was to be involved in this admission. I also spoke with the cardiologist. He requested that the patient be sent to a hospital with ability to perform stat ECHO and pericardial drain, if necessary. The patient has been hypotensive throughout his emergency Department stay. This was discussed with the cardiologist. We called bed control who obtained a CCU bed. We requested a cardiac ultrasonography at the bedside when patient arrived. We were told that this would be arranged. We also arranged for translation services to be available. Family was told that this patient is in critical condition. There is a male member from the mother's side of the family and two children present.
- **At 18:41** an ativan drip was started for sedation.
- **At 18:45** while awaiting transfer, the patient remained hypotensive, so a levophed drip was started.

RESULTS: *ECG at 16:19 follows*:

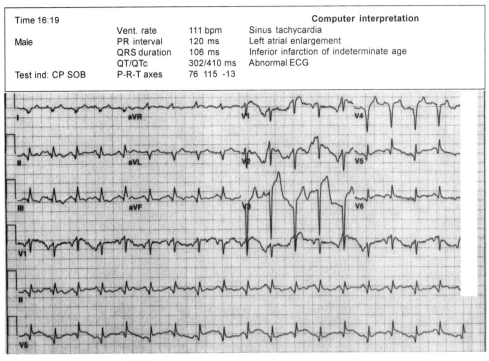

Time 16:19

Male

Test ind: CP SOB

Vent. rate   111 bpm
PR interval   120 ms
QRS duration   106 ms
QT/QTc   302/410 ms
P-R-T axes   76 115 -13

Computer interpretation
Sinus tachycardia
Left atrial enlargement
Inferior infarction of indeterminate age
Abnormal ECG

ReExam (documented at 19:47)

General: Pt is orally intubated

Neck: Continued marked JVD

Card: Regular rate and rhythm. With control of respiratory distress, it is noted that the pt has a harsh holosystolic murmur heard throughout precordium

Resp: Breath sounds clear and equal bilaterally.

RESULTS:

Test	Flag	Value	Units	Ref. Range
WBC	H	15.6	K/uL	4.6-10.2
HGB		13.2	G/DL	12.0-16.0
PLT	L	105	K/uL	142-424
NA	L	124	MMOL/L	135-144
K		4.6	MMOL/L	3.5-5.1
CL		92	MMOL/L	98-107
AGAP	H	32	MMOL/L	6.0-18.0
CO2	L	5	MMOL/L	22-29
BUN		17	MG/DL	7-18
CREAT	H	2.9	MG/DL	0.6-1.3
GLUCOSE	H	460	MG/DL	70-110

(continued on next page)

Test	Flag	Value	Units	Ref. Range
CKMB	H	7.9	NG/ML	0.0-5.0
TROPI		0.17	NG/ML	.00-.27
ALB	L	2.2	G/DL	3.2-4.6
TP		5.0	GM/DL	6.4-8.2
BILT	H	3.1	MG/DL	.0-1.0
BILD	H	2.3	MG/DL	0.0-0.3
BILI		0.8	MG/DL	.0-1.0
ALT	H	2476	U/L	22-65
ALP	H	167	U/L	42-144
AST	H	8712	U/L	10-34
AMY		51	U/L	25-115
LIP		96	U/L	114-286
LACTIC ACID	H	14.9	MMOL/L	0.4-2.0
D-dimer	H	>1000	NG/ML	<500

ABG (17:00):

PH	L	7.069		7.350-7.450
PCO2	L	15.6		32.0-48.0
PO2	H	237		83.0-108.0
FI O2		100		

RADIOLOGY: Portable chest: Comparison with previous studies, the last taken earlier the same day, reveals now an endotracheal tube in good position well above the carina. There is persistent cardiomegaly. There is no evident change since the recent previous study.

DIAGNOSIS:
1. Hypotension
2. Distress - respiratory, acute
3. Hypoglycemia
4. Acidosis
5. Rule out pericardial tampanode

DISPOSITION: Nursing report was called to the receiving hospital at 19:02 and the patient was discharged from the ED at 19:55.

HOSPITAL COURSE AT RECEIVING HOSPITAL:

Hospital course: He received a cardiac ECHO which showed severely reduced left ventricular systolic function with EF 15%. Evidence of apical akinesis and probable remnant of apical thrombus. Moderate mitral insufficiency. Doppler evidence of severely increased right-sided pressures.

He was maintained on a vent for the first 13 days of his hospital course without significant improvement. Repeat ECHO showed that EF remained at 15%. He was seen by cardiology, nephrology and ID. Despite aggressive interventions, he remained poor. Diagnoses included severe left ventricular systolic function, severe hypoperfusion with lactic acidosis, ischemic hepatopathy, multisystem organ failure and adult respiratory distress syndrome (ARDS). The patient was seen for evaluation for palliative care and a decision was made to take him off the ventilator and discontinue the pressors.

FINAL DISCHARGE DIAGNOSIS: Cardiomyopathy of uncertain etiology, resolved acute renal failure, shock liver, bilateral foot ischemia secondary to prolonged levophed and/or DIC, encephalopathy, MRSA pneumonia-resolved.

Disposition: He was subsequently discharged to skilled ECF with tube feedings and DNR status.

Additional comments by Gregory L. Henry:

I do not believe there is anything specific that should have been done differently during the initial visit. His return at 36 hours, and the subsequent diagnosis of heart failure, could not have been predicted initially.

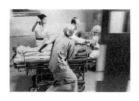

EVALUATION OF SHORTNESS OF BREATH, DIAGNOSIS AND MANAGEMENT OF HEART FAILURE

Michael B. Weinstock, MD

I. SUMMARY OF CASE

On the patient's first ED visit, his main symptoms were cough and sore throat. His primary care physician had prescribed a cough medicine and antibiotic, but we don't know when or why. It is noted that the patient refused an intrepretor, but the quality of the communication was not documented. In the ED, he specifically denied shortness of breath (SOB) on review of symptoms. In a busy ED, it is easy to string together a long list of ROS questions, and if the patient answers "no," to assume they are all negative. It would be interesting to know the patient's understanding of the phrase "shortness of breath." I have often had a patient answer "no" when asked about chest *pain*, but later learned he has chest *pressure*. Possibly he did have dyspnea with exertion, but no SOB at rest—we will never know for sure.

The initial physician did seem to be concerned about heart failure (HF), probably because of the cardiomegaly seen on CXR. A progress note was written just before discharge to justify outpatient testing. If this was a concern (using our retrospectoscope), it may have been helpful to confirm that the history taken was correct. If the patient had been specifically questioned about dyspnea, orthopnea, or dyspnea on exertion just prior to discharge, and if he had answered "yes," the evaluation, as well as the outcome, may have been different. Unfortunately, he was sent home, decompensated quickly, returned less than 2 days later with respiratory distress, and was intubated shortly after his arrival in the ED.

II. INTRODUCTION AND DIFFERENTIAL DIAGNOSES OF DYSPNEA

Patients as well as physicians have different understandings of the term "shortness of breath." [1,4,5,7] The perceived severity is not always proportional to the underlying degree of illness, and anxiety or fear may amplify the sensation of dyspnea.[5] Dyspnea is defined in the textbook *Emergency Medicine: A Comprehensive Study Guide* (by Judith Tintinalli) as, "a subjective feeling of difficult, labored, or uncomfortable breathing." [1]

The evaluation of dyspnea requires consideration of a diverse range of possible causes (Table 1). In the emergency department, this process begins by first evaluating for life-threatening causes with a thorough history and physical exam. Dyspnea can be categorized into upper airway causes, cardiac and pulmonary causes, systemic causes, and central causes. If the diagnosis is not obtained in the ED, and and the life-threatening causes have been reasonably excluded, then the work-up may be continued as an outpatient.

Table 1. Differential Diagnoses of Dyspnea

Upper airway causes	Cardiac causes	Pulmonary causes	Systemic causes	Central causes
1. Angioedema/anaphylaxis 2. Abscess (retropharyngeal, peritonsillar) 3. Tracheal obstruction (mass, foreign body, mucus plug, tracheomalacia) 4. Infectious – Epiglottitis, croup, pharyngitis	1. Myocardial ischemia/angina 2. Heart failure 3. Pericarditis, pericardial effusion/tamponade 4. Valvular disease 5. Cardiac arrhythmias	1. Pneumonia 2. Obstructive lung disease: Asthma, chronic bronchitis, emphysema 3. Pneumothorax 4. Pleural effusion 5. Lung masses, metastatic disease 6. Pulmonary embolism (PE) 7. Pulmonary hypertension 8. Adult respiratory distress syndrome (ARDS) 9. Restrictive lung diseases: Kyphoscoliosis, obesity, diaphragmatic dysfunction, abdominal distention , infiltrative process (sarcoidosis, amyloidosis, pulmonary fibrosis), pneumonectomy, parenchymal process	1. Sepsis/fever 2. Anemia or hemoglobinopathies 3. Diabetic ketoacidosis 4. Shock, metabolic acidosis 5. Gastroesophageal reflux (GERD) 6. Thyroid disorders 7. Deconditioning	1. Psychogenic – Panic disorder, anxiety, hyper-ventilation syndrome 2. Cheyne-Stokes breathing – seen in coma due to intracerebral pathology 3. CNS/systemic neuromuscular disorders – Guillain-Barré, myasthenia gravis 4. Carbon mon-oxide toxicity 5. Drug withdrawal

III. HISTORY AND PHYSICAL EXAM

The history will direct the evaluation and will often yield a diagnosis. Schmitt, et al., evaluated 146 hospitalized dyspnic patients with the examining physician blinded to the patient's diagnosis. The diagnosis was determined with history alone 74% of the time[4]. Other studies have found rates of 73–92%.[5]

During the history, it is important to ask the patient what they mean by "shortness of breath." Several studies, evaluating a total of 222 patients, asked them to describe their breathlessness. It was found that although descriptions overlapped for similar conditions, there were several clusters. Patients with asthma described their breathing as "heavy, requiring extra work, tight or wheezy," or "breathing that did not go all the way out." Patients with heart failure described "rapid breathing," and "a smothering or suffocating sensation." Those with obstructive lung disease described "a hunger for breath" or "inability to get enough air."[5]

Some of the important elements of the history include the following: Does the patient experience painful respirations, which may be seen with a pulmonary embolus (PE)? Is the dyspnea present at rest or exertion only, and what was the acuity of onset? Upper airway symptoms including stridor or difficulty swallowing are concerning for obstruction or infection. An acute onset of SOB may signify a PE, and a prolonged onset (several weeks or months) may suggest an opportunistic infection, such as pneumocystis pneumonia. Dyspnea at night, with exertion, exposure to cold or other environmental triggers, may stem from asthma. Associated symptoms include: fever, suggesting pneumonia or sepsis; peripheral edema, suggesting heart failure; hyperglycemic symptoms, suggesting diabetic ketoacidosis (DKA); hemoptysis, suggesting PE or tuberculosis; and weight loss due to cancer.

The past medical history often is the most important piece of information, particularly in patients with a history of COPD, HF, asthma, spontaneous pneumothorax, coronary ischemia/MI, DKA, or panic disorder. Past causes of dyspnea are often the reason for their current dyspnea; if a different etiology is found, this should be discussed in a progress note.

Other important features of the history include smoking, use of home oxygen, and exposure to other ill persons. New medications may cause allergic reactions or may yield clues about recent treatment by the primary physician. Inquire about risk factors for PE, including prolonged immobilization, lower extremity injury, recent surgery, history of thromboembolic disease, or cancer.

Continuous oximetry may reveal intermittent desaturations and help to gauge response to therapy. Examination of the oropharynx may reveal edema or abscess formation. The neck exam may show elevated jugular venous pressure, suggesting HF, pericardial tamponade, or tension pneumothorax. Unilateral leg swelling suggests deep venous thrombosis (DVT) with possible PE.

The lung exam may be misleading. At least one study found that wheezing was not helpful for predicting asthma, and another found that peripheral edema, jugular venous distention (JVD), and gallop heart rhythms were not helpful in distinguishing cardiac versus pulmonary origin. Crackles on lung exam had a positive predictive value of 0.79 for interstitial lung disease if the pretest probability was 14%.[5] Two tests shown to be suggestive of cardiac disease are a positive response to the valsalva maneuver and the abdominojugular reflux.[5]

IV. EVALUATION OF DYSPNEA

The various modalities available in the ED to evaluate dyspnea include pulse oximetry, arterial blood gas, peak expiratory flow rates, laboratory evaluation, chest x-ray, ECG, cardiac ECHO, chest CT, and ventilation perfusion scan. These should be ordered based on the patient's symptoms and signs, and the pretest probability of subsequent diagnoses.

Pulse oximetry, the "fifth vital sign," is noninvasive and provides information on oxygenation in a "real time" basis, helping to monitor for deterioration in a patient's condition. False readings may occur from hemoglobinopathy (carboxyhemoglobinemia, methemoglobinemia), intravenous dyes (such as methylene blue), signal artifact (ambient light, nail polish), hypotension, vasoconstriction, hypothermia, and anemia (especially in the presence of hypoxia and most pronounced with saturation less than 80%).[6] A healthy patient should have a saturation of 95% or higher, but patients with chronic lung disease may have lower baseline saturations.

The ABG provides information not available from oximetry reading, including pH, CO_2 level, CO level, pO_2, and the ability to calculate the arterial-alveolar gradient. Obtaining a CO level can also be done with a venous stick, which may be less uncomfortable to the patient. One study of 779 patients (280 with angiographically proven PE), found that 11–23% of the patients with PE had a normal A-a gradient.[9] Indications for ABG include altered mental status, persistent hyperventilation, critically ill patients, and those with impending respiratory failure.[7]

It is useful to know if the patient monitors peak flow rates at home and if the peak flow has changed. The national asthma guidelines recommend obtaining a peak flow measurement before and after bronchodilator therapy.[8]

Laboratory evaluation of SOB should be tailored to the suspected etiology. This may include a CBC (anemia, sepsis/infection), glucose (DKA), beta-naturetic peptide (BNP—heart failure—see below), d-dimer (PE), and cardiac enzymes (myocardial infarction).

On the second visit, our patient's labs were grossly abnormal. He was initially hypoglycemic with a blood sugar of 20, which rapidly increased to 460 after IV dextrose. His serum bicarbonate level was 5 with a lactate of 14.9, probably indicating hypoperfusion. ABG revealed severe acidemia with a pH of 7.069, with an unsuccessful attempt at respiratory compensation—pCO_2 was 15. Liver enzymes were extremely elevated from hepatic congestion—the ALT was 2,476, the AST was 8,712.

The chest x-ray provides helpful information: pneumothorax, infiltrate, pleural effusion, cardiomegaly, aortic dissection, mediastinal air, or free abdominal air. Positive findings are often helpful, but may not necessarily be the source of the patient's current complaints—comparison with old x-rays is important. A negative chest x-ray may be helpful, but radiographic findings may lag behind clinical findings. A negative x-ray in a severely dyspneic patient is strongly suggestive of pulmonary embolism.[3] Additional discussion of cardiomegaly and the diagnosis of HF is discussed below.

The ECG may reveal an etiology of dyspnea, such as ischemia, tachyarrhythmias, bradyarrhythmias, left ventricular hypertrophy, or pericarditis. Additional discussion below.

Bedside ECHO may reveal hypoineses of myocardium, pericardial effusion, or aneurysm, but is often difficult to obtain in the ED, as seen with our patient. Evaluation of PE with CT angiogram, ventilation perfusion (V/Q) scan, or pulmonary angiogram is discussed at length in other chapters.

When this patient initially presented, he had been prescribed antibiotics for his cough by his primary care provider. It would be interesting to see the office diagnosis. It was probably acute bronchitis or upper respiratory infection, and in young adults, the etiology of acute bronchitis is almost always viral and antibiotics are not recommended.[2] At the first presentation, this information did not seem important; when he returned, the information was unobtainable. The patient was also taking Zantac; gastroesophageal reflux disease is one of the main reasons (along with post nasal drip and asthma) for chronic cough.[9]

V. EPIDEMIOLOGY AND DEFINITION OF HEART FAILURE
Though the incidence of coronary heart disease and myocardial infarction have decreased approximately 50% over the last several decades, the incidence and prevalence of heart failure (HF), and resulting morbidity and mortality, has dramatically increased. Deaths from HF have increased 6 fold from 1955 to 1992. The reasons are likely multifactorial; prolonged survival from coronary heart disease and hypertension, aging of the population, and increased prevalence of diabetes mellitus. There are 4.7 million Americans with HF, 400,000 new cases per year, and almost 40,000 deaths per year. Heart failure affects 1% of Americans per year over 65 and 2–3% per year from 85–94. Mortality ranges from 9–12% at 1 year for NYHA class I and II HF, and 31-52% for class III-IV HF.[11]

HF may result from any structural or functional disorder that prevents the ventricle from filling or emptying blood (see differential diagnosis below). HF is a clinical diagnosis, characterized by symptoms of dyspnea and fatigue, and signs including fluid retention. A general classification divides HF into systolic dysfunction, diastolic dysfunction, and mixed. Systolic dysfunction is characterized by a dilated chamber with reduced wall motion, decreased ejection fraction (EF), and adequate filling. Diastolic dysfunction is characterized by a normal sized chamber with normal emptying, but impaired filling—the EF is maintained. A poor correlation often exists between ejection fraction and clinical symptoms.[11]

The etiology of HF is coronary artery disease (CAD) in almost 70% of patients, related to recurrent episodes of myocardial ischemia and myocardial stunning.[12] Other causes include hypertension, valvular disease (including endocarditis), alcohol, diabetes, myocarditis, restrictive pericarditis, pericardial tamponade, drug toxicity, thyroid disorders, pulmonary hypertension and infiltrative disease (sarcoidosis, hematochromatosis, amyloidosis, and TB).

VI. DIAGNOSIS OF HEART FAILURE
A. History and physical
The primary reasons patients with undiagnosed HF seek medical attention are dyspnea (at rest or exertion) and fatigue.[10] Other symptoms include leg or abdominal swelling, orthopnea, and paroxysmal nocturnal dyspnea. Important historical clues may be obtained by directing questions toward the possible underlying cause of the heart failure; e.g., symptoms of myocardial ischemia when looking for coronary artery disease. For patients with a diagnosis of HF, common precipitants of decompensation are non-compliance with medications or diet, new medications, recurrent myocardial ischemia, infections, elevated blood pressure, and arrhythmias.

Findings on physical examination may include tachycardia, jugular venous distention (JVD), crackles and/or wheezing on lung auscultation, presence of a third heart sound, abdomino-jugular reflux, or dependent edema. Patients who are not ambulatory may manifest their edema in the sacral area, rather than the pretibial area.

B. ECHO, CXR, ECG
The best diagnostic test is a 2-dimensional echocardiogram, which provides information on the pericardium, myocardium, valves and systolic/diastolic function. Patients with EF < 40% are considered to have systolic dysfunction.[10]

The most common finding on chest x-ray is cardiomegaly, and other findings may include interstitial or alveolar edema, dilated upper lobe vessels, pleural effusion, and Kerley-B lines. Cardiac enlargement is defined as a cardiothoracic ratio (CTR) ≥ 0.5. The heart size may be normal (CTR < 0.5) in up to one-third of patients with HF, and an enlarged heart may not indicate HF. One study (Coronary Artery Surgery Study investigators) found a normal left ventricular EF in 66% of 1,397 patients with CTR > 0.5. Even though the heart size is not diagnostic, it does have prognostic value. In patients with HF, a CTR > 0.5 is a predictor of progression to NYHA class IV HF, increased mortality, and response to therapy.[13]

A normal ECG is helpful in excluding HF. A 1996 study by Davie, et al., examined 534 patients, age 17–94, of which 96 were found to have HF. ECG findings in those with HF included atrial fibrillation, previous MI, left ventricular hypertrophy, bundle branch block or left axis deviation. In this study, none of the patients with HF had a normal ECG. The remaining 438 patients had normal LV systolic function, though 169 had major ECG changes.[14]

C. Beta naturetic peptide (BNP)

BNP is secreted from the ventricles in response to elevated LV pressure. Its 2 clinical uses are 1) to differentiate cardiac etiologies of dyspnea and 2) for use as a prognostic tool. A 2002 study (BNP, "breathing not properly") by Maisel, et al., evaluated 1,586 patients who presented to 7 different ED's from 1999–2000 with a primary complaint of dyspnea. The BNP level was measured on presentation, but the ED physicians were blinded to the results. Patients with AMI, renal failure, and a diagnosis obviously not HF (trauma, cardiac tamponade) were excluded. The final diagnosis was HF in 47%, noncardiac causes with history of LV dysfunction in 5%, and no HF in 49%. After the final diagnosis was obtained, the BNP levels were evaluated and were found to be more accurate than history and physical exam. Patients with HF had a mean BNP of 675 (± 450) pg/ml, those without HF had a mean BNP of 110 (± 225) pg/ml and those with history of LV dysfunction, but without acute exacerbation of HF, had a mean BNP of 346 (± 390) pg/ml. At a cutoff of 100 pg/ml, the diagnostic accuracy was 83.4%. The negative predictive value with BNP < 50 pg/ml was 96%.[15]

Morrison, et al., performed a similar study with 321 patients and also concluded that BNP should be helpful in differentiating pulmonary from other causes of dyspnea. Patients with HF had a BNP of 759 ±798 pg/ml and those with pulmonary disease had BNP 61 ± 10pg/ml. Specific results by diagnosis are displayed in Table 2.[16]

Table 2. BNP Levels by Diagnosis

Diagnosis	BNP level (pg/ml)
CHF	758 (± 798)
COPD	54 (± 71)
Asthma	27 (± 40)
Acute bronchitis	44 (± 112)
Pneumonia	55 (± 76)
Tuberculosis	93 (± 54)
Lung cancer	120 (± 120)
Acute pulmonary embolism	207 (± 272)

Adapted from Morrison LK, Harrison A, Krishnaswamy P, et al., Utility of a rapid β-natriuretic peptide assay in differentiating congestive heart failure from lung disease in patients presenting with dyspnea. J Am Coll Card 2002;39:202-9.

Finally, in 2004, Schwam looked at 6 studies, including the 2 cited above, and summarized that when the pretest probability of HF, as determined by emergency physicians (blinded to the results of the BNP tests), was thought to be 95–100%, then the actual rate of HF was 95%. When the pretest probability was thought to be 0–4%, the actual rate of HF was 7%. In these 2 situations (where the emergency physician thought the patient had a very high or very low risk of HF), the clinical judgment was better than the BNP levels. But for the pretest probabilities in the middle (5–94%), clinical judgment alone was not adequate and other testing was necessary. In these patients, a BNP level of 50–80 pg/ml basically rules out HF, a level of 400–1,000 has a moderate ability to rule in HF, and if the BNP level is > 1,000, there is a large likelihood of HF. They concluded that BNP levels between 80–400 are not helpful in the diagnosis of HF.[17]

Other causes of BNP levels > 1,000 include PE, sepsis, pulmonary hypertension, cor pulmonale, left ventricular hypertrophy, renal failure, lung cancer, circulatory overload, acute coronary syndrome and atrial fibrillation.[17]

VII. MANAGEMENT OF HEART FAILURE

Cardiogenic shock has been defined as an acute deterioration in heart function which causes systemic hypoperfusion and tissue hypoxia resulting in cellular and organ dysfunction.[18] This description clearly fits our patient when he returned 36 hours later. One study reviewed 23,180 patients with cardiogenic shock and found a mortality rate of 70%[19] Another study quoted a rate of 50–80%.[20]

The mainstay of acute therapy for heart failure in patients without hypotension is nitrates. Sublingual nitroglycerin (SL NTG) 0.4mg can be given every 5–10 minutes and IV NTG is started at 0.3–0.5mcg/kg/min (which is 20–35mcg/min for a 70 kg patient) and titrated. Blood pressure should remain > 95–100.[21] Though starting with a NTG drip seems more aggressive than SL NTG, if this is done at 10mcg/min and not titrated, it will take 40 minutes to infuse 400mcg of NTG—the same amount administered in 1 standard sublingual dose. IV NTG may be titrated up to 200mcg/min. If unsuccessful, IV nitroprusside may be attempted. Contraindications include right ventricular infarction, aortic stenosis, hypertrophic cardiomyopathy, use of sildenafil (Viagra), volume depletion, and hypotension. Our patient was not a candidate for nitrate therapy since he presented for his second visit with a systolic BP of 85. Finally, nesiritide has been shown to increase mortality in some patients and cannot currently be recommended.

IV Furosemide (lasix) is given double the home dose and administered IV. Start with 40mg IV if the patient is not already on furosemide. If the urine output is inadequate, the dose may be doubled; it may be given as an IV drip starting at 20–40mg/hour, or another diuretic such as torsemide (Demadex), bumetanide (Bumex) or chlorothiazide (Diuril) may be attempted.[21] Given his hypotension, our patient was not a candidate for diuretics.

Morphine sulfate may be used in 2–5mg IV doses for symptomatic control of anxiety and chest pain in concurrent acute MI, but has not been shown to improve outcomes.[1]

Angiotension converting enzyme (ACE) inhibitors may be started acutely in patients who have not responded to nitrates and diuretics, provided they have an adequate blood pressure. The dose of enalapril (Vasotec) is 1.25mg IV over 5 minutes or captopril (Capoten) 12.5–25mg PO or SL. Avoid ACE inhibitors in patients with hyperkalemia, pregnancy, renal artery stenosis, or ACE induced angioedema.[21] Our patient was not a candidate for ACE inhibitors either.

Initially, our patient required 3 things; airway control, blood pressure support, and transfer for definitive diagnosis and management. Continuous positive airway pressure (CPAP) has been helpful in some patients with HF and may prevent the need for intubation. However, at this point in his management, a diagnosis had not been established—pericardial tamponade remained at the top of the differential. Our patient was too unstable for CPAP. He was given IV versed and succinylcholine, and underwent emergent airway control with endotracheal intubation.

Pressure support was initiated with dopamine at 17:08 and then norepinephrine (Levophed) at 18:45 with a slight increase in BP from 81 to 89 mm Hg just prior to transfer. Ionotropes such as dobutamine at 2.5–15 mcg/kg/min may be attempted. Intra-aortic balloon counterpulsation is indicated in patients with left ventricular failure or cardiogenic shock from myocardial infarction, myocarditis, severe myocardial contusion, or septic shock. Balloon pump is contraindicated in patients with severe aortic valvular insufficiency, aortic dissection, severe peripheral vascular disease, or brain death.[22]

Despite multiple attempts, the ED physician was unable to get a stat cardiac ECHO to evaluate for pericardial tamponade. Some time between 17:42 and 18:41, transfer was arranged. The ECHO at the receiving hospital showed cardiomyopathy with an ejection fraction (EF) of 15%, but no tamponade.

VIII. SUMMARY

This patient had an extremely unusual presentation of heart failure. Could it have been diagnosed at the initial ED visit? The only objective clue was the cardiomegaly found on CXR. Often, positive findings on physical exam or testing will require additional history from the patient; re-questioning the patient about SOB or dyspnea with exertion may have yielded a different answer, prompting an ECG or BNP level at the initial visit.

The ECG would likely have shown changes, though probably would not have been diagnostic. Cardiac enzymes would have probably been negative. The BNP would have been elevated, and may have prompted earlier intervention, with a diagnosis of new onset HF and admission to the hospital for monitoring and echocardiogram.

Documentation on the initial chart of the follow up plan is important for medicolegal reasons and was well done in this case. Unfortunately, this documentation did not help the patient. He had an atypical presentation of an extremely serious illness, and it is difficult to speculate if anything could have been done to change the eventual outcome.

TEACHING POINTS ABOUT CASE 15:
- An interpreter should be offered to patients who are not able to communicate their history adequately.
- Positive unexpected findings on the physical exam or with other testing will often require further history. This should be documented in the chart with times recorded.
- Patients and physicians may have different understanding of "shortness of breath." Just as we ask patients about chest *discomfort* in addition to chest *pain*, we may want to ask patients about *dyspnea* in several different ways.

REFERENCES
1. Stapczynski JS. Respiratory distress. In: Tintinalli J, ed. Emergency medicine: a comprehensive study guide. 6th ed. New York:McGraw-Hill, 2004:437-45.
2. Gonzales R, Bartlett JG, Besser RE, et al. Principles of appropriate antibiotic use for treatment of acute respiratory tract infections in adults: background, specific aims, and methods. Ann Intern Med 2001; 134: 479-86.

3. Stein PD, Willis PW, DeMets DL, et al. History and physical examination in acute pulmonary embolism in patients without preexisting cardiac or pulmonary disease. Am J Cardiol 1981; 47:218-23.

4. Schmitt B, Kusher M, Wiener S. The diagnostic usefulness of history of the patient with dyspnea. J Gen Intern Med 1986; 1:386-93.

5. Mulrow C, Lucey C, Farnett L. Discriminating causes of dyspnea through the clinical examination. J Gen Intern Med 1993; 8:383-92.

6. Sinex JE. Pulse oximetry: principles and limitations. Am J Emerg Med 1999; 17:59-67.

7. Kline JA. Dyspnea: fear, loathing, and physiology. Emerg Med Prac 1999;1:1-20.

8. National Asthma Education and Prevention Program Expert Panel Report 2: Guidelines for the diagnosis and management of asthma. NIH pub. No. 02-5074, June 2003.

9. D'Urzo A, Jugovic P. Chronic cough: three most common causes. Can Fam Physician 2002; 48:1311.

10. Hunt SA, Baker DW, et al. ACC/AHA guidelines for the evaluation and management of chronic heart failure in the adult: a report of the American College of Cardiology/American Heart Association task force on practice guidelines (Committee to revise the 1995 guidelines for the evaluation and management of heart failure). 2001. American College of Cardiology web site. Available at: http://www.acc.org/clinical/guidelines/failure/hf_index.htm

11. Massie BM, Shah NB. Evolving trends in the epidemiologic factors of heart failure: Rationale for preventive strategies and comprehensive disease management. Am Heart J 1997; 133:703-12.

12. Gheorghiade M, Bonow RO. Chronic heart failure in the United States: a manifestation of coronary artery disease. Circulation 1998; 97:282-9.

13. Petrie MC. It cannot be cardiac failure because the heart is not enlarged on the chest x-ray. Eur J Heart Fail 2003; 5:117-9.

14. Davie AP, Davie AP, Francis CM, et al. Value of the electrocardiogram in identifying heart failure due to left ventricular systolic dysfunction. BMJ 1996; 312(7025):222.

15. Maisel AS, Krishnaswamy P, Nowak RM, et al. Rapid measurement of b-type natriuretic peptide in the emergency diagnosis of heart failure. N Engl J Med 2002; 347:161-7.

16. Morrison LK, Harrison A, Krishnaswamy P, et al, Utility of a rapid b-natriuretic peptide assay in differentiating congestive heart failure from lung disease in patients presenting with dyspnea. J Am Coll Card 2002; 39:202-9.

17. Schwam E. B-type natriuretic peptide for diagnosis of heart failure in emergency department patients: a critical appraisal. Acad Emerg Med 2004;11:686-91.

18. Ander DS, Jaggi M, Rivers E, et al. Undetected cardiogenic shock in patients with congestive heart failure presenting to the emergency department. Am J Cardiol 1998; 82:888-91.

19. Barron HV, Every NR, Parsons LS, et al. Investigators in the National Registry of Myocardial Infarction 2. Am Heart J 2001; 141:933-9.

20. Hollenberg SM, Kavinsky CJ, Parrillo JE. Cardiogenic shock. Ann Intern Med 1999; 131:47-59.

21. Kosowsky JM, Kobayashi L. Acutely decompensated heart failure: diagnostic and therapeutic strategies for the new millennium. Emerg Med Prac 2002; 2:1-28.

22. Overwalder PJ. Intra Aortic Balloon Pump (IABP) Counterpulsation. Internet J Thor Cardiovascular Surg. 1999; 2(2). Available at http://www.rjmatthewsmd.com/Definitions/IABP_Counterpulsation.htm

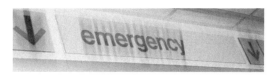

CASE16
46 YEAR OLD MALE WITH NECK & UPPER BACK PAIN

Commentary:
Gregory L. Henry, MD, FACEP

CEO, Medical Practice Risk Assessment, Inc., Ann Arbor, Michigan
Clinical Professor, Department of Emergency Medicine,
   University of Michigan Medical School, Ann Arbor, Michigan
Past President, American College of Emergency Physicians (ACEP)

Discussion:
Ed Boudreau, DO, FACEP, FAAEM

Vice President, Medical Affairs
Chief Medical Officer
Attending Physician Emergency Department
   Mount Carmel St. Ann's Hospital
   Westerville, Ohio

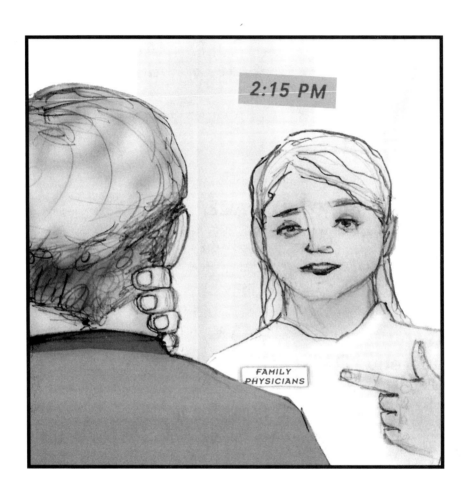

46 YEAR OLD MALE WITH
NECK & UPPER BACK PAIN

—Initial Visit*—

*Authors' Note: The history, exam and notes are the actual documentation of the physicians and providers, including abbreviations (and spelling errors)

CHIEF COMPLAINT (at 23:28): Back pain

VITAL SIGNS

Time	Temp	Pulse	Resp	Syst	Diast	Pain
23:30	96.4	87	18	166	94	7-8
01:22		80	18	146	86	

HISTORY OF PRESENT ILLNESS (at 00:28): Pt has had left sided neck and trapezius pain for two days now. He thinks he slept on it "funny". He has not had any direct trauma. No numbness, tingling, or weakness of the extremities. He saw his family doctor today who prescribed Skelaxin and Bextra for a muscle spasm. He has taken these without any relief. No fever, wt. change, visual changes, cp, sob, edema, cough, n/v/d, abd. pain, urinary symptoms, HA, weakness, loc, rash.

PAST MEDICAL HISTORY/TRIAGE:
  Medications: Bextra, Skelaxin, Percocet, Valium
  Allergies: No known allergies.
  PMH: None
  PSH: Cholecystectomy, Tonsillectomy
  SocHx: Tobacco use: (+), Alcohol use: (+)

EXAM (at 00:29):
  General: Alert and oriented X3, well-nourished, well appearing, in no apparent distress
  Head: Normocephalic; atraumatic.
  Eyes: PERRL
  Neck: Increased muscle spasm left trapezius region, no midline neck tenderness, no step off or crepitance. No ecchymosis or erythema.
  Nose: The nose is normal in appearance without rhinorrhea
  Resp: Normal chest excursion with respiration; breath sounds clear and equal bilaterally; no wheezes, rhonchi, or rales
  Card: Regular rhythm, without murmurs, rub or gallop
  Abd: Non-distended; non-tender, soft, without rigidity, rebound or guarding
  Skin: Normal for age and race; warm and dry; no apparent lesions

ORDERS:
C-spine series, Ibuprofen 600mg PO, Lortab 5mg PO to go, Valium 5mg PO to go

RESULTS:

Cervical spine series, five views: Degenerative findings at C4-5 and C5-6. No acute osseous abnormalities are identified.

DIAGNOSIS (at 01:27): Acute Cervical/trapezius strain

DISPOSITION: The patient was discharged to Home ambulatory accompanied by self with prescriptions for Vicodin (12) and Valium (10). After care instructions for cervical strain. Follow up with PCP in 2 days. He was released from the ED at 01:45.

Gregory L. Henry comments:

"Plain x-rays of the cervical spine may go the way of the nickel coke and the buffalo"

This patient's chief complaint is common. Aching in the neck and upper back area is often due to a musculoskeletal etiology. Who amongst us has not gotten up in the morning and felt some mild soreness in the back or neck? The history was well taken with a good review of symptoms including numbness, tingling, and weakness. Lack of response to muscle relaxants is not uncommon. The patient had no other systemic complaints, which makes a definitive diagnosis very difficult.

The evaluation seems typical for an emergency department. He has very little in his past medical history to suggest a more serious illness.

Parenthetically, the ordering of C-spine films seems useless. He had no neurologic findings or neurologic complaints. Without trauma, it is unlikely that any useful information will be obtained from plain x-rays. In addition, x-rays can be misleading; mild degenerative changes do not necessarily equate to specific neck symptoms. We are entering an era where plain films of the neck are probably a waste of time; if you believe that someone may have an occult fracture, the CT scan is a much better study. Also, if there is thought of spinal cord involvement, MRI is the study of choice. Plain x-rays of the cervical spine may go the way of the nickel coke and the buffalo.

I think "diagnosis" would be much better phrased as a "diagnostic impression," or "current impression," because the final diagnosis is rarely made in the emergency department. This visit seems like a typical musculoskeletal visit - the patient was well evaluated and given reasonable therapy. Documentation is good and the follow-up time of two days is excellent.

- Thoroughness of documentation: 9 out of 10.

- Thoroughness of patient evaluation: 10 out of 10.

(Additional comments and risk management ratings follow...)

46 YEAR OLD MALE WITH NECK & UPPER BACK PAIN

—Second Visit: 3 Days Later—

CHIEF COMPLAINT (at 14:49): Back pain

VITAL SIGNS

Time	Temp	Pulse	Resp	Syst	Diast	Pain scale
14:51	99.2	121	14	178	100	
16:48	103.2	116	20	160	80	7
17:30	103.1	117	20	180	78	7
19:17		128	16	167	92	
20:02	99.9	108	20	152	78	10
22:22		114	20	160	96	0
23:03	100.9	118	20	159	102	
01:59		104	16	137	84	6

HISTORY OF PRESENT ILLNESS (documented at 05:40 the next morning): This forty-six-year-old white male comes to the emergency dept. complaining of intense upper back pain that radiates down through his low back. He was seen at a local urgent care 2 days ago and diagnosed with cervical muscle spasm and cervical arthritis and prescribed Percocet. He was seen again at urgent care yesterday and had a normal CXR and was diagnosed with a back strain and prescribed Valium. He states that approximately three days ago he had onset of atraumatic back pain between his shoulders that seemed to radiate around to the right side along the lateral aspect of his neck. It has progressively worsened and radiates across his shoulders with pain and numbness down to his elbows bilaterally but no farther. His pain also radiates down his back to his low back. He also states that he had some saddle anesthesia, although he has had no loss of bowel or bladder function or weakness in his legs. He states that he has had chills, but no documented fever. He rates his pain at 10 out of 10 at this time, sharp, stabbing, constant. He was seen by his family doctor three days ago and had neck and back x-rays which were unremarkable. He has had Percocet and Valium, which has given him minimal relief. He states that he does have a headache at this time, but his primary pain is in his upper back. He has had some nausea, but no vomiting. No photophobia, rash, chest pain, shortness of breath, cough or hemoptysis, abdominal pain, diarrhea, bloody or black stool. He denies any loss of function in his extremities, but his pain seems minimally worsened when he moves his arms, but he states that it is so intense there is little he can do to get into a comfortable position. He has never had any problems like this before. He denies any history of trauma. He has had no recent travel. No preceeding illnesses. Has an MRI scheduled in 5 days per his PCP.

PAST MEDICAL HISTORY/TRIAGE (at 14:52):
Medications: Bextra, Skelaxin, Percocet, Valium

Allergies: No known allergies.
PMH: None
PSH: Cholecystectomy, Tonsillectomy
SocHx: Tobacco use: (+), Alcohol use: (+)

EXAM (documented at 05:40 the next morning):

General: This is a forty-six-year-old white male who is awake, alert, conversant, and sitting up in bed. He is wincing in pain, clearly uncomfortable. He is not able to really get comfortable in bed. He is able to answer my questions, but is clearly distracted by his pain.

HEENT: Head is normocephalic and atraumatic.

Ears: Clear. No hemotympanum.

Eyes: Pupils equal, round, and reactive to light. EOM grossly intact.

Nose: Symmetric and nontender.

Nares: Patent.

Mouth: Oropharynx is clear. Uvula is midline. Airway is patent. No evidence of dysphonia.

Neck: Supple. He has tenderness along the left lateral aspect of his neck. There is some minimal swelling, but no lymphadenopathy noted. He is nontender over the midline posteriorly in the cervical spine, except for some tenderness just at the base of the neck.

Cardiovascular: Rate and rhythm are regular. No murmurs, rubs or gallops.

Lungs: Clear. No wheezes or rales. He has good air movement to the lateral bases.

Abdomen: Soft and nontender. He has good bowel sounds.

Integumentary: He is quite tan. He has been in a tanning booth apparently.

Neurologic: Cranial nerves II-XII are grossly intact. He is able to move all extremities without difficulty, although he does have pain. He has negative pronator drift with good finger-to-nose coordination. He is able to ambulate. He has 5/5 grip upper arm and lower extremity strength and is able to differentiate between sharp and dull sensation through his upper extremities.

INITIAL ORDERS:

At 15:58 Dilaudid 2mg and phenergan 12.5mg

RESULTS (at 16:51):

Test	Flag	Value	Units	Ref. range
WBC		8.5	K/uL	4.6-10.2
HGB		14.8	G/DL	13.5-17.5
PLT		170	K/uL	142-424
NA		140	MMOL/L	135-144
K		4.3	MMOL/L	3.5-5.1
CL		102	MMOL/L	98-107
CO2		27	MMOL/L	22-29
BUN		8	MG/DL	7-18
CREAT		1.1	MG/DL	0.6-1.3

(continued on next page)

```
Test    Flag   Value    Units       Ref. range
CKMB           0.2      NG/ML       0.0-5.0
TROPI          11       NG/ML       .00-.27

WSR     H      30       MM/HR       0-15
```

UNENHANCED BRAIN CT: There is some nonspecific, small, focal lacunar-type low density areas in the right basal ganglia and periventricular white matter.

PROGRESS NOTES (at 16:59): Recheck of temperature at 103.2 degrees. Will start rocephin 1 gram IVPB and give tylenol 975mg PO

(at 17:37): Discussed with radiology obtaining MRI. Pt. in excruciating pain of the cervical, thoracic, and lumbar spine. I called primary care physician and discussed obtaining MRI - he requests cervical, thoracic, and lumbar MRI to evaluate for transverse myelitis. I was informed by MRI that they would not do all three segments. I had lengthy discussion with radiology, and he indicates no emergent indication for the same and states to do lumbar MRI to evaluate possible cord compression. I spoke with the neurologist twice, PCP once, ID consultant once and neurosurgeon once. In addition, I spoke with radiology multiple times, eventually convincing them to perform MRI scans as previously stated.

RADIOLOGY (at 21:05):

MRI of the thoracic spine: There is a tiny, left T9-10 disc protrusion.

MRI of the lumbar spine: Degenerative disc disease is present at L5-S1 with this contributing to some mild to moderate lateral recess stenosis bilaterally.

MRI cervical spine without and with contrast: Very unusual case. There appears to be compression of the cord between approximately C3 and C6 by a mixture of pathology including degenerative change, possible disk protrusions, but also some inflammatory change (less likely neoplastic change), which is resulting in fairly prominent epidural enhancement circumferentially in the canal and also is probably related to the prevertebral soft tissue swelling and enhancement that is present in the back of the pharynx from about C1 to C6.

ADDITIONAL PROGRESS NOTES (at 22:15): After return of the MRI results, I have started Clindamycin 900mg, Decadron 10mg and given additional dilaudid 1mg.

DIAGNOSIS
1. Spinal cord compression
2. Acute paravertebral soft-tissue infection versus abscess

DISPOSITION: Transferred to the OR at 02:07.

HOSPITAL COURSE:

Per neurosurgeon: An emergent cervical spine MRI showed spinal cord compression from what appeared to be a cervical epidural abscess. In the ER, he progressed to develop fever up to 103 despite a normal white count. While in the ER, he progressed also with left-sided weakness and at that time, I talked to his wife and him about surgery to decompress his spinal cord emergently. I told them I thought this most likely was an abscess, although I did not know the source and it may not indeed be abscess. I talked to them about the risks of surgery including paralysis, transient or permanent, failure to diffuse, breakage of instrumentation, and need for further surgery. They requested that we proceed.

Postoperative diagnosis: Cervical epidural abscess C3-C4, C4-C5, C5-C6 with spinal cord compression, myelopathy, left hemiparesis. The patient was extubated in surgery and awoken moving all 4s. His left-sided weakness appeared to be stronger than preoperatively, although he remains with some mild hand weakness.

Infectious disease consultation: Blood cultures returned positive for staph and it is sensitive to everything except penicillin. Intraoperative aerobic and anaerobic cultures of the abscess have all returned negative. Patient denied any skin lesions, recent infections or recent travel. He does relate now that he had fractured his toe approximately three weeks ago on the left foot, fifth toe. He states that this was red and swollen.

Disposition: He left the hospital in good condition with minimal residual left sided weakness.

FINAL DIAGNOSIS: Cervical peidural abscess with spinal cord compression

Additional comments by Gregory L. Henry:

The second visit three days later is nothing short of excellent; the ED physician immediately picked up on the saddle anesthesia. Despite the lack of urinary tract symptoms, they were properly impressed with both the fever and the anatomic nature of the complaints, and proceeded with an MRI. This patient owes his neurologic functioning to the rapid work of the emergency physicians who stepped up to the plate. This is a once-in-a-lifetime case.

The patient denied drug use; in my experience drug shooters are the most likely group to have these problems. The number of times you will pick up an epidural abscess, particularly in a non-drug user, is incredibly small. Whether a previous cut on his toe actually had anything to do with this is impossible to say, but my congratulations to the emergency physicians who turned in a superior performance.

Rare disease occurs rarely. This patient is one of the luckier people alive. It was only through the persistence of good emergency personnel that his problem was discovered and appropriately managed.

- **Risk of Serious Illness Being Missed:** Initially high-risk, but fortunately made low-risk by persistent examination.

- **Risk Management Legal Rating:** Potentially high-risk case.

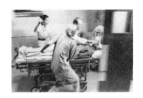

ATRAUMATIC NECK PAIN AND DIAGNOSIS/MANAGEMENT OF SPINAL EPIDURAL ABSCESS

Ed Boudreau, DO, FACEP, FAAEM

I. OVERVIEW

Who hasn't seen a patient presenting like the first visit? This case typifies the randomness of our specialty. The outcome of the second visit could have been very different; whoever picked up that second chart was pulled into a swirling rush that could have easily gone down the drain. Only a consistent and methodical approach to the evaluation of neck pain prevented a disastrous outcome.

A second, but equally important, point is the importance of patient advocacy—demonstrated by the ED physician during the second visit. The difficulty in obtaining the appropriate diagnostic test is highlighted in the documentation; pursuit of appropriate evaluation is often our most frustrating work. Emergency physicians must be positioned to obtain appropriate testing before the patient walks in the door; time spent negotiating with technologists and other physicians when life or limb are on the line is time wasted.

II. EPIDEMIOLOGY AND DIFFERENTIAL DIAGNOSIS OF NONTRAUMATIC NECK PAIN

The annual incidence of neck pain ranges from 11% to 18%. Short and long term morbidity are difficult to predict—within 12 months one third of patients will experience complete resolution while another one-third will have partial resolution. Women are 1.7 times more likely to suffer neck pain than men, and are also more likely to have persistent pain.[1] Causes of non-traumatic neck pain are listed in Table 1:

Table 1. Differential Diagnosis of Non-traumatic Neck Pain

Biomechanical	Infectious	Referred	Neurologic	Rheumatologic	Neoplastic	Other
Neck strain	Osteomyelitis	Thoracic outlet	Brachial	Rheumatoid arthritis	Osteoblastoma	Sarcoidosis
Herniated disc	Discitis	syndrome	plexus injury	Ankylosing spondylitis	Osteochondroma	Paget's
Spondylosis	Meningitis	Pancoast's	Peripheral	Psoriatic arthritis	Giant cell tumor	disease
Myelopathy	Herpes zoster	tumor	entrapment	Reiter's syndrome	Hemangioma	
	Lyme disease	Esophagitis	Neuropathies	Polymyalgia rheumatica	Metastases	
	Thyroiditis	Angina	Reflex	Fibromyalgia	Multiple myeloma	
	Epidural abscess	Vascular	sympathetic	Myofascial pain	Chordoma	
		dissection	dystrophy		Gliomas	
			(RSD)		Chondrosarcoma	
					Syringomyelia	
					Neurofibroma	

Adapted from Borenstein DG. Management of neck pain: a primary care approach. Hospital practice. George Washington University. Available at http://72.14.207.104/search?q=cache: SJfKK-SB0boJ:www.hosppract.com/issues/1998/10/boren.htm+&hl=en&lr=&strip=1

III. EVALUATION OF NECK PAIN—HISTORY

The evaluation begins with a careful history; key features include time of onset, location, character, duration, and exacerbating and relieving factors. Patients are commonly vague about the onset of their pain and should be specifically questioned about a history of trauma or strenuous activity (occupation, hobbies, athletic activities). Inquire about history of similar discomfort, results of previous evaluations, and success or failure of previous therapies.

Neurologic symptoms including weakness, paresthesias, or change in gait may be present. Ask about radiation of pain (Table 2), fever, anorexia, and weight loss. Past history should include history of arthritis, cancer, infections, recent surgical procedures, endocarditis, and diabetes. Social history may reveal history of injection drug use.

IV. EVALUATION OF NECK PAIN—PHYSICAL EXAM

Physical examination begins with observation of the patient. The facial expression often reveals the level of discomfort. During normal conversation most people will move their head and neck in a characteristic manner, but with substantial neck pain movement may be reduced or absent. Inspection may reveal presence of zoster.

Passive range of motion for flexion, extension, and rotation establishes the level of flexibility. Palpation of the neck may reveal presence of neck mass, lymphadenopathy, thyroid masses or enlargement, tenderness of the carotid artery, and areas of maximal tenderness in the neck. Check for carotid pulses, bruits, or palpable thrills. Palpation should also include the parotid glands, submandibular glands, and the clavicular and cranial insertions of the sternocleidomastoid muscles. Range of motion testing for the temporomandibular joint may elicit crepitus, pain, or some evidence of joint malfunction. The cervical paraspinal musculature may elicit areas of focal tenderness or spasm. Cranial nerves should also be evaluated.

Interestingly, an examination of the upper extremities was not documented on this patient's first visit. Both upper and lower extremities should be tested for weakness, pain or light touch sensation, reflex abnormalities, and position sense. Vibratory sensation may play an important role in assessing potential metabolic abnormalities.

The completion of the neurologic evaluation may include detailed lower extremity evaluation. Gait abnormalities, proprioceptive difficulties, or sensory abnormalities may help focus decision making. Changes in sensation should be identified and mapped to the dermatome involved (Table 2). Changes in bowel or bladder habits, or abnormal sensation of the perineum, should prompt a rectal exam for evaluation of sphincter tone.

Table 2. Signs and Symptoms of Cervical Radiculopathy

Disk Space	Cervical Root	Pain Complaint	Sensory Abnormality	Motor Weakness	Altered Reflex
C1-C2	C2	Neck, scalp	Scalp		
C4-C5	C5	Neck, shoulder, upper arm	Shoulder	Infraspinatus, deltoid, biceps	Reduced biceps reflex
C5-C6	C6	Neck, shoulder, upper medial, scapular area, proximal forearm, thumb, index finger	Thumb and index finger, lateral forearm	Deltoid, biceps, pronator teres, wrist extensors	Reduced biceps and brachioradialis reflex
C6-C7	C7	Neck, posterior arm, dorsum proximal forearm, chest, medial third of scapula, middle finger	Middle finger, forearm	Triceps, pronator teres	Reduced triceps reflex
C7-T1	C8	Neck, posterior arm, ulnar side of forearm, medial inferior scapular border, medial hand, ring, and little fingers	Ring and little fingers	Triceps, flexor carpi ulnaris, hand intrinsics	Reduced triceps reflex

Source: Frohna W. Neck pain. In Tintinalli JE, ed. Emergency medicine: a comprehensive study guide. 6th ed. New York:McGraw-Hill, 2004;1769-73. Used with permission.

Because the case under consideration involves atraumatic neck pain, it seems reasonable to focus on this arm of the evaluation algorithm (figure 1). The reader interested in evaluating cervical trauma is referred to the following references:

- Hoffman JR, et al. Validity of a set of clinical criteria to rule out injury to the cervical spine in patients with blunt trauma. N Engl J Med 2000;343:94
- Dickinson G, et al. Retrospective application of the nexus low-risk criteria for cervical spine radiography in canadian emergency departments. Ann Emerg Med 2004; 43:507

V. EVALUATION OF NECK PAIN—DIAGNOSTICS

History and physical should answer the following questions: Is the pain acute or chronic? If the pain is chronic, then is the pain stable? If the pain is stable, then pain management should be the goal. If the pain is acute, or different then their chronic pain, ask the question: "Is there a medical condition contributing to the neck pain?" which may include extra-axial causes such as pulmonary, cardiac or gastrointestinal diseases.[5] Infectious causes include vertebral osteomyelitis, diskitis, paraspinal abscesses, and epidural abscess. Patients with infections of the vertebral spine and/or diskitis (when present without an epidural abscess) usually will not manifest spinal cord symptoms such as radiculopathy and weakness. Patients with unexplained fever and back pain should have an MRI to rule out a spinal infection, as MRI is more sensitive than CT.[10] If infection is suspected, blood cultures, lumbar puncture, and presumptive antibiotic therapy should be considered. If a cardiac or pulmonary etiology is suspected, directed evaluation should be performed.

If radicular symptoms or spinal cord dysfunction is present, imaging is the next critical step. In selecting an imaging modality, access and cost, as well as the speed at which the patient may deteriorate, are critical decision-making factors. MRI is superior to CT or myelography for identification of spinal cord compression.[10] Lesions are often seen before irreversible neurologic events occur, allowing preservation of function with intervention. Spinal cord compression is the most common indication for emergent MRI.[6] Clearly, the days of plain radiographs to evaluate neck pain are passing, but CT and myelography may continue to play a role when MRI is not readily available.

Figure 1. Evaluation of neck pain algorithm

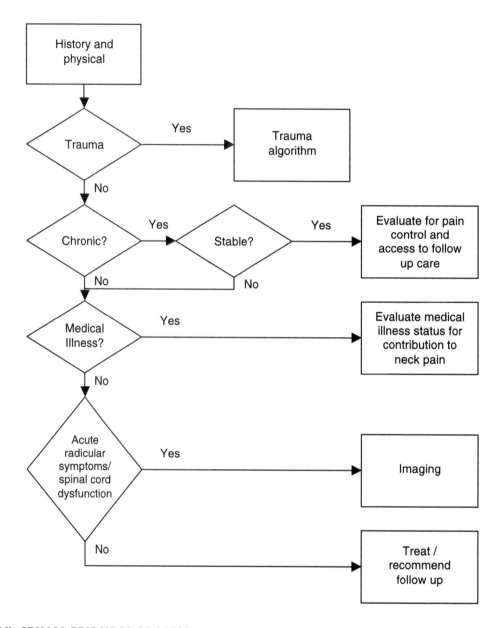

VI. SPINAL EPIDURAL ABSCESS

The emergency physician on the second visit could finish his shift knowing that their tenacity saved this patient further disability or even death. This patient had epidural compression caused by spinal abscess; other causes of epidural compression include spinal canal hemorrhage, tumors, and massive midline disk herniation.[3]

Spinal epidural abscess is a rare ailment, thought to occur in 0.2 to 1.2 cases for every 10,000 hospital admissions, but increasing since 1988 due to the increase in intravenous drug use and invasive spinal procedures.[11] Advances in technology have enabled identification of small lesions that may have gone unrecognized previously. Though initially described in the 16th century, the classic presentation of epidural abscess was presented by Heusner in 1948, and his observations regarding progression remain viable today.[7]

In a 1999 study by Rigamonti et al., a records review of 75 patients diagnosed with spinal epidural abscess at the University of Maryland from 1983-1992, found 64% of patients were male, with an average age of 50.7 years (range of 3 months to 83 years). Concomitant conditions included intravenous drug use (33%), diabetes mellitus (27%), and prior spinal surgery (17%).[11] Other predisposing factors include history of malignancy, obesity, HIV/AIDS, end-stage renal disease, urinary tract infection, cellulitis, endocarditis, dental abscess, pneumonia, and chronic steroid use.[4]

Reviews as far back as 1975 site *Staphylococcus aureus* as a predominant organism in epidural abscess, seeded by hematogenous spread. Khana in 1996 also listed *Streptococcus viridans, Streptococcus pyogenes,* and *Escherichia coli* as causative organisms.[4] Kaufman et al.,[9] reported that Mycobacterium tuberculosis accounts for 25% of infections. H. parainfluenzae and Brucella species have also been reported. Those who are immunocompromised are at risk of developing Cryptococcus, Aspergillus, or Blastomyces.[10]

Distinguishing factors on history and physical exam include back or neck pain, progressive neurologic deficit, and low grade fever, but presentations vary. Fever is present in 30% to 60% of cases. In the series by Rigamonti, 29% of the patients had no motor deficit at presentation.[11] Urinary retention with overflow incontinence has a sensitivity of 90% and specificity of 95%.[12] Sciatica in one or both legs, weakness of the extremities, gait difficulty, or abnormal straight leg raise testing may be present[3]. The patient may have symptoms for weeks to months before the correct diagnosis is established.

The "classic triad" of localized back pain, progressive neurological deficit and fever is not commonly encountered; one series reported its presence in only 37% of cases.[11] McKenzie states that "spinal pain and fever are usually the only symptoms present before a precipitous neurologic deterioration occurs, and were the only features in two of our patients."[10]

As with many clinical illnesses, the value of the total white blood cell count is highly variable. However, the erythrocyte sedimentation rate (ESR) is very often elevated.[3,8,13] In the large series by Rigamonti, ESR was elevated in all patients with an acute presentation, with a mean ESR of 51 (2 patients with a chronic clinical course had normal ESR).[13] Blood cultures are positive in over 40% of patients with abscess.[3] It is unusual to have a spinal infection without either a fever or elevated ESR. An epidural abscess is best visualized by MRI. Additionally, the soft tissues, spinal cord, intervertebral discs and paraspinal muscles are well visualized.

Prognosis is heavily dependent on comorbid conditions. Advanced patient age and degree of thecal sac compression are associated with poor outcome.[4] Early diagnosis and appropriate management (surgery and antibiotics) are associated with improved prognosis, though symptom duration is not a fool proof predictor of outcome. Patients with neurologic deficits over 12 hours old rarely recovered, and those with paralysis over 36 hours often died. The mortality rate is approximately 14%.[10]

The cornerstone of management is acute surgical intervention followed by IV antibiotics, however, some patients can be managed without surgery.[13]

VII. SUMMARY

Though the physician encountered resistance in obtaining the necessary diagnostic testing, persistence paid off for this patient. If they had not stood their ground, and sent the patient home with a prescription for symptom relief, this case would likely have had a catastrophic outcome. A high index of suspicion for spinal epidural abscess needs to be maintained for patients with severe back or neck pain with a fever or markedly elevated ESR.

TEACHING POINTS ABOUT CASE 16:

- You will see a spinal epidural abscess in your career; pain out of proportion to the physical findings should heighten your suspicion for this diagnosis.
- These patients are not all febrile, though ESR is almost universally elevated.
- Do not let the radiologist tell you " no," when your gut tells you "yes."

REFERENCES

1. Cote P, Cassidy JD, Carroll LJ, et al. The annual incidence and course of neck pain in the general population: a population-based cohort study. Pain 2004; 112:267-73.
2. Borenstein DG. Management of neck pain: a primary care approach. Hospital practice. George Washington University. Available at http://72.14.207.104/search?q=cache:SJfKK-SB0boJ:www.hosppract.com/issues/1998/10/boren.htm+&hl=en&lr=&strip=1
3. Della-Giustina D, Coppola M. Thoracic and lumbar pain syndromes. In: Tintinalli J, ed. Emergency medicine: a comprehensive study guide. 6th ed. New York:McGraw-Hill, 2004;1769-73.
4. Khanna RK, Malik GM, Rock JP, et al. Spinal epidural abscess: evaluation of factors influencing outcome. Neurosurgery 1996; 39:958-64.
5. Gerber O, Heyer EJ, Vieux U. Painless dissections of the aorta presenting as acute neurologic syndromes.Stroke1986;17:644-7.
6. Quint DJ. Indications for emergent MRI of the central nervous system. JAMA 2000; 283:853-55.
7. Baker AS, Ojemann RG, Swartz MN, et al. Spinal epidural abscess. N Engl J Med 1975; 293:463-8.
8. Sampath P, Rigamonti D. Spinal epidural abscess: a review of epidemiology, diagnosis, and treatment. J. Spinal Disorders 1999; 12:89-93.
9. Kaufman, DM. Infectious agents in spinal epidural abscess. Neurology 1980; 30:844-50.
10. Mackenzie AR, Laing RB, Smith CC, et al. Spinal epidural abscess: the importance of early diagnosis and treatment. J Neurol Neurosurg Psychiatry 1998; 65:209-12.
11. Rigamonti D, Liem L, Sampath P, et al. Spinal epidural abscess: contemporary trends in etiology, evaluation, and management. Surg Neuro 1999; 52:189-97.
12. Deyo RA, Rainville J, Kent DL. What can the history and physical examination tell us about low back pain? JAMA 1992; 268:760-5.
13. Frohna W. Neck pain. In Tintinalli JE, ed. Emergency medicine: a comprehensive study guide. 6th ed. New York:McGraw-Hill, 2004;1769-73.

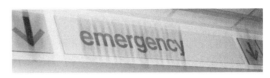

CASE 17
82 YEAR OLD FEMALE WITH GENERALIZED WEAKNESS

Commentary:
Gregory L. Henry, MD, FACEP

CEO, Medical Practice Risk Assessment, Inc., Ann Arbor, Michigan
Clinical Professor, Department of Emergency Medicine
   University of Michigan Medical School, Ann Arbor, Michigan
Past President, American College of Emergency Physicians (ACEP)

Discussion:
Ryan Longstreth, MD, FACEP

Attending ED Physician
   Mt. Carmel St. Ann's Emergency Department, Westerville, Ohio
Assistant ED Director, St. Ann's Emergency Department

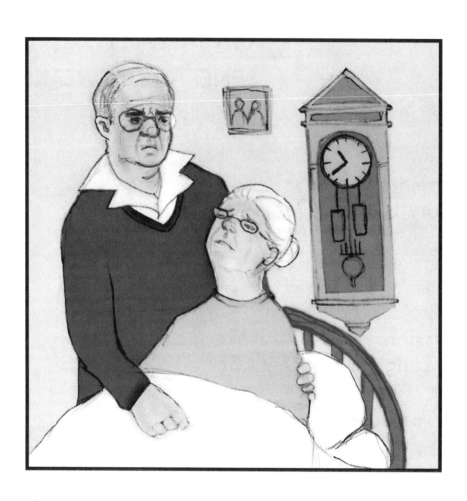

82 YEAR OLD FEMALE WITH GENERALIZED WEAKNESS

—Initial Visit*—

*Authors' Note: The history, exam and notes are the actual documentation of the physicians and providers, including abbreviations (and spelling errors)

CHIEF COMPLAINT (at 20:22): Weakness

Time	Temp(F)	Rt.	Pulse	Resp	Syst	Diast	Pos.	O2 sat	O2%
20:28	97.6	T	92	22	146	65	L	100	RA
21:25			86		129	59	L	100	RA
22:15			86	20	124	59	L	100	RA
00:07			92	20	135	58	L	100	RA

HISTORY OF PRESENT ILLNESS (at 20:53): 82 y/o female presents with generalized weakness for past week. She lives with her husband and she has not been able to get out of bed for last 5 days. Family states she has not eaten in 5 days. Her mental status is slightly depressed compared with baseline per family members here. She does complain of SOB. No CP, abdominal pain, vomiting, diarrhea, fever, chest pain, cough, rhinorrhea, dysuria, HA, rash, blurred vision, LAN.

PAST MEDICAL HISTORY/TRIAGE:
Allergies: NKDA
Current meds: Prinivil, Metoprolol, Lisinopril, and Nitroglycerin
Past medical history: Negative. Past surgical history: Hemorrhoidectomy.
Social history: She drinks 2 beers daily.

EXAM (at 20:57):
General: Alert and oriented X 2, appears dehydrated and mildly cachectic
Head: Normocephalic; atraumatic.
Eyes: PERRL
Nose: The nose is normal in appearance without rhinorrhea
Resp: Normal chest excursion with respiration; breath sounds clear and equal bilaterally; no wheezes, rhonchi, or rales
Card: Regular rhythm, without murmurs, rub or gallop
Abd: Non-distended; non-tender, soft, without rigidity, rebound or guarding
Skin: Normal for age and race; warm and dry; no apparent lesions
Neurological: Patient is alert and oriented times 2. Cranial nerves III-XII are intact. Sensory and motor functions are intact. Strength is 5/5 for flexion and extension in all 4 extremities. Patellar DTRs are equal and intact. Finger to nose testing is equal and normal bilaterally.

RESULTS (at 21:42)

Test	Flag	Value	Units	Ref. Range
WBC	H	11.8	K/uL	4.6-10.2
HGB		12.9	G/DL	12.0-16.0
PLT		312	K/uL	142-424

Test	Flag	Value	Units	Ref. Range
NA	L	129	MMOL/L	135-144
K	L	3.4	MMOL/L	3.5-5.1
CL	L	95	MMOL/L	98-107
AGAP	H	24.4	MMOL/L	6.0-18.0
CO2	L	13	MMOL/L	22-29
BUN	H	51	MG/DL	7-18
CREAT	H	1.4	MG/DL	0.6-1.3

Test	Flag	Value	Units	Ref. Range
CKH		310	U/L	21-232
CKMB	H	12.0	NG/ML	0.0-5.0
REL IND		3.9		0.0-4.0
TROP I		.01	NG/ML	.00-.27

Liver function tests: WNL

Accudata: Fingerstick blood sugar - 95.

Test	Flag	Value	Units	Ref range
DDIMERQUNT	*	>1000	NG/ML	<500
BNP		99	PG/ML	0-100
TSH CAS		1.66	uIU/ML	.34-4.82

Urinalysis - WNL

CXR: No acute cardiopulmonary disease.

Lung-vent/perf scan: No findings of pulmonary emboli are appreciated.

COMPUTED TOMOGRAPHY OF THE ABDOMEN WITH IV CONTRAST:
1. Large hiatus hernia with fundus of the stomach in the chest.
2. Nodule at the posterior left lung base behind the descending thoracic aorta, seen on only one image, of uncertain etiology.
3. Low position and slight malrotation to the right kidney seen in the upper pelvis.
4. No evidence for inflammatory bowel change. There is dilated rectum filled with stool, possibly indicating fecal impaction.
5. Soft tissue density related to the cecum but there is respiratory motion present. Cannot evaluate for possible mass.

DIAGNOSIS: 1. Dehydration, 2. Acidosis – metabolic, 3. Elevated CK - ?Rhabdo - vs - Acute Coronary Syndrome

DISPOSITION (at 22:33): Admit the patient to Telemetry bed

Gregory L. Henry comments:

"A confused patient constitutes a danger to themselves or others"

Nothing is worse than the elderly patient who is weak and dizzy… except a patient who has been weak and dizzy since 1917! Fortunately, this patient had a short interval of weakness and mental status change. These are difficult cases in the best of circumstances.

The history is taken from the husband as well as the patient. The evaluation of this patient is reasonable, except that we do not know the level of delirium or encephalopathy based on the documentation provided. Documentation states she is "alert and oriented X 2". What exactly does this mean? With an altered mental status, more specific documentation should be provided. No one has observed the patient's gait to see why she is having difficulty with ambulation. The documentation recorded: "Sensory and motor functions are intact. Strength is 5/5 for flexion and extension in all 4 extremities." This does not comport with someone who is supposedly weak.

The laboratory evaluation is thorough, supporting the maxim that the laboratory may bail you out of trouble, particularly in an elderly patient with a confused and indistinct story.

The physician did the right thing in admitting this patient; with an elevated BUN, creatinine, anion gap, and hyponatremia, further investigation is going to be required. A confused patient constitutes a danger to themselves or others.

- Thoroughness of documentation: 7 out of 10.

- Thoroughness of Patient Evaluation: 8 out of 10.

- Risk of Serious Illness Being Missed: Low risk.

- Risk Management Legal Rating: Low risk.

HOSPITAL COURSE:

********** Discharge Summary Report **********

The patient was admitted and was in the hospital for 7 days. Additional history revealed that for some time she had been taking large amounts of salicylate for hip pain and right ribcage pain. She came in with obtundation, mental status changes. She was found to be severely dehydrated and acidotic. Admitting blood work revealed anion-gap acidosis and a salicylate level which was 5 times normal. We hydrated her aggressively and, due to the fact that this was a chronic ingestion issue, we elected not to use activated charcoal at the time of her admission. Her anion-gap acidosis did improve over the ensuing 3-4 days with aggressive hydration. Her kidney function remained stable and intact. Her hyponatremia and renal failure also improved significantly with aggressive IV fluid administration. She had some elevated cardiac enzymes upon admission. Cardiology consultation was placed, but it was thought that these elevations were more likely to be due to muscular tissue breakdown. Two-dimensional echo was obtained and was unremarkable. Lower extremity venous doppler examination was normal. Her mental status was slow to improve. We started her on Zyprexa and had Psychiatry follow her while she was in the hospital. Their impression was that the delirium was multifactorial and that she may have an underlying baseline dementia.

She eventually became completely oriented and alert and was responding appropriately. Consultation was placed to Physical Therapy, who recommended short-term ECF for physical therapy.

FINAL DIAGNOSIS: Delerium secondary to chronic salicylate toxicity

Additional comments by Gregory L. Henry:

During the ED visit, she does not list aspirin as one of her medications. Families and patients should be specifically queried as to nonprescription medications. Patients often feel that, unless they have purchased a prescription drug, they are not truly on medication. Nothing could be further from the truth!

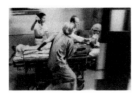

EVALUATION OF THE POISONED PATIENT, MANAGEMENT OF ACETAMINOPHEN AND SALICYLATE TOXICITIES

Ryan Longstreth, MD, FACEP

I. GENERAL APPROACH TO THE POISONED PATIENT

In 1999, there were approximately 2.2 million toxic exposures reported to the American Association of Poison Control Centers.[1] Approximately 75% were exposures in the home, and over 50% of these were in patients under the age of 18. Between 1985 and 1999, the incidence of toxin related deaths in the US increased by over 300%.[2]

What makes a "poison" poisonous? A toxin may produce its effects by altering normal cellular or organ function or by interfering with an organism's ability to uptake substances for normal body processes.

As with all potentially ill patients, the initial management must start with the ABCs. The patient's airway, breathing, and circulation must first be stabilized before further managing the specific ingestion.

If the patient is noted to have an altered mental status, then remember **"DONT"** (the coma cocktail), which stands for **D**extrose, **O**xygen, **N**arcan, and **T**hiamine. In this case, the first interventions performed were an Accucheck and a pulse ox. If the patient is hypoglycemic, then the average adult may be given one ampule of D50. A rough pediatric estimate is 1 ampule of D10 for the neonate, and 1 ampule of D20 for the older child.

The patient's hypoxia is treated with 100% oxygen per nonrebreather mask. Narcan, given as a 0.4–2 mg intravenous bolus, is a safe and effective antidote for opiate toxicity. The dose of IV or IM thiamine is 100mg, and should be given before dextrose. Flumazenil (benzodiazepine antagonist) is not part of the coma cocktail since it may induce life-threatening seizures in the chronically benzodiazepine dependent patient. Table 1 provides a good overview for the management of the poisoned patient.

Table 1. Guide to the Management of Poisoned Patients

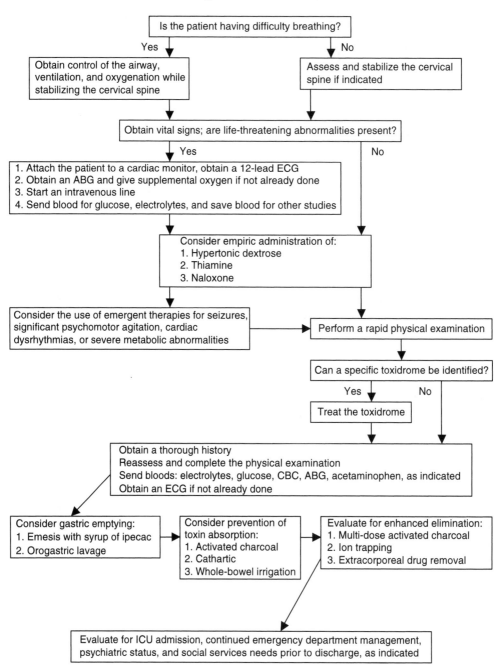

Is the patient having difficulty breathing?

Yes → Obtain control of the airway, ventilation, and oxygenation while stabilizing the cervical spine

No → Assess and stabilize the cervical spine if indicated

Obtain vital signs; are life-threatening abnormalities present?

Yes:
1. Attach the patient to a cardiac monitor, obtain a 12-lead ECG
2. Obtain an ABG and give supplemental oxygen if not already done
3. Start an intravenous line
4. Send blood for glucose, electrolytes, and save blood for other studies

No

Consider empiric administration of:
1. Hypertonic dextrose
2. Thiamine
3. Naloxone

Consider the use of emergent therapies for seizures, significant psychomotor agitation, cardiac dysrhythmias, or severe metabolic abnormalities

Perform a rapid physical examination

Can a specific toxidrome be identified?

Yes → Treat the toxidrome

No

Obtain a thorough history
Reassess and complete the physical examination
Send bloods: electrolytes, glucose, CBC, ABG, acetaminophen, as indicated
Obtain an ECG if not already done

Consider gastric emptying:
1. Emesis with syrup of ipecac
2. Orogastric lavage

Consider prevention of toxin absorption:
1. Activated charcoal
2. Cathartic
3. Whole-bowel irrigation

Evaluate for enhanced elimination:
1. Multi-dose activated charcoal
2. Ion trapping
3. Extracorporeal drug removal

Evaluate for ICU admission, continued emergency department management, psychiatric status, and social services needs prior to discharge, as indicated

Source: Goldfrank L. Goldfrank's toxicologic emergencies. 7th ed. New York:McGraw-Hill, 2002:38. Used with permission.

II. HISTORY AND PHYSICAL EXAM

Once the patient has been stabilized, a focused history should be obtained. Important aspects of the history include: 1) the type of toxin or toxins involved; 2) the time of exposure and whether it was acute or chronic; 3) the route of exposure (ingestion, inhalation, intravenous, etc.); and 4) the reason for the exposure (euphoria, suicide, medication error, etc.). The case presented here was one of chronic salicylate ingestion, which is managed much differently than the single, acute ingestion. A good rule of thumb when managing the poisoned patient is to assume the patient is lying to you until proven otherwise. The paramedics, witnesses, pharmacists, primary care physicians, or others may provide additional history.

Many toxidromes are based on alterations in vital signs. Table 2 provides a useful mnemonic for diagnosing various toxicities based on vital sign abnormalities. If the patient presents with dilated pupils, consider sympathomimetic or anticholinergic toxicity. If the pupils are constricted, consider an opiate ingestion. Horizontal nystagmus may be seen with ingestions of ethanol, lithium, anti-seizure medications, and various tranquilizers. Patients with anticholinergic ingestions will present with dry skin; sympathomimetic ingestions present with diaphoresis. Needle tracks are noted with opiate use, bullous lesions with barbiturate ingestion, and flushing with anticholinergic syndrome. Seizures may be induced by lithium, tricyclic antidepressants, anticholinergics or benzodiazepine withdrawal. Tremors may occur with lithium or methylxanthines (i.e., Theophylline) ingestion.

Table 2. Diagnosing Toxicity from Vital Signs

Bradycardia (PACED)	Hypothermia (COOLS)	Hypotension (CRASH)	Rapid respiration (PANT)
Propranolol or other beta-blockers, poppies (opiates), propafenone, phenylpropanolamine Anticholinesterase drugs Clonidine, calcium-channel blockers Ethanol or other alcohols Digoxin	Carbon monoxide Opiates Oral hypoglycemics, insulin Liquor Sedative-hypnotics	Clonidine, calcium-channel blockers Reserpine or other antihypertensive agents Antidepressants, aminophylline Sedative-hypnotics Heroin or other opiates	PCP, paraquat, pneumonitis (chemical) ASA and other salicylates Non-cardiogenic pulmonary edema Toxin-induced metabolic acidosis
	Hyperthermia (NASA) Neuroleptic malignant syndrome, nicotine Antihistamines Salicylates, sympathomimetics Anticholinergics, antidepressants	**Hypertension (CT SCAN)** Cocaine Thyroid supplements Sympathomimetics Caffeine Anticholinergics, amphetamines Nicotine	**Slow respiration (SLOW)** Sedative-hypnotics (including GHB) Liquor Opiates, sedative-hypnotics Weed (marijuana)
Tachycardia (FAST) Free base or other forms of cocaine Anticholinergics, antihistamines, amphetamines Sympathomimetics (cocaine, amphetamines), solvent abuse Theophylline			

Source: Erickson TB, Aks SE, Gussow L, et al. Toxicology update: a rational approach to managing the poisoned patient. Emerg Med Practice 2001; 3(8):4. Used with permission.

Toxidromes are useful in identifying the specific toxin and will help guide management. Table 3 lists various toxidromes.

Table 3. Toxidromes

Toxidrome	Representative Agent(s)	Most Common Findings	Additional Signs and Symptoms	Potential Interventions
Opiod	Heroin Morphine	CNS depression, miosis, respiratory depression	Hypothermia, bradycardia. Death may result from respiratory arrest, acute lung injury	Ventilation or naloxone
Sympathomimetic	Cocaine Amphetamine	Psychomotor agitation, mydriasis, diaphoresis, tachycardia, hypertension, hyperthermia	Seizures, rhabdomyolysis, myocardial infarction Death may result from seizures, cardiac arrest, hyperthermia	Cooling, sedation with benzodiazepines, hydration
Cholinergic	Organophosphate insecticides Carbamate insecticides	Salivation, lacrimation, diaphoresis, nausea, vomiting, urination, defacation, muscle fasciculations, weakness, bronchorrhea	Bradycardia, miosis/mydriasis, seizures, respiratory failure, paralysis Death may result from respiratory arrest from paralysis, bronchorrhea, or seizures	Airway protection and ventilation, atropine, pralidoxine
Anticholinergic	Organophosphate insecticides Carbamate insecticides	Altered mental status, mydriasis, dry/flushed skin, urinary retention, decreased bowel sounds, hyperthermia, dry mucous membranes	Seizures, dysrhythmias, rhabdomyolysis Death may result from hyperthermia and dysrhythmias	Physostigmine (if appropriate), sedation with benzodiazepines, cooling, supportive management
Salicylates	Aspirin Oil of wintergreen	Altered mental status, respiratory alkalosis, metabolic acidosis, tinnitus, hyperpnea, tachycardia, diaphoresis, nausea, vomiting	Low-grade fever, ketouria Death may result from acute lung injury	MDAC, alkanization of the urine with potassium repletion, hemodialysis, hydration
Hypoglycemia	Sulfonylureas Insulin	Altered mental status, diaphoresis, tachycardia, hypertension	Paralysis, slurring of speech, bizarre behavior, seizures Death may result from seizures, altered behavior	Glucose containing solution intravenously, and oral feedings if able, frequent capillary blood for glucose measurement, octreotide
Serotonin syndrome	Meperidine or dextromethorphan and MAOI; SSRI and TCA; SSRI/TCA/MAOI and amphetamines; SSRI alone	Altered mental status, increased muscle tone, hyperreflexia, hyperthermia	Intermittent whole-body tremor Death may result from hyperthermia	Cooling, sedation with benzodiazepines, supportive management, theoretical benefit—cyproheptadine

Abbreviations: CNS = central nervous system; MDAC = multidose activated charcoal; MAOI = monoamine oxidase inhibitor; SSRI = selective serotonin reuptake inhibitor; TCA = tricyclic antidepressant

Source: Tintinalli JE, ed., et al. Emergency medicine: a comprehensive study guide, 5th ed. New York: McGraw-Hill, 2000:1018. Used with permission.

III. ED EVALUATION OF OVERDOSE

Recommendations for initial evaluation include ECG and cardiac monitoring to identify arrhythmias and ECG interval changes unique to various ingestions. Patients with tricyclic overdose may have QRS widening and a terminal R-wave in lead aVR. Serum electrolytes may reveal anion gap metabolic acidosis due to salicylate, methanol, ethylene glycol, or iron ingestion. The anion gap acidosis encountered in this case was secondary to salicylate toxicity.

The use of qualitative toxicology screens are somewhat controversial. Many clinicians indiscriminately order tox screens on all poisoned patients, even though numerous studies have shown that in adults and children they rarely, if ever, change patient management or outcome.[3,4] Under certain circumstances, however, quantitative toxicology levels may be helpful; elevated levels of acetaminophen, aspirin, or digoxin may lead to treatment with a specific antidote or intervention.

IV. MANAGEMENT OF POISONED/OVERDOSE PATIENTS

In the past, Ipecac was used to induce emesis in all poisoned patients. Recently, its use has fallen out of favor due to lack of benefit in clinical trials. Some argue that there may be a role for Ipecac use in the home. Gastric lavage has also fallen out of favor in recent years—some experts feel it may still be helpful when a patient presents within 1 hour of a potentially life-threatening ingestion.[5]

The current standard of care for most poisonings includes administration of activated charcoal, which works by absorbing toxin within the bowel lumen, making it less available for absorption and thus enhancing GI elimination. It is often given with a cathartic, such as sorbitol, at a dose of 1 g/kg (or 50 g in the average adult patient) PO, or by nasogastric tube in the obtunded or uncooperative patient. Numerous studies have proven the efficacy and safety of charcoal.[6] The patient's airway must be protected, and it is contraindicated if endoscopy is being considered, as in the case of a caustic ingestion. Many experts have suggested the routine use of multiple dose activated charcoal, given every 4–6 hours. However, data to support this practice is lacking.

Whole bowel irrigation using polyethylene glycol will produce a rapid catharsis; the pediatric dose is 25 cc/kg and adult dose is 1–2 L. Indications include body packing or specific ingestions of substances not bound by activated charcoal, such as heavy metals. Contraindications include pre-existing diarrhea, bowel obstruction, or absent bowel sounds.

Urinary alkalinization is achieved by administration of intravenous sodium bicarbonate to achieve a urine pH of 7.5 to 8, causing "ion trapping," and enhancing urinary secretion. Indications include salicylate and methanol ingestions. As our patient had chronic salicylate toxicity, hemodialysis was not indicated.

Hemodialysis is used with life-threatening ingestions of dialyzed soluble substances, such as salicylate, theophylline, lithium, and methanol ingestion. As our patient had chronic salicylate toxicity, hemodialysis was not indicated.

Antidotes exist for specific toxins. (Table 4)

Table 4. Antidotes and Their Indications

Antidote	Toxin
N-acetylcysteine	Acetaminophen, possibly carbon tetrachloride
Ethanol/4-MP	Methanol/ethylene glycol
Oxygen/HBO	Carbon monoxide
Naloxone/nalmefene	Opioids
Physostigmine	Anticholinergics
Atropine/pralidoxime	Organophosphates
Methylene blue	Methemoglobinemia
Nitrites and thiosulfate, hydroxycobalamin	Cyanide
Deferoxamine	Iron
BAL (chelating agent)	Arsenic
Succimer (chelating agent)	Lead, mercury, arsenic
Fab fragments	Digoxin, colchicine, crotalid
Glucagon	ß-blockers
Sodium bicarbonate	Tricyclic antidepressants and other sodium-channel blockers
Calcium/Insulin/dextrose/glucagon	Calcium-channel antagonists

Source: Erickson TB, Aks SE, Gussow L, et al. Toxicology update: a rational approach to managing the poisoned patient. Emerg Med Practice 2001; 3(8):19. Used with permission.

V. ACETAMINOPHEN TOXICITY

Acetaminophen, easily accessible, has become one of the most commonly encountered toxic ingestions in the US. In 1996, the Toxic Exposure Surveillance System estimated that 5% of all toxic exposures and 11% of reported fatalities were directly related to acetaminophen.[7]

Acetaminophen is metabolized by the liver. At therapeutic dosages, normal metabolism produces an insignificant amount of NAPQI. However, with a toxic ingestion of acetaminophen, high levels of NAPQI are formed, resulting in hepatic toxicity[8] with pathognomonic findings of hepatic centrilobular necrosis.[9] The therapeutic dose of acetaminophen is 10–15 mg/kg, while a single toxic dose is over 140 mg/kg—a known ingestion below this amount does not require further testing.

Acetaminophen toxicity is traditionally broken down into four stages.[8] Stage I is from time zero (time of ingestion) until 24 hours post-ingestion; during this time, the patient may present to the emergency department with no evidence of liver toxicity. The patient may be asymptomatic or complain of generalized malaise, nausea, or vomiting. This is a critical stage, since prompt treatment may prevent fulminant hepatic failure. Stage II is 24–72 hours after ingestion and may include early signs of hepatic failure, such as right upper quadrant abdominal pain. Lab work may demonstrate liver transaminase elevation, hyperbilirubinemia, or coagulopathy. Stage III is 72–96 hours after ingestion with signs of fulminant hepatic failure, including GI hemorrhage, acute renal failure, hepatic encephalopathy, or coma. Indicators of poor prognosis include an elevated bilirubin, elevated creatinine, elevated protime, and metabolic acidosis. Patients with a protime >100, a pH < 7.3, and a creatinine > 3.3 are likely to die unless there is a liver transplant.[9] Death usually occurs due to multisystem organ failure, sepsis, ARDS, or cerebral edema. Stage IV is known as the recovery phase. If the patient survives stage III, they are likely to recover completely without any long-term hepatic problems.

Diagnosis of acetaminophen toxicity is determined by history and laboratory findings; it is one of the few ingestions we face in emergency medicine in which laboratory testing plays a critical role.[10] The initial presentation is extremely nonspecific and acetaminophen levels will guide therapy. Interpretation of measured acetaminophen level is based on the Rumack-Matthew nomogram.[11] The nomogram (Table 5) was originally based on a single injection of regular acetaminophen (it excludes multiple ingestions or extended release preparations). Correlating the acetaminophen level with the time of ingestion and placing this value on the nomogram will determine whether or not liver toxicity may occur. Patients with acetaminophen levels above the treatment line have a 60% risk of developing AST > 1000, 1% risk of acute renal failure, and 5% risk of death if untreated.[12] Patients with levels below the treatment line have a risk of hepatic toxicity that is close to or equal to zero. The Rumack-Matthew nomogram is one of the most sensitive tools we have in medicine today.[13]

Table 5. Rumack-Matthew nomogram

Source: Rumack BH, Matthew H. Acetaminophen poisoning and toxicity. Pediatrics 1975; 55:871, 873). © 1975 by the American Academy of Pediatrics. Used with permission.

Management of acetaminophen toxicity includes GI decontamination with activated charcoal since there is always the possibility of co-ingestion. The antidote for acetaminophen toxicity is N-acetylcysteine (NAC) which works by prevention of NAPQI binding to hepatic proteins and reduction of NAPQI conversion back to acetaminophen. The dose of NAC is 140 mg/kg, easily remembered since it is the same as the toxic dose of acetaminophen 4 hours post ingestion. The initial dose of 140 mg/kg is followed by 70 mg/kg every 4 hours for a total of 17 doses. If administered within 8 hours of ingestion, it is nearly 100% effective in preventing hepatotoxicity.[14] An IV form has been used worldwide for years, but has only recently been given FDA approval in the US—it is most often utilized in patients with persistent vomiting who cannot tolerate oral NAC. It has also been hypothesized that the IV form may be more effective than the oral form.

VI. SALICYLATE TOXICITY

Historically, salicylate toxicity has been one of the most common toxicological causes of morbidity and mortality. In 1996, according to the American Association of Poison Control Centers Toxic Exposures Surveillance System (AAPCC/TESS), there were 25,281 exposures, with 12,385 cases requiring treatment in a health care facility (49%), resulting in 48 deaths.[15] Salicylates have consistently ranked number 2 behind acetaminophen in analgesic-related deaths per year. In recent years, however, the incidence of unintentional toxicity has decreased due to better safety packaging, increased use of various NSAID's, and the use of acetaminophen to avoid Reye's Syndrome.[16] The presentation and management of salicylate toxicity varies between acute and chronic ingestions.

Once ingested, acetyl salicylic acid (ASA) is hydrolyzed to salicylate, which is responsible for both the therapeutic and toxic effects of ASA. Salicylate stimulates the respiratory center in the brainstem, resulting in hyperventilation and a subsequent respiratory alkalosis in a toxic ingestion. It will also cause a wide anion gap metabolic acidosis. A mixed acid-base picture is the classic finding of salicylate toxicity; over 50% will manifest a respiratory alkalosis and anion gap metabolic acidosis.[17]

Patients with *acute* salicylate toxicity present with a sudden onset of nausea and vomiting since salicylate acts as a direct stomach irritant. Other symptoms include hyperthermia and/or profound tachypnea resulting in respiratory alkalosis. Various neurological symptoms include tinnitus, vertigo, ataxia, delirium and seizures.

Chronic salicylate toxicity is much more subtle. Patients are often elderly with multiple medical problems and typically manifest a more gradual onset of symptoms. The symptoms may be similar to acute toxicity, but less severe, and include nausea, vomiting, dyspnea, tinnitus, hallucinations and seizures. These symptoms are attributed to other comorbidities, making the diagnosis more challenging. Chronic salicylate toxicity must be considered in the presence of an unexplained anion gap metabolic acidosis (as was the case in this patient).[18]

Multiple strategies, but no specific antidote, are available for managing salicylate toxicity. Salicylate levels should be drawn, but should not guide management. A nomogram based on serum salicylate levels was developed to determine which patients should be dialyzed; however, this was developed for healthy pediatric patients with a single acute ingestion, and should not be extrapolated to all clinical scenarios.[19] The patient's clinical condition and the entire picture should guide therapy. Urine alkalinization will result in an increased urinary excretion of salicylate—3 amps of sodium bicarbonate are added to a liter of D5W, starting at 1.5 × maintenance rate, with a goal of keeping urine pH > 7.5. Indications include a metabolic acidosis within 18 hours of salicylate ingestion. Contraindications include pH > 7.55, pulmonary or cerebral edema, or oliguric renal failure.

Many studies have addressed multi-dose charcoal in salicylate toxicity, but have found little convincing evidence that multiple doses of charcoal are any better than a single dose.[20] Fluid replacement is important since the patient is often volume-depleted from vomiting, hyperthermia, and an increased metabolic state. Forced saline diuresis (fluid resuscitation beyond simple replacement) has been used in the past, but has not proven more effective than simple PO fluids.[21]

Indications for hemodialysis include renal failure, noncardiogenic pulmonary edema, seizures/coma, and clinical deterioration despite supportive care and urinary alkalinization.[22] Some authorities also recommend dialysis with an ASA level > 100 mg/dL after a single ingestion.

VII. SUMMARY

This patient presented with unexplained mental status changes. Her initial management, including stabilization of her ABCs, and initial determination of blood glucose and pulse ox, were solid. She did have an unexplained wide anion gap metabolic acidosis on her initial assessment, and was eventually diagnosed with chronic salicylate toxicity—this should always be considered in an elderly patient with mental status changes and an AG acidosis. This history was discovered during the hospitalization, but not during the initial ED encounter.

At this point, it is difficult to know if this information was available during the initial ED encounter, but it does not seem that it was specifically inquired about. Though medication reactions are often from prescription meds, they can occur from over-the-counter meds as well as herbal medications. Natural substances taken in pharmacologic doses are no longer natural!

Definitive therapy of the salicylate toxicity was delayed, but the eventual outcome was acceptable. It would be difficult to say if quicker therapy would have made a difference.

TEACHING POINTS FOR CASE 17:
- Consider chronic salicylate toxicity in elderly patients with confusion and AG acidosis.
- Patients (or family) may not mention over-the-counter or herbal medications unless specifically questioned.
- A mixed anion gap metabolic acidosis and respiratory alkalosis is highly suspicious for salicylate toxicity.
- A salicylate level is only useful for a single acute ingestion, and is not helpful in guiding chronic toxicity management.
- Fluid replacement and urinary alkalinization with sodium bicarbonate are cornerstones of therapy for acute salicylate toxicity. Management should be based on the entire clinical picture and not solely on the ASA level.
- The toxic dose of acetaminophen and the therapeutic dose of n-acetyl cysteine are both 140mg/kg. A 4 hour acetaminophen level below the treatment threshold of the nomogram rules out potential liver toxicity.
- The mneumonic "DONT" (dextrose, oxygen, narcan, thiamine) helps in the initial management of altered mental status.

REFERENCES

1. Litovitz TL, Klein-Schwartz W, White S, et al. 1999 annual report of the American Association of Poison Control Centers Toxic Exposure Surveillance System. Am J Emerg Med. 2000; 18:517-74.

2. Tintinalli JE, ed. Emergency medicine: a comprehensive study guide. 6th ed. New York:McGraw-Hill, 2004.

3. Belson MG, Simon HK, Sullivan K, et al: The utility of toxicologic analysis in children with suspected ingestions. Pediatr Emerg Care 1999;15:383-7.

4. Brett AS. Implications of discordance between clinical impression and toxicology analysis in drug overdose. Arch Intern Med 1988;148:437-41.

5. Kulig K, Bar-Or D, Cantrill SV, et al: Management of acutely poisoned patients without gastric emptying. Ann Emerg Med 1985; 14:562-7.

6. Levy G. Gastrointestinal clearance of drugs with activated charcoal. N Eng J Med 1982; 307:676-8.

7. Litovitz TL, Smilkstein M, Felberg L, et al. 1996 annual report of the American Association of Poison Control Centers Toxic Exposure Surveillance System. Am J Emerg Med 1997; 15:447-500.

8. Linden CH, Rumack BH. Acetaminophen overdose. Emerg Clin North Am 1984; 2:103-19.

9. O'Grady JG, Alexander GJ, Hayllar KM, et al: Early indicators of prognosis in fulminant hepatic failure. Gastroenterology 1988; 87:439-45.

10. Ashbourne JF, Olson KR, Khayam-Bashi H. Value of rapid screening for acetaminophen in all patients with intentional drug overdose. Ann Emerg Med 1989; 18:1035-8.

11. Rumack BH, Matthew H. Acetaminophen poisoning and toxicity. Pediatrics 1975; 55:871-6.

12. Prescott LF. Paracetamol overdosage. Pharmacological considerations and clinical management. Drugs 1983; 25:290-314.

13. Smilkstein MJ, Douglas DR, Daya MR. Acetaminophen poisoning and liver function. N Engl J Med. 1994;331:1310-1.

14. Smilkstein MJ, Knapp GL, Kulig KW, et al: Efficacy of oral N-acetylcysteine in the treatment of acetaminophen overdose. N Engl J Med 1988;319:1557-62.

15. Litovitz TL, Smilkstein M, Felberg L, et al. 1996 Annual report of the American Association of Poison Control Centers Toxic Exposure Surveillance System. Am J Emerg Med 1997; 14:447-500.

16. Belay ED, Bresee JJ, Holman RC et al. Reye's Syndrome in the United States from 1981 through 1997. N Engl J Med 1999; 340:1377-82.

17. Gabow PA, Anderson RJ, Potts DE, et al. Acid-base disturbances in the salicylate poisoning in adults. Arch Intern Med 1978; 138:1481-4.

18. Gabow PA. How to avoid overlooking salicylate intoxication. J Crit Illness 1986; 1:77-85.

19. Done AK. Treatment of salicylate poisoning: review of personal and published experiences. Clin Toxicol 1968; 1:451-67.

20. American Academy of Clinical Toxicology and European Association of Poison Centers and Clinical Toxicologists. Position statement and practice guidelines on the use of multi-dose activated charcoal in the treatment of acute poisoning. J Toxicol Clin Toxicol 1999; 37:731-51.

21. Prescott LF, Balali-Mood M, Critchley JA, et al: Diuresis or urinary alkalinization for salicylate poisoning. Br Med J 1982;285:1383-6.

22. Jacobsen D, Wiik-Larsen E, Bredesen JH. Haemodialysis or haemoperfusion in severe salicylate poisoning? Hum Toxicol 1988;7:161-3.

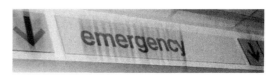

CASE18

10 YEAR OLD MALE WITH EYE PAIN

Commentary:
Gregory L. Henry, MD, FACEP

CEO, Medical Practice Risk Assessment, Inc., Ann Arbor, Michigan
Clinical Professor, Department of Emergency Medicine
   University of Michigan Medical School, Ann Arbor, Michigan
Past President, American College of Emergency Physicians (ACEP)

Discussion:
Grace J Kim, MD, FAAP

Assistant Professor, Attending Physician
   Pediatric Emergency Medicine
   Loma Linda University Medical Center
   Loma Linda, California

Lance Brown, MD, MPH, FACEP, FAAEM

Chief, Division of Pediatric Emergency Medicine
   Associate Professor of Emergency Medicine and Pediatrics
   Loma Linda University Medical Center and Children's Hospital
   Loma Linda, California
Editor-in-Chief, Pediatric Emergency Medicine Practice
Speaker of the Year—2004 USC Essentials of Emergency Medicine
Associate Editor, Canadian Journal of Emergency Medicine
Member ACEP Pediatric Emergency Medicine Committee

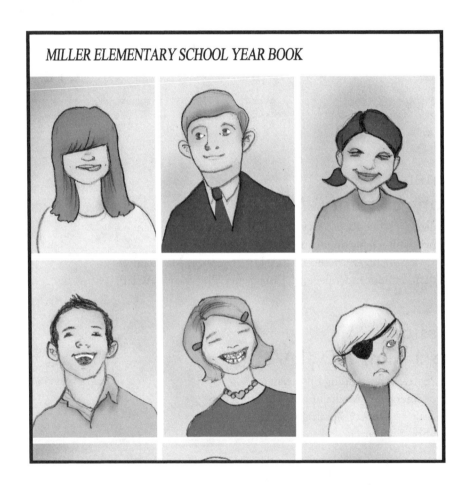

MILLER ELEMENTARY SCHOOL YEAR BOOK

10 YEAR OLD MALE WITH EYE PAIN

—Initial Visit*—

*Authors' Note: The history, exam and notes are the actual documentation of the physicians and providers, including abbreviations (and spelling errors)

CHIEF COMPLAINT (at 20:19): Eye pain

```
VITAL SIGNS
Time      Temp    Pulse   Resp   Syst   Diast
20:30     97.5    69      16     133    85
```

HISTORY OF PRESENT ILLNESS (at 21:21): This pt is a 10 y/o male who presents with OS pain s/p direct, blunt trauma to eye approx 1pm this afternoon. The pt reports playing "rubber" darts with friends at home when one accidentally struck him in OS centrally from direct throw. Now experiencing mod pain, photophobia, and tearing in OS. He does have redness and blurred vision. The pt reports no previous h/o eye injury or trauma. Denies any other ROS

PAST MEDICAL HISTORY/TRIAGE:
  Medications: None
  Allergies: No known allergies.
  PMH: None
  PSH: none
  SocHx: Tobacco use: (-), Alcohol use: (-)
  Visual acuity (at 20:38): Left eye: totally blind; Right eye: uncorrected 20/20,
  Immunizations: The infant/child's immunizations are current

EXAM (at 21:26):
  General: Well-appearing; well nourished; A&O X 3, in no apparent distress.
  Head: Normocephalic; atraumatic.
  Skin: Normal for age and race; warm and dry; no apparent lesions
  Eyes: Fundoscopic exam attempted, unable to visualize anything. No pupillary constriction on exam.
  Visual acuity 20/20 OD, contrary to triages notes, vision was 20/30 after alcaine eye drops instilled to OS; Visual fields are abnormal by confrontation. Extraocular muscles are intact. Pupils are unequal and OS is nonreactive to light. The irises are abnormal. Unable to visualize the Retina and disc margins due to injury. Lids, lashes and puncta are normal. Everted lids are normal. Cornea is not clear with abrasion noted and no foreign bodies. The anterior chamber is not clear

with abnormal depth. Conjunctiva and sclera are abnormal with injection. Slit lamp exam with Fluroscein stain reveals no foreign body, increased dye uptake, abrasion w/o rust ring. ? sidels sign. Noted in ant chamber clear and bloody fluid intermixed.

ORDERS (at 21:38):
CT Brain and Orbits, Homatropine 2% ophth drops OS Q12 hours. Given to take home

RESULTS:

CT OF THE BRAIN AND CT OF THE ORBITS, TWO PROJECTIONS (at 22:36): Dedicated thin sections through the orbits obtained in the coronal and axial projection show no evidence of bone injury in the orbits or sinuses. Several small bubbles are seen in the anterior space of the orbits, presumably due to eye examination. The globes themselves appear to be intact, at least as far as morphology and internal architecture. The extraocular muscles and lacrimal glands are normal in appearance.

IMPRESSION: Normal CT examination of the orbits.

PROGRESS NOTES (at 23:06): This patient presented after a rubber dart struck his left eye - dart thrown by his sibling. His acuity is 20/30. His eye does reveal a hyphema. EOMI. CT reveals no globe rupture. I discussed this with the ophthalmologist on call who recommends Homatropine, Ocuflox, Predforte, analgesics, eye shield, head elevation, no anticoagulants. I gave him the patient's home phone number - he will call him tomorrow to be seen tomorrow in his office.

DIAGNOSIS:
   1. Eye injury, contusion
   2. Eye pain
   3. Corneal abrasion
   4. Visual disturbance

DISPOSITION (at 00:04): Discharged to home ambulatory for ophthalmologist examination the next day. Sent home with homatropine drops. Prescriptions for predforte 1%, ocuflox drops, and Tylenol elixir with codeine. Aftercare instructions for hyphema. Eye patch applied to the left eye.

Gregory L. Henry comments:

"Considering that the laws of fluid dynamics are applicable in virtually all situations, the pressure transmitted to the front of the eye is transmitted equally to the back."

When a child presents with a traumatic eye injury, the questions are obvious, "Is there an injury that has disturbed the integrity of the globe itself? Has enough pressure been transmitted to cause an injury to the lens, retina, or other supporting structures of the eye?"

The history in this case is relatively straightforward and is adequately recorded. A blow from a "rubber dart" to the eye can have the same consequences (damage directly to the cornea) as a blow from any other instrument. Considering that the laws of fluid dynamics are applicable in virtually all situations, the pressure transmitted to the front of the eye is transmitted equally to the back. Structures in all planes of the eye have the potential for injury.

Initial evaluation by the nursing staff leaves something to be desired. When stated, "Left eye is totally blind," this is almost never the case. The patient may not be able to read the eye chart, but nearly always has light perception. If a patient has light perception, hand movement or count fingers may also detected. Therefore, it is unlikely that the eye is totally blind. The examination performed by the physician seemed to cover the correct areas, but some of the conclusions drawn were incorrect.

The administration of a small amount of anesthetic in the eye is essentially never contraindicated. The patient is much more relaxed and easier to examine when pain has been taken out of the equation. Once the pain medication was given, the patient's visual acuity was recorded as 20/30. It is also noted that the visual fields are abnormal by confrontation. What does this mean? It is unlikely that a patient who has a trauma to one eye has an visual field defect or a hemianopsia that would indicate a lesion posterior to the optic chiasm. When it is noted that the left pupil is non-reactive to light, we must assume that this is not secondary to a neurologic deficit, but present from local involvement of the iris itself. The physician properly notes that the iris is involved and the retina cannot be visualized due to injury. The slit lamp examination found increased dye uptake, but does not specify whether this occurs in a linear fashion or if there is diffusion into the deeper layers of the eye. This can be an early indication of a globe penetration.

Initial CT scans of the eye may be inaccurate. They are excellent for finding metallic foreign bodies, fractures of the boney supporting structures, and retro orbital blood and pus, but not definitive in deciding whether globe penetration or retinal detachment has occured. The physician's evaluation showing a post-traumatic hyphema with disruption of the uveal tract is correct; questions remain about the degree of retinal involvement and the possibility of globe penetration. These questions will not be answered in an emergency department and require further consultation.

It is interesting that the ophthalmologist, aware a severe traumatic hyphema had occurred, chose to see the patient the next day. I would have liked to visualize the ophthalmologist in the department that night. But in all truth, it is unlikely that the outcome or management would have changed.

Documentation on this case is reasonably good, but a discrepancy exists between the nursing evaluation and the physician's evaluation—this needs to be commented upon.

Principal concerns in this case involve timing of intervention; if a true penetration of the globe is in question, then questions about timing of surgery become paramount.

- **Thoroughness of Documentation:** 6 out of 10.

- **Thoroughness of Patient Evaluation:** 5 out of 10.

- **Risk of Serious Illness Being Missed:** Medium risk.

- **Risk Management Legal Rating:** Medium risk.

10 YEAR OLD MALE WITH EYE PAIN

—Follow up with Ophthalmology: The Next Day—

PROGRESS NOTES (the next day): Patient was seen by the ophthalmologist the next day in his office and was diagnosed with a complete globe rupture with partial retinal detachment. At that point, the visual acuity in the left eye was 'light perception' only, suggesting the nursing documentation of the visual acuity was more accurate than the physician's – the documented OS 20/30 visual acuity was probably because he was 'peeking' from his other eye.

He was taken to surgery that same day and the corneal laceration was repaired and he underwent a partial lens resection. He was then sent to a retina specialist who performed a complete lens removal and vitrectomy.

On the last office check, his visual acuity had improved to 20/100 in the left eye.

Per the ophthalmologist; if he has no further improvement, then he may be a candidate for a corneal transplant.

FINAL DIAGNOSIS: Acute traumatic globe rupture.

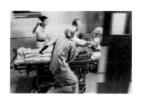

EVALUATION AND MANAGEMENT OF EYE INJURIES IN CHILDREN

Grace J Kim, MD, FAAP
Lance Brown, MD, MPH, FACEP, FAAEM

I. INTRODUCTION

Eye complaints are relatively common in the emergency department. Most cases of pediatric eye complaints are from relatively benign causes, such as minor corneal abrasions or conjunctivitis. Eye pain may arise from traumatic and nontraumatic causes. A wide range of conditions, including pseudotumor cerebri and sarcoidosis, may present with eye pain. Fortunately, these conditions are relatively uncommon and rarely present with isolated eye complaints. Pediatric eye trauma, however, is relatively common.[1] Because children may be struck in the face with a variety of objects, or fall and strike their faces, emergency physicians are frequently called upon to evaluate children for clinically significant eye injuries.

II. DEFINITIONS OF EYE INJURIES

Reading the literature regarding severe eye injuries can be confusing due to the authors' varying definitions of key terms. Prior to the mid-1990's, there were no accepted definitions used to describe eye injuries. In 1996, Kuhn and colleagues proposed standardized trauma-specific terms for eye injuries.[2] These terms have been endorsed by multiple ophthalmologic societies including the International Society of Ocular Trauma, The United States Eye Injury Registry, The American Academy of Ophthalmology, The Vitreous and Retina Societies, and The Hungarian Eye Injury Registry.[3] Recent and future studies may offer more easily interpretable data if these terms are widely accepted and used by researchers. Definitions of some of the terms pertinent to our case include the following:

- **Eye wall**—The rigid structures of the sclera and cornea
- **Rupture**—Blunt force to the eye wall leading to a rapid increase in intraocular pressure and a subsequent full-thickness disruption of the eye wall from an "inside-out" force (may or may not occur at the site of injury)
- **Laceration**—Force from a sharp object that results in a full-thickness wound of the eye wall at the site of injury, an "outside-in" force
- **Open-globe injury**—Full thickness wound to the eye
- **Closed-globe injury**—Direct injury to the eye without a full-thickness wound
- **Contusion**—A closed-globe injury from a blunt object

For our case, it is clear that the child had an open-globe injury. It is not clear whether "rubber" darts are blunt or sharp objects. Given that the child sustained an open-globe injury due to a corneal laceration presumably at the site of injury, it would appear that, however the dart was constructed, it acted like a sharp object. The emergency physician diagnosed the child as having a closed-globe injury and appears to have properly used the term eye "contusion" as the initial diagnosis.

Unfortunately, this was the wrong diagnosis. In retrospect, the child actually had open-globe injury from an eye laceration.

III. EPIDEMIOLOGY

Fortunately, although eye injuries of all kinds are relatively common,[4] pediatric open-globe injuries are relatively uncommon. In the United States, eye injuries have an annual incidence of over 2 million, about half of which are in children younger than 18 years old.[1] Based on the available data, about 2% of these eye injuries (42,000) are related to sports and recreational activities.[5] It is estimated that about 18,000 of these injuries occur in children younger than 15 years old and about 3,300 occur in children younger than 8 years old. Although studies have limitations due to varying terminology, the proportion of eye-injured children who sustain open-globe injuries and present for medical attention is probably around 1– 2%.[6,7] This rough analysis suggests a few hundred open-globe injuries in children occur in the entire United States each year. The number of children struck in the eye who do not seek medical attention is unknown.

Maw and colleagues recently completed a meta-analysis of open-globe injuries in children younger than 18 years old.[8] They reviewed 5 major studies and pooled data from them.[9-13] Combined, these studies reported on 447 eye injuries in children. These authors report that patients in these studies were predominantly male (79%). Nearly half of the children (47%) were in the 6–12 year age cohort, 32% were in the ≤ 5 year group, and 20% were adolescents. Sharp objects caused the injuries in the majority of cases (75%), and the majority of cases occurred during sports, hobbies or play (59%). The cornea was the site of the wound most of the time, either in isolation (54%) or in combination with corneoscleral wounds (28%). Other findings and their frequency included iris prolapse (58%), hyphema (44%), flat anterior chamber (44%), uveal prolapse (40%), vitreous hemorrhage (21%), retinal detachment (10%), and afferent pupillary defect (see below) (9%). Although the authors did not use formal statistical methods to assess this, they reported that children with poorer outcomes (in terms of final, post-operative visual acuity) tended to have larger wounds, wounds that involved the sclera, wounds caused by BB guns, and worse visual acuity on presentation. Unfortunately, the authors do not report on the time from initial identification of the open-globe injury to operative care. Of the 118 children who presented with an initial visual acuity worse than 5/200 (i.e., can't read large letters even at a distance of only 5 feet rather than the typical testing distance of 20 feet), 28 (24%) had nearly normal post-operative visual acuity, 29 (25%) had moderate persistent visual loss, and 61, more than half, (51%) had persistently poor vision (worse than 5/200). Of the 30 children who presented with near normal visual acuity (up to 20/50), all but 1 maintained near normal visual acuity following treatment. Although the meta-analysis is quite useful in understanding eye injuries, Maw and colleagues were not comprehensive in their study of open-globe injuries, and they did not present their selection criteria in the article.[14-19] There are a few articles that describe serious eye injuries specifically due to darts, but too few cases are reported to make any generalizations about this type of injury.[20-22]

IV. HISTORY AND EXAMINATION

In most cases of blunt eye trauma, the history of present illness is straightforward and unambiguous —this is nicely demonstrated in our case; the child said he was hit in the eye with a "rubber" dart. At times, other historical features may be helpful,[1,2,3] particularly when a child has had prior eye surgery or other previous ophthalmologic problems. (Table 1)

Table 1. Historical Features That May Be Useful in Evaluating a Child with an Eye Injury[1,23]

- Time of injury
- Mechanism of injury:
  o Blunt
  o Penetrating
  o Missile
- Visual changes:
  o Acuity
  o Photophobia
  o Diplopia
- Any initial intervention
- Possibility of retained foreign body:
  o Organic vs. inorganic
  o Magnetic vs. non-magnetic
- Assessment of pain:
  o Pain scale
  o Characteristics of pain (sharp, throbbing, dull, constant, episodic)
  o Onset (acute, subacute or chronic)
  o Factors exacerbating pain (eye movement, lights)
  o Palliating factors
- Pertinent medical and ocular history:
  o Baseline vision
  o History of ocular surgery
  o Corrective lenses
  o Previous ocular trauma
  o History of amblyopia or previous visual decrease
  o History of pupillary abnormalities
- Medications:
  o Eye drops (specifically dilating drops)
  o Pain medications

The examination of the injured pediatric eye in the emergency department can be quite challenging. There are several published reviews of the evaluation of the eye-injured child in the emergency department and ambulatory setting.[24-28] School-aged children may be emotionally distraught by the event and unable to cooperate with the examination. Even relatively gross examination techniques, such as lifting a swollen eye lid to assess visual acuity, may cause a child sufficient distress as to make the assessment intolerable and inaccurate. If sedation is needed to facilitate the elevation of a swollen eyelid, the child may then be able to tolerate the examination, but then be too sedated to participate with visual acuity testing. The process can be very frustrating for the patient, family, and emergency physician. If at all possible, painless parts of the examination should be done first. An ambulatory child can usually participate in visual acuity testing which is painless and does not typically invoke fear. Other gross features of an eye assessment that can be done painlessly include evaluating eye movements, pupillary light response, and inspection of the orbits. Since attempting to open the lids forcibly may worsen the injury, if this is necessary to visualize the eye, it is best to stop the examination and let the ophthalmologist take the patient to the operating room where an adequate evaluation may be carried out under controlled circumstances.

Besides gross inspection and visual acuity testing, the 2 tests most helpful in assessing a potential open-globe injury are the swinging flashlight test and Seidel's test. The swinging flashlight test is performed to determine if an afferent pupillary defect is present.[28,29] In this test, a flashlight is shined in 1 eye and then the other. If an afferent pupillary defect is present, both eyes will constrict when light is directed into the unaffected eye, but both pupils will dilate when light is directed into the injured eye. In the setting of a potential open-globe injury, an afferent pupillary defect typically is present when there is opacification of structures in the line of sight or neurologic involvement of the optic nerve. The swinging flashlight test will not be of much value in an eye with obvious damage, such as hyphema, corneal laceration, or vitreous hemorrhage. In one study, this finding was part of a group of features that had 100% sensitivity in detecting an open-globe injury.[6] (Table 2)

Seidel's test assesses the integrity of the globe more directly than the swinging flashlight test.[30-32] Although initially used to assess the adequacy of post-operative globe closure,[33] Seidel's test has been adapted for use in the setting of eye trauma. To perform Seidel's test, fluorescein dye is applied to the surface of the injured eye. When applied to a closed globe in room light, fluorescein leaves a dull yellow-orange color on the surface of the globe. If aqueous fluid is leaking from the cornea or sclera, the aqueous fluid dilutes the fluorescein and changes the color from dull yellow-orange to bright green. The Seidel test evaluates the integrity of the cornea and requires use of the slit lamp for accurate evaluation. In a severely damaged eye such as this, it has minimal value. Although corneal abrasions may appear bright green, the discoloration associated with corneal abrasions is relatively fixed whereas the changes associated with a fluid leak should move about with the fluid. The Seidel test will show a "stream" of green coming from leaking aqueous fluid through a corneal laceration.

Table 2. Clinical Findings Found to be 100% Sensitive for Identifying a Ruptured Globe[6]

In cases in which globe rupture is not obvious, the patient should demonstrate one feature from each group.

A. Evidence of intraocular or periocular hemorrhage
- hemorrhagic chemosis
- hyphema
- vitreous hemorrhage

B. Poor function
- visual acuity with only 'light perception' or worse
- abnormal anterior chamber depth
- low intraocular pressure (< 6 mm Hg) if tested*
- inability to view the fundus due to opacification of line of sight structures

*The measurement of eye pressures typically involves pressing on the globe. In cases where ruptured globe is suspected, applying pressure to the globe is contraindicated.

Adapted from Kylstra JA, Lamkin JC, Runyan DK. Clinical predictors of scleral rupture after blunt ocular trauma. Am J Ophthalmol 1993; 115:530-5.

V. DIAGNOSTIC TESTING FOR OPEN-GLOBE INJURIES

As a diagnostic adjunct for identifying open globes, computed tomography (CT) scanning[34-36] and ocular ultrasound[37] have been studied. Proponents of CT scanning for identifying open globe injuries may report good inter-relater reliability, and a 95% positive predictive value (i.e., if the CT scan is read as positive for an open globe, there is a 95% chance that there actually is an open-globe).[34] This study included 375 readings of 200 CT scans by 3 radiologists. The authors reported a 95% positive predictive value, but did not report a negative predictive value at all.[34] Using the authors' data for calculations, the negative predictive value is only 74%. In other words, if the CT scan does not reveal an open-globe injury, there is still a 26% chance that an open-globe injury is present. Although there are studies evaluating the test characteristics of CT scanning to detect intraocular foreign bodies, we identified only 2 other studies evaluating CT scanning to evaluate potential open-globe injuries and they included too few subjects from which to draw meaningful conclusions.[35,36] At this point, ocular ultrasound should probably be considered experimental, with too little data to evaluate the test characteristics. In addition, the risk of applying external pressure to the globe, which may cause extrusion of the globe contents through the wound, has not been adequately evaluated.[37] In our case, the emergency physician obtained a negative orbital CT scan, but should not have been reassured by this. From the available information, there still remained a 1 in 4 chance that the child had an open-globe injury.

VI. MANAGEMENT OF OPEN-GLOBE INJURIES

Iimportant issues to consider for suspected open-globe injuries include: avoiding increased intra-ocular pressure, the administration of tetanus prophylaxis, and the administration of antibiotics. In addition, pain management and sedation are important issues in the evaluation and management of children with suspected open-globe injuries. These factors become particularly important not only for the examination but for management as well. Maneuvers that increase intraocular pressure (the Valsalva maneuver, flexion of the head, coughing, crying, vomiting, rubbing the eyes, etc.) have the potential to increase the amount of globe contents extruded through the wound.[38] Therefore, these problems should be anticipated and children with suspected globe rupture should be treated with anti-emetics, analgesia, and sedatives as necessary. Given the rarity of clinical tetanus, it is difficult to study the utility of tetanus prophylaxis for eye injuries. There is some reasonable animal data to suggest that although corneal abrasions do not seem to place mice at risk for tetanus, open-globe injuries do pose some risk.[39] Therefore, tetanus prophylaxis would be indicated for this child if his tetanus immunization was not up to date. Although serious infections such as post-traumatic endophthalmitis[40] may follow trauma, there is insufficient data to make specific recommendations regarding prophylactic antibiotics for "clean" injuries, such as being hit in the eye by a "rubber" dart.

VII. MEDICAL-LEGAL ISSUES AND SUMMARY

Although a recent study of 2,283 closed malpractice claims, involving children in emergency departments and urgent care centers, did not have eye injuries listed in the top ten most common diagnoses,[41] our case raises some interesting medical-legal issues. The patient had a corneal abrasion with a questionable Seidel's test. This is very worrisome for an open-globe injury, especially in the setting of a dart injury with a hyphema, abnormal irises, an obscured view of the retina, and an anterior chamber with an abnormal depth. It appears that the emergency physician was inappropriately reassured by the negative orbital CT scan. Even if the plan would have remained the same (follow up in the morning with the ophthalmologist), acknowledgement by the emergency physician, ophthalmologist, and the family that an open-globe injury was likely present may have done quite a bit to avoid potential litigation.

TEACHING POINTS ABOUT CASE 18:
- One of the primary goals of evaluating a child who has sustained eye trauma is to assess for an open-globe injury.
- Visual acuity should be as accurate as possible; if the patient is not able to read the chart, assess for "finger counting" or "light perception."
- When fluorescein staining is performed, if an area seems to change from dull yellow-orange to bright green (a positive Seidel's test), an open-globe injury should be presumed. Abnormal anterior chamber depth may indicate a substantial deformity of the globe, again indicating probable open-globe injury.
- A CT scan is helpful if positive, but has insufficient negative predictive value to rule out an open-globe injury.
- If a globe rupture is suspected, avoid any increased intraocular pressure or manipulation of the eye and contact an ophthalmologist for determination of the next step.

REFERENCES
1. Levine LM. Pediatric ocular trauma and shaken infant syndrome. Pediatr Clin North Am 2003;50: 137-48.
2. Kuhn F, Morris R, Witherspoon D, et al. A standardized classification of ocular trauma. Ophthalmology 1996;103: 240-3.
3. Pieramici DJ, Sternberg P Jr, Aaberg TM, et al. A system for classifying mechanical injuries of the eye (globe). Am J Ophthalmol 1997;123: 820-31.
4. Smith D, Wrenn K, Stack LB. The epidemiology and diagnosis of penetrating eye injuries. Acad Emerg Med 2002;9: 209-13.
5. American Academy of Pediatrics Committee on Sports Medicine and Fitness. Protective eyewear for young athletes. Pediatrics 2004;113:619-22.
6. Kylstra JA, Lamkin JC, Runyan DK. Clinical predictors of scleral rupture after blunt ocular trauma. Am J Ophthalmol 1993;115:530-5.
7. Joseph E, Zak R, Smith S, et al. Predictors of blinding or serious eye injury in blunt trauma. J Trauma 1992;33:19-24.
8. Maw R, Pineda R, Pasquale LR, et al. Traumatic ruptured globe injuries in children. Int Ophthalmol Clin 2002;42: 157-65.
9. Sternberg P Jr, de Juan E Jr, Michels RG. Penetrating ocular injuries in young patients: initial injuries and visual results. Retina 1984;4:5-8.
10. Alfaro DV, Chaudhry NA, Walonker AF, et al. Penetrating eye injuries in young children. Retina 1994;14: 201-5.
11. Rostomian K, Thach A, Isfahani A, et al. Open globe injuries in children. JAAPOS 1998;2: 234-8.
12. Baxter RJ, Hodgkins PR, Calder I, et al. Visual outcome of childhood anterior perforating eye injuries: prognostic indicators. Eye 1994;8: 349-52.
13. Rudd JC, Jaeger EA, Freitag SK, et al. Traumatically ruptured globes in children. JPOS 1994;31:307-11.

14. Scharf J, Zonis S. Perforating injuries of the eye in childhood. J Pediatr Ophthalmol 1976;13: 326-8.
15. MacEwen CJ, Baines PS, Desai P. Eye injuries in children: the current picture. Br J Ophthalmol 1999;83: 933-6.
16. Grin TR, Nelson LB, Jeffers JB. Eye injuries in childhood. Pediatrics 1987;80: 13-7.
17. Luff AJ, Hodgkins PR, Baxter RJ, et al. Aetiology of perforating eye injury. Arch Dis Child 1993;68: 682-3.
18. Patel BCK. Penetrating eye injuries. Arch Dis Child 1989;64: 317-20.
19. LaRoche GR, McIntyre L, Schertzer RM. Epidemiology of severe eye injuries in childhood. Ophthalmology 1988;95: 1603-7.
20. Patel BC, Morgan LH. Serious eye injuries caused by darts. Arch Emerg Med 1991;8: 289-91.
21. Cole MD, Smerdon D. Perforating eye injuries caused by darts. Br J Ophthalmol 1988;72: 511-4.
22. Thill-Schwaninger M, Marquardt R. [Perforating eye injuries caused by darts]. Klin Monatsbl Augenheilkd 1988;192: 699-702.
23. Lee AG, Beaver HA, Brazis PW. Painful ophthalmologic disorders and eye pain for the neurologist. Neurol Clin 2004;1: 75-97.
24. Juang PSC, Rosen P. Ocular examination techniques for the emergency department. J Emerg Med 1997;15: 793-810.
25. Sit M, Levin A. Direct ophthalmoscopy in pediatric emergency care. Pediatr Emerg Care 2001;17: 199-204.
26. Khaw PT, Shah P, Elkington AR. Injury to the eye. BMJ 2004;328: 36-8.
27. Levin AV. Eye emergencies: Acute management in the pediatric ambulatory care setting. Pediatr Emerg Care 1991;7: 367-77.
28. Young TA, Levin AV. The afferent pupillary defect. Pediatr Emerg Care 13: 61-5; 1997.
29. Glazer-Hockstein C, Brucker AJ. The detection of a relative afferent pupillary defect. Am J Ophthalmol 2002;134: 142-3.
30. Seidel's test. (available at http://www.nova.edu/hpd/otm/otm-c/seidel.html)
31. Romanchuk KG. Seidel's test using 10% fluorescein. Can J Ophthal 1979;14: 253-6.
32. Cain W Jr, Sinskey RM. Detection of anterior chamber leakage with Seidel's test. Arch Ophthalmol 1981;99: 2013.
33. Seidel E. Weitere experimentelle Untersuchungen uber die Quell und den Verlauf der intraokularen Safstromung: XII. Ueber den manometrischen Nachweis des physiologischen Druckgefalles zwischen Voderkammer und Schlemmschem Kanal. Arch Ophthalmol 1921;107: 101.
34. Joseph DP, Pieramici DJ, Beauchamp NJ. Computed tomography in the diagnosis and prognosis of open-globe injuries. Ophthalmology 2000;107: 1899-906.
35. Lee HJ, Jilani M, Frohman, et al. CT of orbital trauma. Emerg Radiol 2004;10: 168-172.
36. Weissman JL, Beatty RL, Hirsch WL, et al. Enlarged anterior chamber: CT finding of a ruptured globe.1995;AJNR 16: 936-8.
37. Blaivas M, Theodoro D, Sierzenski PR. A study of bedside ocular ultrasonography in the emergency department. Acad Emerg Med 2002;9:791-9.
38. Holloway KB. Control of the eye during general anaesthesia for intraocular surgery. Br J Anaesth 1980;52: 671-9.

39. Benson WH, Snyder IS, Granus V, et al. Tetanus prophylaxis following ocular injuries. J Emerg Med 1993;11:677-83.
40. Essex RW, Yi Q, Charles PGP, et al. Post-traumatic endophthalmitis. Am Acad Ophthalmol 2004;111:2015-22.
41. Selbst SM, Friedman MJ, Singh SB. Epidemiology and etiology of malpractice lawsuits involving children in US emergency departments and urgent care centers. Pediatr Emerg Care 2005;21:165-9.

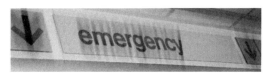

CASE19
57 YEAR OLD MALE WITH HEART FLUTTERING & LIGHTHEADEDNESS

Commentary:
Gregory L. Henry, MD, FACEP

CEO, Medical Practice Risk Assessment, Inc., Ann Arbor, Michigan
Clinical Professor, Department of Emergency Medicine
    University of Michigan Medical School, Ann Arbor, Michigan
Past President, American College of Emergency Physicians (ACEP)

Discussion:
Sandy Craig, MD, FACEP

Adjunct Assistant Professor, Department of Emergency Medicine
    University of North Carolina at Chapel Hill
Associate Program Director, Department of Emergency Medicine
    Carolinas Medical Center, Charlotte, North Carolina

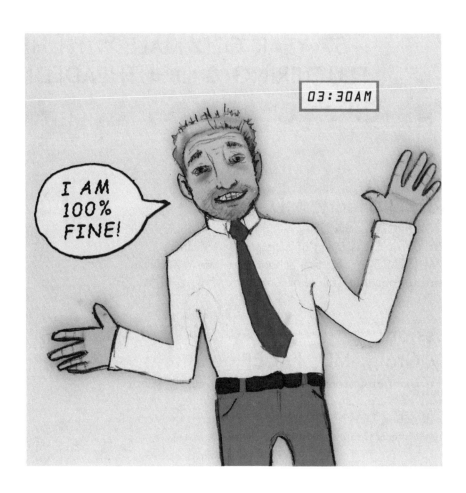

57 YEAR OLD MALE WITH HEART FLUTTERING & LIGHTHEADEDNESS

—Initial Visit*: New Year's Eve—

*Authors' Note: The history, exam and notes are the actual documentation of the physicians and providers, including abbreviations (and spelling errors)

CHIEF COMPLAINT (at 23:37): Heart beat rapid

```
VITAL SIGNS
Time    Temp(F)  Rt. Pulse  Resp  Syst  Diast  Pos  O2   sat O2%
23:42   98.3  Oral  147      20    176   127    S    99
01:19                158      16    149   94     S    99    2L
02:25                111      20    137   82     S    98
03:08                125      16    142   71     S    99
04:10                114      16    133   68     S    97
```

HISTORY OF PRESENT ILLNESS (at 00:27): Pt. states heart flutter for 3 days, lightheaded with standing. Has intermittent left chest pain which beg. gradually 3 days ago. The pain is mild with rad to left lateral ribs and upper arm. Has tingling left fingers. Hx of panic attacks, did not have any all summer but has been having increasing attacks that have been present the last 3 days with fluttering. Has been on paxil last winter for panic attacks. No prev. hx. of heart problems. Last summer with left upper arm pain, was eval at another local hospital (tertiary care center) and had negative stress test done at that time. Denies syncope, peripheral edema, fever, SOB, cough, diahoresis, abd. Pain, nausea. Hx of high triglycerides, no longer on meds for same. Had Hepatitis C last summer, resolved. Has had anxiety and panic attacks. Pt is otherwise healthy, watches weight, workouts regularly.

PAST MEDICAL HISTORY/TRIAGE:

Allergies: No known allergies.
Current meds: Names of medications unknown.
Past surgical history: Herniorrhaphy
Past medical history: Hypertension, panic attacks
Social history: D/C ETOH 15 yrs ago after pancreatitis/pseudocysts. Smokes 3 cigs per day for 15 yrs., Drug use: (-)
Family history: Father with MI age 70. No hx HTN, DM, DVT, CVA

EXAM (at 01:00):

General: Well-appearing; well-nourished; A&O X 3, in no apparent distress
Head: Normocephalic; atraumatic
Eyes: PERRL
Nose: The nose is normal in appearance without rhinorrhea

Neck: No JVD or distended neck veins

Resp: Normal chest excursion with respiration; breath sounds clear and equal bilaterally; no wheezes, rhonchi, or rales

Card: Regular rhythm, tachycardia, without murmurs, rub or gallop

Abd: Non-distended; non-tender, soft, without rigidity, rebound or guarding, no pulsatile mass

Chest: No pain with palpation

Skin: Normal for age and race; warm and dry without diaphoresis ; no apparent lesions

Extremities: Pulses are 2 plus and equal times 4 extremities, no peripheral edema or calf muscle pain

ORDERS: At 00:42: Ativan 1mg IVP, **At 01:18:** Ativan 1mg IVP

RESULTS:

Time 00:11			Computer interpretation
	Vent. rate	153 bpm	Undetermined rhythm
Male	PR interval	* ms	Left axis deviation
	QRS duration	80 ms	Marked ST abnormality, possible inferior subendocardial injury
	QT/QTc	262/418 ms	Abnormal ECG
Technician:	P-R-T axes	61 -36 -83	
Test ind: RAPID HEART RATE			**ED Dr. interpretation:** Suspect rate related

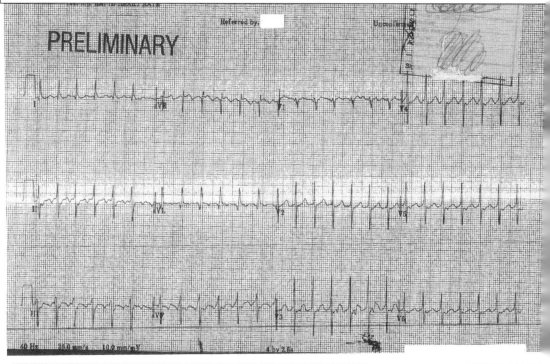

Test	Flag	Value	Units	Ref. Range
WBC		6.9	K/ul	4.6-10.2
HGB		16.6	G/DL	13.5-17.5
PLT		220	K/uL	142-424

(continued on next page)

Test	Flag	Value	Units	Ref. Range
NA		141	MMOL/L	135-144
K		3.5	MMOL/L	3.5-5.1
CL		101	MMOL/L	98-107
CO2		29	MMOL/L	22-29
BUN	H	20	MG/DL	7-18
CREAT		1.0	MG/DL	0.6-1.3

Test	Flag	Value	Units	Ref. Range
CK	H	233	U/L	21-232
CKMB	H	5.9	NG/ML	0.0-5.0
RELIND		2.5		0.0-4.0
TROPI		.06	NG/ML	.00-.27

Accudata: Fingerstick blood sugar -150

RADIOLOGY: PORTABLE CHEST. IMPRESSION: Normal portable chest.

ECG at 02:43: *ECG #2 follows*

Time 02:43		**Computer interpretation:**	
Male	Vent. rate	114 bpm	Unusual P axis, possible ectopic atrial tachycardia with undetermined rhythm irregularity
	PR interval	* ms	Left axis deviation
	QRS duration	78 ms	ST & T wave abnormality, consider lateral ischemia
Technician:	QT/QTc	320/441 ms	Abnormal ECG
Test ind: CP	P-R-T axes	263 -41 -33	
			ED Dr. interpretation: Doubt ischemia—no CP during EKG

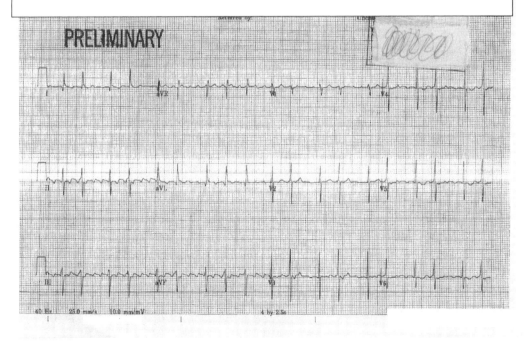

Progress Note (at 03:42): I spoke with this patient at length. He says he feels "100% better" about 03:30 AM. He has been stable throughout his stay in sinus tach w/o ectopy. The pressure he described earlier to the physician asistant is not reproducible with exertion. He regularly exercises and does not experience chest pain. He states he does not use cocaine. He had a negative stress test within the last year. Overall I believe his symtpoms are more consistent with anxiety and am very comfortable sending him home.

DIAGNOSIS (at 03:45):
1. Chest pain - atypical
2. Anxiety
3. Tachycardia - supraventricular

DISPOSITION: The patient was discharged to Home ambulatory accompanied by spouse. Follow-up with primary care physician in 2 days. AfterCare Instructions for anxiety. Prescription for Ativan (lorazepam) 1mg. Sixteen (16). Take one tablet by mouth every eight hours as needed for anxiety. Released from the ED at 04:22, New Years Day.

Gregory L. Henry comments:

"If there are orthostatic symptoms and an abnormal heart rate, assume they are related until proven otherwise"

The function of the heart is to supply blood to the brain. If there are orthostatic symptoms and an abnormal heart rate, assume they are related until proven otherwise.

The road to hell is paved with a diagnosis of panic attacks. A patient with a history of panic attacks is not protected against other disease entities, and a prior normal stress test does not protect a patient from ischemic cardiac disease.

A chief complaint of rapid heart rate can be confusing. Keep it simple; the patient has an abnormal heart rate with neurologic symptoms. It should be assumed that the abnormal heart rate is the cause of the lightheadedness. A pulse rate of 158 is rapid, even during a panic attack, and should be considered abnormal.

The evaluation of this patient was seriously flawed. The initial EKG showed tachycardia at approximately 150 beats per minute. It is impossible to say from the EKG whether we are looking at atrial flutter or an accelerated atrial, or perhaps even a junctional, rhythm. In addition, the marked S-T abnormality has to be taken seriously. The improvement in heart rate after Ativan should not have reassured the ED physician. I believe discretion would have been the better part of valor.

The documentation in this case is reasonable, but the multiple EKG abnormalities should have prompted consultation with cardiology, and admission would have been most appropriate. The most common cause of death in 57 year old American males is still cardiac disease; to disrespect this fact shows lack of familiarity with the current nature of litigation in emergency medicine.

Finally, the diagnosis of psychiatric disease, such as hysterical conversion reaction and panic disorders, should be very carefully thought out before being placed on the chart. Assume an organic cause until proven otherwise; it is hard to go wrong with that bit of philosophy.

- Thoroughness of Documentation: 7 out of 10.

- Thoroughness of Patient Evaluation: 6 out of 10.

- Risk of Serious Illness Being Missed: High risk.

- Risk Management Legal Rating: High risk.

57 YEAR OLD MALE WITH HEART FLUTTERING & LIGHTHEADEDNESS

—Second Visit: Same Day (New Year's Day)—

Note: *Per established protocol, all ECG's reviewed by the ED physician on the following shift. It was decided that the patient had atrial fibrillation/flutter and he was called to return to the ED.*

CHIEF COMPLAINT (at 17:05): Called to return for abnormal ECG

| VITAL SIGNS | | | | | | | | | O2% | Pain |
Time	Temp(F)	Rt.	Pulse	Resp	Syst	Diast	Pos.	O2	sat	scale
17:35	98.5	T	166	24	157	114	S	96	ra	0
18:30			90	14	140	98	S	95	2L/NC	0
20:22			88	16	156	109	S	99	2L/NC	0
21:06			90	12	168	104	S	98	2L/NC	
22:20			90	16	160	98	S	99	2lnc	0

HISTORY OF PRESENT ILLNESS (at 18:13): The patient presents as he was asked to return after a review of his ECG from last PM which seemed to show a fib. He is a difficult historian. He does have complaints of fluttering in his chest which has not improved with the ativan prescribed last PM. He also has mild chest pain that began 6 month(s) ago. The symptoms are intermittant. The symptoms longest duration was 2 minute(s). The discomfort is currently 0/10. The discomfort was previously 3/10. It is a tight pain located in the left chest area. The pain radiates to the left arm. Patient denies chest discomfort with exertion. There was no prior treatment. Patient complains of diaphoresis. The patient denies peripheral edema, fever, SOB, abd. pain, nausea or vomiting, lightheadedness, calf muscle pain

PAST MEDICAL HISTORY/TRIAGE: Same as initial visit, plus; The negative stress test was 4 months ago. Stopped his BP medicine 1 month ago. Takes many herbal medicines. PMH: HTN, hepatitis C, high cholesterol

EXAM (at 18:16):

General: Alert and oriented X3, well-nourished, well appearing, in no apparent distress

Head: Normocephalic; atraumatic.

Eyes: PERRL

Nose: The nose is normal in appearance without rhinorrhea

Resp: Normal chest excursion with respiration; breath sounds clear and equal bilaterally; no wheezes, rhonchi, or rales

Card: Regular rhythm, gallop, without murmurs or rub

Abd: Non-distended; non-tender, soft, without rigidity, rebound or guarding

Skin: Normal for age and race; warm and dry; no apparent lesions

RESULTS: *ECG #3 at 18:00 follows*

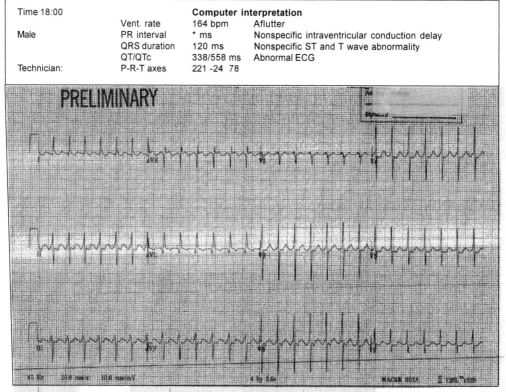

Time 18:00			**Computer interpretation**
	Vent. rate	164 bpm	Aflutter
Male	PR interval	* ms	Nonspecific intraventricular conduction delay
	QRS duration	120 ms	Nonspecific ST and T wave abnormality
	QT/QTc	338/558 ms	Abnormal ECG
Technician:	P-R-T axes	221 -24 78	

ORDERS:

At 17:48: Aspirin 325mg PO

At 18:02: Cardizem 20mg IVP, then cardizem drip 10mg/hour (Note: see vital signs, pulse decreased to 90 at 18:30)

At 20:23: Lovenox 1mg/kg

Test	Flag	Value	Units	Ref. Range
WBC		7.3	K/uL	4.6-10.2
HGB		16.4	G/DL	13.5-17.5
PLT		211	K/uL	142-424

Test	Flag	Value	Units	Ref. Range
TSH		4.35	uIU/ML	.34-4.82

Test	Flag	Value	Units	Ref. Range
NA		141	MMOL/L	135-144
K		3.8	MMOL/L	3.5-5.1
CL		104	MMOL/L	98-107
CO2		25	MMOL/L	22-29
BUN		15	MG/DL	7-18
CREAT		0.9	MG/DL	0.6-1.3

Test	Flag	Value	Units	Ref. Range
CKMB		4.4	NG/ML	0.0-5.0
TROPI		.05	NG/ML	.00-.27

CONSULTATION(at 20:22): I spoke with his PCP to discuss case. I also spoke with the hospitalist for admission and a cardiologist for consultation

DIAGNOSIS (at 20:23): New onset atrial flutter with RVR, chest pain

DISPOSITION: Pt. was admitted to tele bed and left the ED for the floor at 23:34.

INPATIENT COURSE:

Treadmill stress test: Patient completed exam and remained in normal sinus rhythm

Inpatient ECG: (displayed on next page)

********** **Nuclear Medicine Report** **********
IMPRESSION: 1. No evidence for ischemia or infarction. 2. Normal wall motion exam.

********** **Echocardiogram Report** **********
CONCLUSION: Generally normal exam although the mitral E:A ratio is slightly elevated.

********** **Cardiology consultation** (condensed report) **********
This 57-year-old male works construction. He states he runs jack hammers and helps fix basements. On the day in question (New Year's Eve), the patient had a chest discomfort with heart fluttering that he had noticed for a couple of days. However, he also has panic attacks and therefore tried to handle the whole situation with biofeedback. He had been on Paxil for the panic attacks in the past. He was seen in the ED and sent home with a diagnosis of anxiety. His ECG was reviewed by the next ED

physician who diagnosed atrial flutter/fibrillation and he was called to return for admission. His EKG shows T waves that are inverted 1-1.5 mm laterally and inferiorly. When compared to the EKG from a year ago, it is thought that the changes are qualitatively similar and just a little more pronounced now. Troponin, however, is normal x 2, as is CPK. All those tests were run on the first of January. Total CPK is noted to be slightly elevated, actually, at 233, but the index and MB are normal.

ASSESSMENT AND PLAN:
1. Apparently this is a flutter episode, or actually looks like fibrillation. We will let him go home on Toprol 50 mg QD
2. History of hypertension and hepatitis C
3. History of pancreatitis with pseudocyst noted.
4. Abnormal EKG associated with normal stress test result one year ago.

Male		Vent. rate	58 bpm	**Computer interpretation:** Sinus bradycardia with 1st degree AV block
		PR interval	214 ms	Left axis deviation
		QRS duration	84 ms	Minimal voltage criteria for LVH, may be normal variant
		QT/QTc	414/407 ms	ST & T wave abnormality, consider inferior ischemia
Technician:		P-R-T axes	61 -34 -85	ST & T wave abnormality, consider anterolateral ischemia
Test ind: Routine				

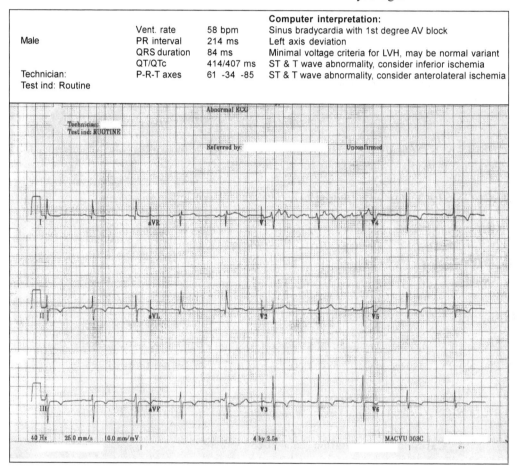

FINAL DIAGNOSIS: New onset atrial fibrillation/flutter

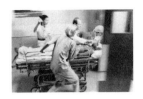

EVALUATION AND MANAGEMENT OF TACHYCARDIAS AND ATRIAL FLUTTER

Sandy Craig, MD, FACEP

I. INTRODUCTION

This patient presents with chief complaint of rapid heart beat, relating 3 days of palpitations and orthostasis. His past medical history is significant for panic attacks, with an increase in anxiety symptoms over the past 3 days. One look at the vital signs, however, would tell the astute emergency physician that this is not likely a simple case of anxiety. The triage heart rate is 147, the initial ECG reveals a rate of 153, and a second set of vital signs reveals a rate of 158. This degree of tachycardia is not typical of a simple anxiety disorder.

II. CATEGORIZATION OF TACHYCARDIA

The differential diagnosis of tachycardia can be simplified greatly by categorizing the rhythm as narrow or wide QRS complex, and then as regular or irregular. A narrow QRS complex is defined as less than 0.10 seconds; our patient has a narrow QRS tachycardia. Regularity in very rapid rhythms may be difficult to detect by auscultation or ECG due to slight variations in the very short R-R interval. Examination of a rhythm strip, in addition to standard 12 lead ECG, may detect irregularities in the rhythm that weren't initially apparent. If it is still not apparent if the rhythm is regular or irregular, obtain a rhythm strip at twice-normal paper speed; this will accentuate the irregular nature of a rhythm.

The physical examination and initial ECG in this patient revealed a regular rhythm. The differential diagnosis of a regular, narrow QRS complex tachycardia includes sinus tachycardia, supraventricular tachycardia (SVT) and atrial flutter.[1] The rate of SVT remains constant from moment to moment, so this patient's presentation is not particularly consistent with SVT. Sinus tachycardia can usually be distinguished because the rate varies from moment to moment, rarely exceeds 150 beats per minute, and is usually associated with acute physiologic stressors such as fever, anemia, pulmonary embolism, hyperthyroidism or toxic ingestion. While this patient's rate is a bit fast for sinus tachycardia, it would be prudent to keep sinus tachycardia in the differential diagnosis, and consider obtaining a rectal temperature, hemoglobin, thyroid function tests, and drug screen, if the etiology remains a mystery after the initial assessment.

III. ATRIAL FLUTTER AND DISCUSSION OF ECG'S AT INITIAL VISIT

Signs and symptoms of atrial flutter include complaints of palpitations, dyspnea, fatigue, chest pain, exercise-induced fatigue or worsening heart failure or pulmonary disease.[1]

Atrial flutter can often be distinguished by the presence of a "saw-tooth" pattern in the isoelectric baseline, apparent especially in leads II and V1. This represents regular atrial depolarizations at a rate of 300–320 beats per minute. (see figure) Typically, two to one conduction through the AV node yields a ventricular rate of 150–160. The saw-tooth pattern is often obscured by the presence of QRS complexes and T waves. Consider the diagnosis of atrial flutter when confronted with a regular narrow tachycardia at a rate of 150-160, even if you cannot appreciate the classic saw tooth pattern.

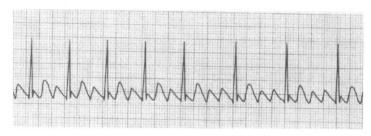

Source: Image from http://www.medibyte.com/cme/tutorial05/arrhyth12.jpg
Used with permission.

A closer look at this patient's initial ECG tells the story. After the sixth QRS complex there is a single RR interval that is longer than the others, a result of 3 consecutive nonconducted atrial depolarizations. This allows us a brief opportunity to see the isoelectric baseline unobscured by QRS complexes. Lo and behold, in leads II and III, we can see the classic saw-tooth pattern of atrial flutter. Is this patient anxious? You bet he is! You'd feel anxious too if your atria were contracting 300 times a minute, pushing your ventricles along at 150 beats per minute.

An hour and a half after the initial ECG, the emergency physician has a second chance to make the correct diagnosis. By this time the patient has received Ativan, the ventricular rate has decreased, and another ECG is obtained. At first glance this second ECG appears to be irregularly irregular and this rhythm could easily be mistaken for atrial fibrillation. But note the saw tooth pattern of P waves in leads II, III, and AVF. And note that every RR interval is a precise multiple of the PP interval. This represents atrial flutter with AV conduction varying from 2:1 to 3:1 throughout the tracing. The diagnosis is once again missed by the emergency physician, and the patient is discharged with diagnoses of anxiety and atypical chest pain.

This case also teaches a valuable lesson about computerized ECG interpretations - they are not to be trusted! In both cases the computerized ECG interpretation missed the diagnosis of atrial flutter. So cover up the computer interpretation, analyze each tracing yourself in a methodical fashion, taking note of rate, rhythm, axes, intervals and morphologies.

Fortunately this emergency department had a quality assurance system in place whereby ECGs were over-read by the next emergency physician on duty. The rhythm was correctly diagnosed and the patient was summoned back to the department for evaluation and treatment of atrial flutter. Happily, there were no adverse events related to the delay in diagnosis.

Atrial flutter is a distinct form of reentrant supraventricular tachycardia, with the reentry circuit typically located around the tricuspid valve annulus. The more common form (present in this patient) features a counterclockwise reentry circuit around the tricuspid valve, giving rise to a saw-tooth pattern of P waves, which appear negative in the inferior leads II, III and aVF and positive in lead I. A less common form features a clockwise circuit around the annulus with saw tooth type P waves appearing positive in the inferior leads and negative in lead I.[1] Regardless of the electrophysiologic subtype, prolonged atrial flutter can result in tachycardia-induced cardiomyopathy, or can degenerate into chronic atrial fibrillation.[8] Prompt diagnosis and treatment is therefore essential for optimal outcome.

IV. ETIOLOGY OF ATRIAL FLUTTER

Atrial flutter has many clinical features in common with atrial fibrillation. Indeed, atrial flutter and fibrillation coexist in many patients, and it has been noted that elimination of atrial flutter often reduces or eliminates atrial fibrillation. Both rhythms are associated with advancing age and underlying disease; atrial flutter is usually associated with cardiovascular or pulmonary disease.[9] Like atrial fibrillation, atrial flutter sometimes occurs in patients with underlying cardiomyopathy, chronic hypoxia, COPD, thyrotoxicosis, pheochromocytoma, pulmonary embolism, or excessive consumption of alcohol (the so-called "holiday heart syndrome"). Atrial flutter is also commonly observed in patients who have had open cardiac surgery involving the atria, when the resulting scar tissue creates an electrophysiologic environment conducive to reentry.

V. MANAGEMENT OF ATRIAL FLUTTER

Despite the fact that the atria are contracting in an organized fashion during atrial flutter, these patients do seem to be at increased risk for atrial thrombus formation (usually in the left atrium or left atrial appendage) and thromboembolic events.[3]

Management of atrial flutter should include:

- A search for underlying cause of the dysrhythmia
- Rate control
- Rhythm control
- Prevention of thromboembolic complications

All patients with newly diagnosed atrial flutter should have thyroid function testing, as atrial flutter can be the lone manifestation of thyrotoxicosis. Chest pain is a common symptom of atrial flutter, given the frequent association with underlying coronary artery disease. consider the possibility of occult coronary artery disease, and maintain a low threshold for ruling out myocardial infarction. Transthoracic echocardiography is of value in detecting underlying cardiomyopathy or valvular dysfunction. Question the patient carefully about use of alcohol—this patient used alcohol extensively in the past. Has he resumed alcohol use, especially in a binge pattern? Shame or denial might prevent him from sharing this information during initial questioning. Finally, consider evaluation for pulmonary embolism or pheochromocytoma if the clinical scenario is compatible with these entities.

VI. RATE CONTROL OF ATRIAL FLUTTER

The approach to rate control is dictated by the hemodynamic stability of the patient. The typical ventricular response rate of 150–160 beats per minute, while well tolerated by most patients, will occasionally cause hypotension, syncope, decompensated congestive heart failure, or rate related cardiac ischemia.[8] One-to-one atrioventricular conduction with ventricular rates of 300–320, though rare, would almost certainly present with cardiovascular collapse. In these cases, emergent electrical cardioversion is indicated. Atrial flutter is relatively sensitive to electrical therapy and can often be converted with as little as 50 joules, but recent literature suggests that a dose of 100 joules is more effective in achieving sinus rhythm, and less likely to result in inadvert conversion to atrial fibrillation.[5] Place the paddles (or electrodes) in the anteroapical or right anterior-left posterior position so as to maximize transatrial delivery of energy. Select synchronous mode on the defibrillator so as to avoid the R-on-T phenomenon with precipitation of ventricular dysrhythmias. Sedation prior to cardioversion is indicated if circumstances permit.[10]

The vast majority of patients will be hemodynamically stable and therefore candidates for pharmacologic rate control. Calcium channel blockers and beta blockers are the drugs of choice and are typically given intravenously so as to achieve prompt rate control and prompt improvement in symptoms. The best studied of these is intravenous diltiazem, given at a dose of 0.25 mg/kg over 2 minutes followed by an infusion of 5–15 mg/hr titrated to a ventricular rate of 60–100 beats per minute. Rate control is typically achieved in less than 30 minutes. Intravenous verapamil is equally effective but associated with a greater incidence of hypotension. Intravenous beta blockers such as inderal, metoprolol or esmolol are effective alternatives to calcium channel blockers. Digoxin and amiodarone are second line drugs, as target heart rates are not achieved for several hours.[8]

When catheter ablation is used for atrial flutter, the recurrence rate is reduced from 93% to 5%, making it more effective than pharmacologic therapy.[8]

VII. CONVERSION TO SINUS RHYTHM

Restoration of sinus rhythm is the ultimate goal, but elective conversion of atrial flutter requires thoughtful consideration of the potential for cardioembolic complications. The edict "First do no harm." certainly applies here. Echocardiographic studies of non-anticoagulated patients with atrial flutter document left atrial or left atrial appendage thrombus in 6–43% of patients. In addition, conversion (spontaneous or induced) to normal sinus rhythm causes transient stunning of the atria, increasing the risk of thromboembolism up to 10 days after conversion.[4] Observational studies document a 1.7 to 7.3% rate of embolic complications in non-anticoagulated patients with atrial flutter who undergo cardioversion.[7] Adequate anticoagulation has been shown to decrease the incidence of post-conversion stroke and peripheral embolic phenomena in atrial fibrillation. As a result, it is generally agreed that patients who have atrial flutter of more than 36–48 hours duration should receive anticoagulation for 4 weeks prior to attempted cardioversion, with continuation of coumadin therapy for 4 weeks after cardioversion. Unless it can be definitively shown that the atrial flutter began less than 36 hours ago, the emergency physician should avoid immediate cardioversion of stable patients and initiate heparin or lovenox therapy.[2] The purpose of admission is to search for underlying pathology and to establish therapeutic coumadin anticoagulation in anticipation of cardioversion 4 weeks later.

If circumstances are such that the patient cannot be anticoagulated for 4 weeks prior to elective cardioversion, the patient should undergo transesophageal echocardiography just prior to planned cardioversion in order to look for atrial thrombus. If thrombus is evident, cardioversion should be deferred if at all possible. Even if no thrombus is seen on TEE, the patient should receive heparin anticoagulation prior to cardioversion and continue coumadin for 4 weeks post cardioversion. Case reports document thromboembolic complications after conversion of atrial fibrillation even in the face of a negative TEE, so this approach is to be used with caution.[2]

Elective restoration of sinus rhythm more often falls under the purview of the cardiologist but is occasionally carried out in the emergency department if flutter is known to be present for less than 36 to 48 hours. Conversion to sinus rhythm can be achieved by electrical direct current cardioversion, atrial overdrive pacing, or pharmacologic techniques. Studies suggest that the most effective pharmacologic agents are the Class III agents ibutilide (Corvert) and dofetilide (Tikosyn). Ibutilide has achieved 63% efficacy in converting recent-onset atrial flutter within 24 hours after a single infusion. The initial dose is 0.01 mg/kg for patients under 60 kg, or 1 mg over 10 minutes in patients over 60 kg. A second dose may be given after 10 minutes if sinus rhythm is not achieved. The average time to conversion is 30 minutes. These agents may precipitate ventricular dysrhythmias, primarily PVCs, in approximately 10% of patients. The most notable dysrhythmia is Torsades de pointes ventricular tachycardia.[8] Although this occurs in less than 2% of patients, the emergency physician should be prepared to treat this complication when using these Class III agents.

VIII. CONTINUATION OF CASE AND SUMMARY

Upon returning to the emergency department, our patient was found to have persistent atrial flutter with a rapid ventricular response rate. He was hemodynamically stable with palpitations present for more than three days. Emergent cardioversion is thus unnecessary and, in fact, would place him at risk for embolic stroke. The emergency physician wisely initiates anticoagulation with lovenox and achieves prompt rate control with intravenous cardiazem. Upon admission to the hospital he is found to be euthyroid with unremarkable transthoracic echocardiogram. Myocardial infarction is ruled out and nuclear scanning is negative for ischemic heart disease. While in the hospital he spontaneously converts to normal sinus rhythm. Problem solved, right?

But wait! Conversion of atrial flutter of greater than 48 hours duration is associated with a risk of acute thromboembolic event regardless of whether the conversion was electrical, pharmacologic or spontaneous. Stunning of the left atrial appendage occurs immediately upon conversion and may persist for weeks. Thromboembolic complications have been noted to occur up to 10 days after conversion. This patient still has a small but elevated risk of thromboembolism which can be mitigated with continued anticoagulation. This author would argue that, in the absence of any contraindication, anticoagulation should have been continued with the goal of maintaining an INR of 2–3 for a period of 4 weeks after conversion.

TEACHING POINTS FROM CASE 19:

- Heart rates over 140 per minute are very likely due to organic illness and should not be attributed to anxiety or functional disorders.
- Emergency department mechanisms for quality assurance are important to protect patient safety.
- A regular narrow QRS tachycardia with a rate of 150–160 per minute is a classic presentation of atrial flutter.
- If there is difficulty in determining the rhythm because of a fast rate, run a rhythm strip at twice the normal paper speed.
- Atrial flutter of more than 36–48 hours is associated with an increased risk of stroke and peripheral embolism. Anticoagulation is indicated prior to cardioversion of the stable patient and should be continued for 4 weeks after conversion to sinus rhythm.
- The diagnosis of psychiatric disease should be very carefully thought out before being placed on the chart. Assume an organic cause until proven otherwise.

REFERENCES

1. Blomström-Lundqvist C, Scheinman MM, Aliot EM, et al. ACC/AHA/ESC guidelines for the management of patients with supraventricular arrhythmias—executive summary: a report of the American College of Cardiology/American Heart Association Task Force on Practice Guidelines, and the European Society of Cardiology Committee for Practice Guidelines (Writing Committee to Develop Guidelines for the Management of Patients With Supraventricular Arrhythmias.). J Am Coll Cardiol 2003;42: 1493–531.

2. Berger M, Schweitzer P. Timing of thromboembolic events after electrical cardioversion of atrial fibrillation or flutter: a retrospective analysis. Am J Cardiol 1998;82: 1545-7, A8.

3. Dunn MI. Thrombolism with atrial flutter. Am J Cardiol 1998;82: 638.

4. Irani WN, Grayburn PA, Afridi I. Prevalence of thrombus, spontaneous echo contrast, and atrial stunning in patients undergoing cardioversion of atrial flutter. A prospective study using transesophageal echocardiography. Circulation 1997;95: 962-6.

5. Pinski SL, Sgarbossa EB, Ching E, Trohman RG. A comparison of 50-J versus 100-J shocks for direct-current cardioversion of atrial flutter. Am Heart J 1999;137: 439-42.

6. Rosenthal L, Ngarmukos T. Atrial Flutter. eMedicine Journal (serial online). 2004. Available at http://www.emedicine.com/med/topic185.htm

7. Seidl K, Hauer B, Schwick NG, et al: Risk of thromboembolic events in patients with atrial flutter. Am J Cardiol 1998;82: 580-3.

8. Fuster V, Rydén LE, Asinger RW, et al. ACC/AHA/ESC guidelines for the management of patients with atrial fibrillation: executive summary: a report of the American College of Cardiology/American Heart Association Task Force on Practice Guidelines and the European Society of Cardiology Committee for Practice Guidelines and Policy Conferences (Committee to Develop Guidelines for the Management of Patients With Atrial Fibrillation). J Am Coll Cardiol 2001;38: 1231-65.

9. Pollock GF. Agtrial fibrillation in the ED: cardioversion, rate control, anticoagulation and more. Emergency Medicine Practice 2002;8: 1-28.

10. American Heart Association. Guidelines 2000 for cardiopulmonary resuscitation and emergency cardiac care. Circulation. 2000;102 (suppl. I): 1-1384.

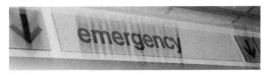

CASE 20

76 YEAR OLD FEMALE WITH SYNCOPE

Commentary:
Gregory L. Henry, MD, FACEP

CEO, Medical Practice Risk Assessment, Inc., Ann Arbor, Michigan
Clinical Professor, Department of Emergency Medicine
   University of Michigan Medical School, Ann Arbor, Michigan
Past President, American College of Emergency Physicians (ACEP)

Discussion:
Wyatt Decker, MD, FACEP

Chair, Department of Emergency Medicine, Mayo Clinic
   Jacksonville, Florida and Mayo Clinic, Rochester, Minnesota
Associate Professor of Emergency Medicine
   Mayo Clinic College of Medicine
Member ACEP Clinical Policies Committee
Member ACEP Subcommittee on MI and Unstable Angina

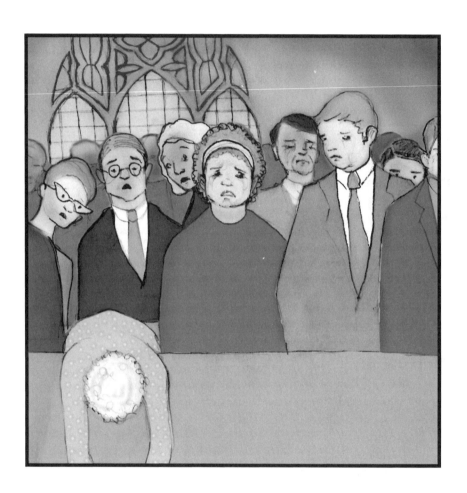

76 YEAR OLD FEMALE WITH SYNCOPE

—Initial Visit*—

*Authors' Note: The history, exam and notes are the actual documentation of the physicians and providers, including abbreviations (and spelling errors)

CHIEF COMPLAINT (at 12:53): Fall

```
VITAL SIGNS
Time     Temp(F)  Rt.   Pulse   Resp   Syst   Diast   Pos.
13:00     97.3     O     96      20     152     96      L
14:00                    76      18     124     78      S
14:35                    76      20     110     60      S
```

HISTORY OF PRESENT ILLNESS (documented at 13:53): The patient may have had a syncopal episode today. She was at a funeral today for her daughter in law. She has not eaten today. She also had to urinate. She fell or passed out. No one is sure. She was alert upon the medics arrival. She denies any pain. She may have a laceration to her scalp. She arrives via EMS in a collar and on a backboard. No fever, chills, nausea, vomiting, chest pain, syncope, SOB, dysuria, HA, or rash.

PAST MEDICAL HISTORY/TRIAGE: Chief complaint/quote: Per EMS, pt was at a funeral and passed out and fell backwards striking her head. Patient arrived by stretcher via EMS in full C-spine immobilization. Finger stick blood sugar (at 12:48), per EMS was 76.
Allergies: No known allergies.
Medications: The patient is not taking medications at this time.
PMH/PSH: No significant medical history. No significant surgical history.

EXAM (documented at 13:54):
Airway: Airway is patent and clear.
Breathing: Unlabored and clear.
Circulation: Carotid and distal pulses normal, capillary refill is brisk.
Neuro: Awake, alert and cooperative, in mild distress, on long spine board with C-collar in place.
Head: laceration posterior scalp.
Eyes: PERRL; EOM intact; normal fundi.
ENMT: TM's normal; normal nose; no rhinorrhea; normal mouth and pharynx.
Neck: C-collar in place, non-tender to palpation.
Card: Normal S1, S2; no murmurs, rubs, or gallops.
Chest/resp.: Normal chest excursion with respiration; breath sounds clear and equal bilaterally, no pain with chest palpation.
Abd: Normal bowel sounds; non-distended; non-tender; no palpable organomegaly.
Ext: Normal ROM in all four extremities; non-tender to palpation; distal pulses are normal.
Skin: Normal for age and race; warm; dry; good turgor; no apparent lesions or exudate.

RESULTS (ordered at 13:03, resulted at 14:00):

Test	Flag	Value	Units	Ref. Range
WBC		7.0	K/uL	4.6-10.2
HGB		12.9	G/DL	12.0-16.0
PLT		276	K/uL	142-424

Test	Flag	Value	Units	Ref. Range
NA		141	MMOL/L	135-144
K		4.0	MMOL/L	3.5-5.1
CL		103	MMOL/L	98-107
CO2		28	MMOL/L	22-29
BUN	H	20	MG/DL	7-18
CREAT		1.0	MG/DL	0.6-1.3

Test	Flag	Value	Units	Ref. Range	Status
CKMB		0.5	NG/ML	0.0-5.0	
TROPI		0.00	NG/ML	.00-.27	

Urine dip stick: WNL except Glucose; Results 50 mg/dL

RESULTS: *ECG at 13:10 follows*:

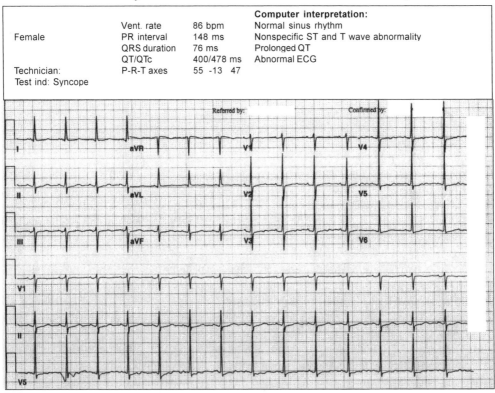

			Computer interpretation:
Female	Vent. rate	86 bpm	Normal sinus rhythm
	PR interval	148 ms	Nonspecific ST and T wave abnormality
	QRS duration	76 ms	Prolonged QT
Technician:	QT/QTc	400/478 ms	Abnormal ECG
Test ind: Syncope	P-R-T axes	55 -13 47	

ED COURSE: Td 0.5cc IM. Laceration repair: The affected area was cleansed with normal saline. The area was anesthetized with 1.5cc's 1% lidocaine with epinephrine. The wound was explored No foreign body. The posterior scalp laceration was closed with 3 staples. Antibacterial ointment

DIAGNOSIS (at 14:00): 1. Syncope, 2. Laceration - scalp

DISPOSITION: The patient was discharged to Home (at 14:47) via wheelchair accompanied by self and family member. Follow-up with primary physician if not improved in 3 days. ACI for Fainting/syncope. Released at 14:47.

Gregory L. Henry comments:

"...elderly patients with their first episode of syncope should be admitted for monitoring and provocative testing to evaluate for arrhythmia"

The etiology of syncope is highly stratified by age. In an older patient with syncope, the underlying problem is decreased blood supply to the brain until proven otherwise.

In this case, the syncopal episode was observed, without obvious tonic clonic activity to suggest a seizure. She was neurologically intact after the event, making a primary brain problem less likely. Arrhythmia causing a momentary decrease in circulation to the brain is the most concerning etiology. Her initial EKG was normal but does not rule out an arrhythmia; further monitoring is usually required.

The evaluation of this patient was thorough. The hemoglobin was checked; other tests should include a stool guaiac to rule out occult bleeding. Most of the other testing is overkill. The fact that the patient is now alert and not complaining of any pain is also important. The tetanus immunization, wound closure, and determination of glucose are within the standard of care.

Now the question is, "How should a patient with syncope and nonspecific findings be handled?" Hindsight is always perfect, but many experts feel that elderly patients with a first episode of syncope should be admitted for monitoring and provocative testing to evaluate for arrhythmia.

- Thoroughness of Documentation: 9 out of 10.

- Thoroughness of Patient Evaluation: 9 out of 10.

- Risk of Serious Illness Being Missed: Medium risk.

- Risk Management Legal Rating: Medium risk.

76 YEAR OLD FEMALE WITH SYNCOPE

—Second Visit: Same Day 5 Hours Later—

CHIEF COMPLAINT (at 19:55): Altered mental status

```
VITAL SIGNS
Time      Temp(F)  Rt. Pulse  Resp   Syst  Diast  Pos.  O2 Sat  O2%
19:57     94.7     Tym. 129   16     119   66     L     97      2L
20:15                                88    42     S
```

HISTORY OF PRESENT ILLNESS (at 20:01): 76yo WF seen earlier today for syncope returns as patient was sleeping and tried to be aroused by family. Was unarousable so medics were called. Patient had bp reportedly of 50/p and was given 600 cc NS bolus with bp in 100/p. Patient arrived alert and appropriate. Denies any pain except in left side area. Describes pain as an 'aching' pain and has gotten better since seen earlier. Denies any headache. Reports generalized weakness/ fatigue. Family at bedside with patient. No chest pain/abdominal pain. No fever, chills, nausea/ vomiting/diarrhea, hematemesis, blood in stool, abd. pain, chest pain, SOB, p. edema, or cough.

PAST MEDICAL HISTORY/TRIAGE: (Per triage RN on arrival at 19:55): Patient arrived by stretcher via EMS transport from Home Pt. seen in ER approx 5hr ago for a syncopal episode and laceration repair to post. head. This evening family states pt was asleep and hard to arouse. Was diaphoretic and pale. On arrival of medics Bp was 50/d given 600cc fluid bolus and pressure increased to 121/ 72. Pt alert and oriented x 3 states feels tired. Also c/o pain to post left back just above hip.
Past medical history: Negative
Social history: Patient does not smoke. Patient denies alcohol use.

EXAM (at 20:05):
General: Sleepy, ill-appearing elderly WF; pale; easily arousable and follows all commands
Head: Normocephalic; atraumatic.
Eyes: PERRL, EOMI
OP: MMM, no exudates/erythema
Ears: bilateral TM's with nl light reflex
Nose: The nose is normal in appearance without rhinorrhea
Resp: Normal chest excursion with respiration; breath sounds clear and equal bilaterally; no wheezes, rhonchi, or rales
Card: Regular rhythm, without murmurs, rub or gallop
Abd: Non-distended; non-tender, soft, without rigidity, rebound or guarding
Ext: 2+ radial/DP pulses bilaterally; no edema; no calf tenderness
Skin: Pale and cool on all extremities

ORDERS:

At 19:50: Immediately on arrival in ED; Finger stick glucose = 494

At 20:09: CXR and labs inc. CBC, lytes BUN/creat, troponin, CK-MB and serum glucose ordered and IV started, but labs not able to be obtained at this time. Head CT ordered.

At 20:21: Brain CT canceled and Abd/pelvis CT to r/o AAA. IVF bolus 250cc NS ordered

```
ADDITIONAL VITAL SIGNS
Time    Temp(F)  Pulse  Resp  Syst  Diast  Pos.  O2 Sat O2%
20:23            80     18    65    P      S
20:45            120          40    0      L
21:10            124          42    0      L
22:12            104          46    0      L
22:45            60     14    40    0      L
23:02            125          56    0      L
```

PROGRESS NOTES:

At 20:35–Patient taken to CT scan and returned (at 20:44) with syncope and agonal respirations. Patient was immediately taken into the main trauma room. Patient responded to sternal rub with 'yes', but remained hypotensive and tachycardic. (At 20:50) dopamine was ordered. The decision was made for intubation. The patient was intubated at 21:05 after administration of lidocaine 150mg and etomidate 10mg. The patient remained hypotensive. A femoral stick was performed for blood draw. (At 21:14), I ordered 2 units of uncrossed blood.

At 21:55–Patient noted to have Hemoglobin 7.1 where had Hemoglobin 12.9 earlier today (lab results below). Patient remained hypotensive. Patient's family was made aware of all the decisions and patient progress. Patient's family have been in the room with the patient. Intensivist was contacted early in the w/u and has been with the patient through the CT scan.

At 22:10–Radiologist call with CT scan report shows leaking AAA with retroperitoneal hematoma (results per radiology below). Spoke with the vascular surgeon again who is on the way. I am consulting the surgical house officer. Patient was noted to become bradycardic. Atropine was given with good response.

At 22:54–Patient noted to have change in rhythm with wide complex tachycardia moving into v-fib. Patient was shocked at 360. Chest compressions started due to asystole. Shocked again x 2 at 360 Patient then received rounds of epinephrine and atropine. Patient went in and out of v-fib requiring shocks. At 22:57 infusion of PRBC was started.

At 23:07–Patient had return of sinus appearing rhythm with a faint left carotid pulse. Vascular surgeon is now in the hospital. Surgery house officer in the room. Patient given two more units of blood. Patient's son in the room during the code and aware of the situation. Spoke with patient's multiple family members who asked questions. Started on levophed per recommendations of house officer. Received a total of 2L normal saline and 4 units of blood.

At 23:14 - Patient taken to OR. Blood bank notified and requested to keep 4 units available at all times.

RESULTS:

Test	Flag	Value	Units	Ref. Range
WBC	H	14.0	K/uL	4.6-10.2
HGB	L	7.1	G/DL	12.0-16.0
PLT	L	129	K/uL	142-424

Test	Flag	Value	Units	Ref. Range
NA		139	MMOL/L	135-144
K		3.9	MMOL/L	3.5-5.1
CL		107	MMOL/L	98-107
CO2	L	16	MMOL/L	22-29
BUN	H	25	MG/DL	7-18
CREAT	H	1.9	MG/DL	0.6-1.3
GLUC	H	356	MG/DL	70-110

Test	Flag	Value	Units	Ref. Range
TROPI		.12	NG/ML	.00-.27
CKMB		1.2	NG/ML	0.0-5.0

Test	Flag	Value	Units	Ref. Range
pH	L	7.308		7.350-7.450
PCO2	L	24.5	MMHG	32.0-48.0
PO2	H	249.0	MMHG	83.0-108.0

RADIOLOGY:
Portable chest #1 (at 20:09): No evidence of acute cardiopulmonary disease
Portable chest #2 (at 21:22): Status post intubation. No evidence of acute disease.

CT scan abdomen with contrast (per radiologist): Leaking abdominal aortic aneurysm with very large left-sided retroperitoneal hematoma. There is an approximately 6-cm abdominal aortic aneurysm, which shows leakage of contrast material toward the left side just above the aortic bifurcation. There is a very large left-sided retroperitoneal hematoma, which displaces the left kidney anteriorly. Contrast opacification of the parenchymal organs of the abdomen is diminished, consistent with the patient's profound hypotension. The hematoma extends into the left side of the pelvis.

DIAGNOSIS: Ruptured AAA

DISPOSITION: Pt. went to OR emergently, unable to obtain clothing list, her watch was given to son at bedside. Released from ED to the OR at 23:14.

HOSPITAL COURSE

OPERATIVE REPORT (summary): (Enter OR at 23:30) The abdomen is prepped with Betadine solution, then (at 23:37) an incision was made from the xiphoid to the pubis in the midline. The retroperitoneum is exposed after placing a T-bar across the proximal aorta. The aneurysm is identified and clamps are placed on the distal aorta at the iliac bifurcation. The neck of the aneurysm is identified at the level of the left renal artery and it was deemed necessary to divide the left renal vein in order to provide adequate exposure. An 18 mm Dacron tube graft was anastomosed to the proximal neck in an end-to-end fashion utilizing a running 3-0 Prolene.

During the course of the dissection, the patient again experienced arrest and ACLS protocol was instituted. Pulse was regained and the surgery proceeded. The graft was measured to satisfactory length and anastomosed to the distal aorta at the iliac bifurcation. The graft was flushed antegrade and the iliacs were flushed retrograde prior to opening the left iliac artery, perfusing the left leg. The patient was deemed to have satisfactory pressure and the right iliac clamp subsequently removed. The skin was closed (at 00:45) and dressing applied. The patient moved from the Operating Room in guarded condition.

DEATH NOTE: The patient had a very stormy postoperative course, was made DNR CC by the family, and subsequently expired later in the morning of the day of surgery. Cause of death determined to be sequelae of ruptured abdominal aortic aneurysm.

FINAL DIAGNOSIS: Ruptured abdominal aortic aneurysm.

Additional Greg Henry comments:

The final outcome of this case is incredibly surprising. Initially, this patient had a normal abdominal examination and was not complaining of abdominal pain. This puts her into a microscopically small group of AAA patients. Her general condition and lack of risk factors also place her in a very low risk group for ruptured aortic aneurysm. It is easy to say that I would have picked this up, but in all honesty, in my hands she would have been admitted to a telemetry unit and, more than likely, gone downhill over the next few hours. Whether we would have picked up the aneurysm earlier is a matter of conjecture.

One point to consider is the extended amount of time during her second visit between ordering the abd/pelvic CT, presumably to look for AAA, and the time she was taken to surgery. It is difficult to tell from the documentation why there was such a long delay. Intubation occurred at 21:05 after she had returned from CT, but the results of the CT were not received by the emergency physician until 22:10. Forty five minutes later she was still in the ED, and arrested.

Additionally, this chart highlights a very important principle in risk management; the ED physician must always read the nurses' documentation. At 19:55 (on arrival) the nurse documented an initial BP (per medics) of 50/d and complaint of pain to "post left back just above hip." The physician documented aching "left side pain." Back pain and hypotension in an elderly patient should immediately raise the possibility of AAA.

To summarize, to have a woman without cardiac disease or abdominal pain, feeling well in the department on her initial visit, near dead in 5 hours from an abdominal aortic aneurysm—this is incredibly rare. I am glad I am not the emergency physician whose name is on the original chart!

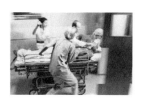

EVALUATION AND MANAGEMENT OF SYNCOPE

Wyatt Decker, MD, FACEP

I. INTRODUCTION

Syncope is a common presenting complaint in the Emergency Department (ED), accounting for up to 3% of ED visits.[1,2] It is usually defined as a sudden loss of consciousness with spontaneous and full recovery.

II. DIFFERENTIAL DIAGNOSIS

It is important to differentiate syncope from conditions which may present in a similar fashion, such as seizures, strokes, and psychiatric conditions. While seizures are usually easily differentiated from syncope by the presence of tonic clonic movements and a postictal period, occasionally the presenting symptoms will be similiar. Clinical studies contrasting these two presenting diagnoses have found that tongue biting and confusion after the episode (postictal phase) are strongly associated with seizures. Neurologic events such as strokes, while often on the forefront in the mind of patients and family members, are seldom related to syncope. A drop attack, caused by disruption of the posterior circulation, is an extremely rare event and is usually described as a sudden 'give way' of muscle strength. Psychiatric causes of syncope (pseudosyncope) are also rare—a diagnosis of exclusion, it is often suspected based on irregular historical features, patient affect, and lack of physical exam findings.

Syncope represents a diagnostic and disposition challenge since often the patient in the ED has a benign exam and feels well, yet may have a life-threatening condition such as an arrhythmia.

III. SYNCOPE AND RUPTURED ABDOMINAL AORTIC ANEURYSM (AAA)

Abdominal aortic aneurysm is on the list of catastrophic vascular events that can include syncope in their presentation. Other vascular events include aortic dissection, massive GI bleed, pulmonary embolus, and subarachnoid hemorrhage.[3,4] The vast majority of these patients will have compelling findings on history or physical exam which direct the provider toward the underlying etiology.

When a ruptured aortic aneurysm causes syncope, one would expect to also find one or more of the following: abdominal pain, flank or back pain, hypotension, palpable abdominal mass, decreased distal pulses, or decreased hemoglobin. In the recently published San Francisco Syncope Study,[5] of the 684 patients with syncope who enrolled and were followed, 12 (1.8%) presented with significant hemorrhage. If combined with other causes of blood loss, such as subarachnoid hemorrhage and PE, 4.1% of syncope patients were found to have one of these diagnoses. In the derivation of the San Francisco syncope decision rule, hematocrit <30 identified 5 of 684 syncope patients with a serious outcome. Other elements of the decision rule for identifying adverse events within 7 days included abnormal ECG, shortness of breath, hypotension and congestive heart failure. Of note, Martin[6] and Kapoors' previous work on making a decision rule for syncope did not include any patients with known aortic pathology.

Table 1. Characteristics of Patients Presenting with Syncope (N=684)*

Characteristic	No. (%)
Age, y, mean (SD) [range]	62.1 (23) [10-102]
Female, No. (%)	403 (58.9)
Admitted	376 (54.9)
Admission length, days, median (IQR) [range]	2 (1-3) [1-19]
1-Day admissions	161 (23.5)
2-Day admissions	74 (10.8)
Syncope as primary complaint	500 (73.1)
Patients with serious outcomes by Day 7[+]	79 (11.5)
Death	5 (0.7)
Cardiac causes	56 (8.2)
Myocardial infarction	21 (3.1)
Non-Q wave myocardial infarction	12 (1.8)
Arrhythmia	30 (4.4)
Structural	5 (0.7)
Pulmonary embolism	5 (0.7)
Significant hemorrhage	12 (1.8)
Gastrointestinal tract bleed	10 (1.5)
Spontaneous ruptured spleen	1 (0.2)
Ruptured ectopic pregnancy	1 (0.2)
Subarachnoid hemorrhage	3 (0.4)
Stroke syndromes	3 (0.4)
Other	5 (0.7)
Sepsis	1 (0.2)
Anemia	2 (0.3)
Readmit	2 (0.3)

IQR, Interquartile range.

* All values are number (%) unless otherwise noted.

[+] Some patients had >1 diagnosis as a cause for a serious outcome.

Source: Quinn JV, Stiell IG, McDermott DA, et al. Derivation of the San Francisco syncope rule to predict patients with short-term serious outcomes. Ann Emerg Med 2004; 43(2):224-32. Used with permission.

IV. DISCUSSION OF CASE

Our patient presented with syncope, but no other signs or symptoms of aortic aneurysm, which is exceptionally rare. Cases such as this are sometimes used to argue for aggressive imaging in all syncope patients. However, the list of catastrophic events that can include syncope is long, and includes virtually all vital organs, making routine imaging unrealistic. A better approach is for the physician to conduct a careful history and physical, with attention to the clues of aortic aneurysm and other potential life-threatening conditions.

V. MANAGEMENT OF SYNCOPE

In the absence of findings of life-threatening conditions, the diagnosis of syncope will not be obtained in approximately half of patients in the ED, and in a full 30% after outpatient work up.[3] If the initial history, physical, and ECG are unrevealing, the focus turns to risk stratification. In addition to the San Francisco syncope rule discussed earlier, one study has determined that clinicians can effectively identify low, intermediate, and high risk patients.[6] Patients at intermediate risk for serious outcomes (based primarily on clinical judgement) were randomized to routine care (admission to a cardiology service) or care in an ED Observation Unit. Those patients cared for in an observation unit had shorter lengths of stay but no difference in event rates. Utilizing an observation unit, rather than hospital admission, may serve as a safe option for a subset of syncope patients.

VI. INITIAL MANAGEMENT

Regarding the initial management of this patient, it appears that the work up was appropriate. The patient's age places her in an intermediate risk category based on Martin's work,[7] which means that admission should be considered but is not mandatory. The use of an ED observation unit as described by Shen and colleagues[6] may represent a lower cost but safe alternative in this type of patient. The primary goal of such an approach is to exclude cardiac arrhythmias— and it is doubtful that even hospital admission would have altered the outcome of this case.

VII. ADMISSION CRITERIA FOR SYNCOPE

The American College of Emergency Physician's (ACEP) Clinical Policy on Syncope recommends hospital admission for syncope patients with any of the following:[8]

1. A history of congestive heart failure or ventricular arrhythmias.
2. Associated chest pain or other symptoms compatible with acute coronary syndrome.
3. Evidence of significant congestive heart failure or valvular heart disease on physical examination.
4. ECG findings of ischemia, arrhythmia, prolonged QT interval, or bundle branch block.

And consideration of admission if:

1. Age older than 60 years.
2. History of coronary artery disease or congenital heart disease.
3. Family history of unexpected sudden death.
4. Exertional syncope in younger patients without an obvious benign etiology for the syncope.

Both decision rules and the ACEP clinical policies are general in nature, and individual patient findings and features are key in decisions on guiding the work up and management of those patients.

TEACHING POINTS ABOUT CASE 20:
- Look for evidence of a hidden life-threatening condition in all patients with syncope.
- Clues to a leaking abdominal aorta aneurysm include:
  - ➢ Abdominal, flank, or back aches
  - ➢ Hypotension
  - ➢ Diminished pulses distally
  - ➢ New anemia
- If you do not feel a patient with syncope needs admission, document a progress note detailing why you do not think a life-threatening condition is occurring.
- Consider an observation unit protocol for intermediate risk syncope patients.
- Discrepancies between nursing and physician notes need to be discussed and resolved.

REFERENCES

1. Sun CV, Emond JA, Camargo CA. Characteristics and admission patterns of patients presenting with syncope to US Emergency Departments, 1992-2000. Acad Emerg Med 2004; 11:1029-34.

2. Soteriades ES, Evans JC, Larson MG, et al. Incidence and prognosis of syncope. N Engl J Med 2002;347: 878-85.

3. Kapoor WN. Evaluation and outcome of patients with syncope. Medicine 1990;69: 160-75.

4. Nallamothu BK, Saint S, Eagle K, et al. Syncope in acute aortic dissection: Diagnosis, prognostic, and clinical implications; Am J Med 2002;113: 468-71.

5. Quinn JV, Stiell IG, McDermott DA, et al. Derivation of the San Francisco syncope rule to predict patients with short-term serious outcomes. Ann Emerg Med 2004;43: 224-32.

6. Shen WK, Decker WW, Smars PA, et al. Syncope evaluation in the emergency department study (SEEDS): A multidisciplinary approach to syncope management. Circulation 2004;110: 3636-45.

7. Martin TP, Hanusa BH, Kapoor WN. Risk stratification of patients with syncope. Ann Emerg Med 1997;29: 459-66.

8. ACEP Clinical Policies Subcommittee on Syncope. Clinical policy: critical issues in the evaluation and management of patients presenting with syncope. Ann Emerg Med 2001; 37: 771-6.

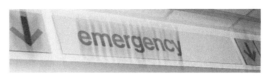

CASE21
47 YEAR OLD FEMALE WITH FLANK PAIN

Commentary:
Gregory L. Henry, MD, FACEP

CEO, Medical Practice Risk Assessment, Inc., Ann Arbor, Michigan
Clinical Professor, Department of Emergency Medicine
    University of Michigan Medical School, Ann Arbor, Michigan
Past President, American College of Emergency Physicians (ACEP)

Discussion:
Patrick Pettengill, MD

Attending ED physician, Department of Emergency Medicine
    Beaumont Hospital, Royal Oak, MI

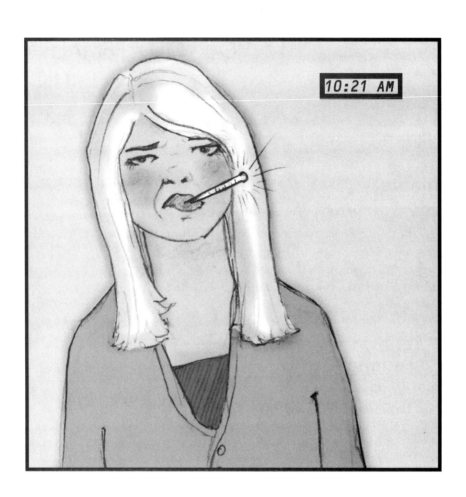

10:21 AM

47 YEAR OLD FEMALE WITH FLANK PAIN

—Initial Visit*—

*Authors' Note: The history, exam and notes are the actual documentation of the physicians and providers, including abbreviations (and spelling errors)

CHIEF COMPLAINT (at 10:17): Flank pain

```
VITAL SIGNS
Time      Temp     Pulse    Resp    Syst   Diast
10:21     100.2     98       24      140     70
```

HISTORY OF PRESENT ILLNESS (at 10:47): 47 year old woman with a PMH significant for DM, CAD, seizures, and kidney stones (by her history) presents with c/o left flank pain with radiation to the left groin which began earlier today. She states this is the same pain that she had when she had kidney stones last summer. She also complains of mild dysuria and some urinary frequency. No nausea or vomiting. Was seen in the ER last night for headache and given Rx for Percocet.

PAST MEDICAL HISTORY/TRIAGE:
Medication, common allergies: Penicillin, Compazine
PMH: Diabetes, CAD, Seizures, Kidney Stones
PSH: Chole, Spinal fusion at L3-4, Left Knee, Right Ankle

EXAM (at 10:49):
Eyes: PERRL
Lungs: CTAB
CV: RRR without M/R/G
Abd: Soft, NT, without R/R/G
Back: No CVAT

ORDERS: At 11:02 she was given dilauded and phenergan. She received 1 L NS.

RESULTS (at 11:37):

```
Test    Flag    Value    Units    Ref. Range
WBC      H      15.7     K/uL     4.6-10.2
HGB             14.0     G/DL     12.0-16.0
PLT             238      K/uL     142-424

Chem-7:    WNL
Glucose:   190
Urinalysis: 25-50 WBC, 0-2 RBC
```

Helical CT (at 11:33): Hydronephrosis and hydroureter on left with a small calcification at left UVJ, probably due to a tiny calculus

PROGRESS NOTES: (At 12:02) she received IV Levaquin 500mg. Will let the stone pass on it's own. Urine strainer. Drink plenty of fluids. She is not able to afford Levaquin and was given a prescription for Macrobid instead. Rx for Percocet. Referral to new urologist (was seen by urology in the past, but requests a new referral)

DIAGNOSIS:
1. Left ureterolithiasis with obstruction
2. Urinary tract infection

DISPOSITION (at 14:17): The patient was discharged to home ambulatory. Follow up with urology. Prescriptions: Percocet and Macrobid.

Gregory L. Henry comments:

"The documentation for this case is adequate. It is the decision making that is problematic."

The evaluation of a patient with a kidney stone revolves around two questions; Do they have a true stone or obstruction, and, are they systemically sick? Many patients present to the ED with recurrent kidney stones; the vast majority are handled on an outpatient basis.

This history in this case suggests that this patient has an infection. She has urinary frequency and was initially febrile in the emergency department.

The evaluation of this patient was perfectly reasonable. Adequate history was obtained, and the history of kidney stones was discovered early in the process. The physical examination, although brief, seems to be to the point. The patient's laboratory workup did show an elevation of the serum white blood cell count and a urinalysis suggested infection. The helical CT showed hydronephrosis and hydroureter, indicating obstruction.

The documentation for this case is adequate. It is the decision making that is problematic. The patient received IV fluids, IV antibiotics and pain medication in the emergency department. The mistake was not consulting a urologist. In a patient with a kidney stone, without hydroureter, and no systemic illness, outpatient management is the therapy of choice. In a patient with fever, elevated white count, obstruction, and obviously infected urine, in-hospital IV antibiotics (until a decision is made about relieving the obstruction) is the most appropriate way to go.

- **Thoroughness of Documentation:** 8 out of 10.
- **Thoroughness of Patient Evaluation:** 9 out of 10.
- **Risk of Serious Illness Being Missed:** Medium risk.
- **Risk Management Legal Rating:** Medium risk.

—Second Visit: Less Than 24 Hours Later—

```
VITAL SIGNS
Time     Temp     Pulse    Resp    Syst    Diast
08:20    101.5     96       20      174      76
```

CHIEF COMPLAINT (at 08:15): Urinary frequency and fever

HISTORY OF PRESENT ILLNESS (at 08:51): Now with complaints of fever and chills, urinary frequency and urgency. Sharp left flank pain. Feels thirsty. Denies any nausea or vomiting, blood in the urine. Requests not to be seen by former urologist, as he told her that she did not have a kidney stone.

EXAM:
General: Shaking with chills and seems uncomfortable.
Lungs: CTAB
Abdomen: WNL
Back: Minimal left CVAT

RESULTS (at 09:59):

```
Test       Flag    Value    Units      Ref. Range
WBC         H      12.7     K/uL       4.6-10.2
HGB                14.7     G/DL       12.0-16.0
PLT                 249     K/uL       142-424


Chem-7:  WNL
Glucose: 140
Urinalysis:25-50 WBC, leukocyte esterase positive, Bacteria 2+
```

PROGRESS NOTES (at 10:25): She received IV fluids. The physician spoke with on call urology, who recommended a repeat helical CT, because if the patient was still obstructed, she would need to have a stent placed. The repeat CT was resulted at 12:02, and showed hydronephrosis and ureteral dilation persists. When the CT was compared with an old CT, the stone seen yesterday seemed to represent a phlebolith (as it was seen on both CT's as well as the old CT). There was stranding around the ureter and kidney, which was consistent with acute obstruction as well as pyelonephritis. When the old records were reviewed, it was discovered that the patient had a ureteral dilation procedure for a distal ureteral stricture by her former urologist about 5 months previously. Urology felt that regardless of the cause of the obstruction (stone or stricture), it would need to be relieved with a stent. Patient was given Levaquin 500mg IVPB, social worker saw the patient about obtaining medications. She will be admitted.

DIAGNOSIS (at 13:13):
1. Left ureteral obstruction
2. UTI with probable pyelonephritis

HOSPITAL COURSE:

Patient went from the ED to the OR and was given spinal anesthesia and underwent cystourethroscopy.
Per urology: Retrograde pyelogram showed no evidence of stricture, stone or extrinsic compression of the ureter. There was some medial deviation of the ureter in the upper lumbar spine at the site of her previous lumbar spine surgery, but no obstruction or tortuosity. Contrast was injected into the ureter and drained back down without difficulty. The ureteral catheter was left in until the next day, and then it was removed. Her antibiotics were changed to Ancef and Gentamicin. Urine culture from the first ED visit grew > 100,000 cfu/ml E. coli, which was sensitive to everything.

FINAL DIAGNOSIS AND DISPOSITION: She left the hospital in 48 hours in good condition with a diagnosis of acute pyelonephritis and a prescription for Cipro bid and Lorcet plus.

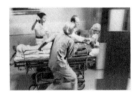

EVALUATION OF FLANK PAIN, DIAGNOSIS AND MANAGEMENT OF URETEROLITHIASIS

Patrick Pettengill, MD

I. INTRODUCTION

In agreement with Dr. Henry, I wonder why a physician who found distal ureteral obstruction, in a patient with diabetes and 25–50 white cells in the urine, did not discuss this with a urologist. The physician ordered a computerized tomography scan looking for something, found it, and then did not act on the results.

II. APPROACH TO THE PATIENT WITH FLANK PAIN

This patient's chief complaint is left flank pain radiating to the left groin. In addition to renal etiologies, the differential diagnoses for flank pain are extensive, including abdominal aortic aneurysm, aortic dissection, mesenteric ischemia, renal infarct, incarcerated hernias, and ovarian torsion.

In this case, a review of the vital signs shows the patient had a mildly elevated temperature, but was otherwise unremarkable. No significant tenderness was found at the costovertebral angle, making the diagnosis of pyelonephritis unlikely. The abdomen was not significantly tender, decreasing the possibility of intra-abdominal pathology. Her pain, by history, was "the same pain" that she had with her previous kidney stone, but this time she also had dysuria and frequency. In considering the cause of her symptoms, one would think of recurrent renal calculus, urinary tract infection, or both.

Pain from renal stones can be gradual or sudden in onset and is usually unaffected by lying still. Classically, pain in the flank radiates anteriorly into the lower abdomen, and into the testicle or labia majora. The pain generated by a calculus can vary depending on the location of the stone. Occasionally, patients may present with nonradiating, dull flank pain, or pain localized in the testicle or labia. If the pain manifests in the upper flank or lumbar region on the right, it can mimic cholecystitis. Mid-ureteral stones can cause mid to lower abdominal pain, and stones that are in the distal ureter typically cause pain in the testicle or labia majora. These pain locations are "typical," but not all kidney stones obey these rules.

III. EVALUATION OF POSSIBLE URETEROLITHIASIS

A urinalysis is the first test that should be ordered. It is helpful to find a large amount of blood in the urine of the patient who has a good history for ureterolithiasis, but the urine can be free of blood in a significant number of patients. Including microscopic evaluation of the urine sample, Bove et al found that 33% of patients with ureterolithiasis had 5 or fewer RBCs, 19% had 3 or fewer, and 11% had none.[1] The presence or absence of hematuria has not been found to correlate with the severity of ureteral obstruction.[2]

Urine culture may be indicated if urease-forming bacteria, such as *Proteus mirabilis, Providencia stuartii* or *Morganella morganii,* is suspected based on the finding of alkali urine (pH>7.6) or if "coffin lid crystals" are found in the urinalysis. These organisms may contribute to the formation of struvite stones (magnesium-ammonium-phosphate stones), accounting for 15% of renal stones.[3] Other indications for culture include suspicion of a sub-clinical infection.

A complete blood count is not always necessary in the evaluation of an uncomplicated renal calculus; however it may be considered if the diagnosis is unclear or when patients have other co-morbidities. Often an elevated white blood count will be found, but is difficult to interpret based on the possibility of demargination secondary to pain and stress. In this case, the patient had a white blood cell count of 15.7, most likely related to infection when considered with the findings of 25–50 white blood cells in the urine.

Electrolytes, BUN, and creatinine are generally not needed unless: 1) a contrast study is contemplated in patients who may have renal insufficiency; 2) there is evidence to support chronic renal insufficiency; or 3) there is a suspicion of chronic obstruction. Acute, complete ureteral obstruction does not immediately affect renal function—the presence of an acute obstruction in one ureter will cause an increase in the glomerular filtration rate in the contralateral kidney. It is generally held that significant damage does not occur to the kidney unless the obstruction has been present for greater than 4 weeks[4,] although Rosen's text suggests that permanent damage may occur with obstruction lasting 1–2 weeks.[5]

I confess that I have probably ordered fewer than 5 IVPs for renal stones and most of the time this was at the urologist's recommendation. I believe, and most EM physicians and radiologists would agree, that a CT is the better choice for imaging in cases of suspected renal colic for several reasons: CT is quick; does not require the administration of contrast, gives information regarding other disease processes; and, even if done after-hours, will be read by a radiologist (see examples at end of chapter). The CT scan has a reported sensitivity of 86–95% with a specificity of 86–98% for the detection of calculi.[6,7,8] In one study, the finding of a significant alternative diagnosis in patients without evidence of calculi was found to be as high as 12%.[6] CT also has the capacity to directly visualize stones that are otherwise considered radiolucent on plain film. One study in the emergency medicine literature showed that emergency medicine clinicians have a high inter-rater reliability with the radiologist in detection of renal tract abnormalities and calculi, but are not as accurate at finding non-renal abnormalities.[7]

Ultrasound can also be helpful in evaluating the presence of renal calculi. It does not involve radiation, making it well suited for children and pregnant patients. However, ultrasound mainly detects secondary indicators of ureterolithiasis, such as hydronephrosis, intrarenal calculi, and possibly a very proximal ureteral calculus. It does not aid in the diagnosis of distal stones without obstruction. Ultrasound is generally considered second-line to non-contrast CTs. The sensitivity and specificity of ultrasound in detecting calculi found on CT has been reported as 24% and 90% respectively.[8]

IV. MANAGEMENT OF URETEROLITHIASIS

Patients with suspected renal colic should receive pain medication expeditiously. Few patients in the emergency department deserve pain medications faster than those with renal colic. Evidence suggests that prostaglandins play an important role in mediating pain caused by ureteral irritation. One randomized, double blinded study evaluating 100-150mg IM meperidine versus 60 mg IM ketorolac showed that ketorolac was significantly better than meperidine in reducing pain, and led to an earlier discharge.[9] In another study, a meta-analysis found that non-steroidal anti-inflammatory medications were as effective as narcotics in treatment of renal colic.[10] I treat patients with a combination of a narcotic (morphine, dilaudid, or Fentanyl) IV, ketorolac IV, and promethazine IV along with one liter of normal saline. Some physicians believe that overly aggressive administration of fluids can cause increased pain whereas some believe it aids in the passage of the stone; there appears to be no clear evidence to support either argument. I provide repeat doses of narcotics as needed. Pain medication is clearly indicated prior to performing a confirmatory imaging study in a patient with a history consistent with renal colic.

A recent and interesting development in the management of ureterolithiasis is the use of alpha-1 receptor blockers. Blocking the α-1 receptors decreases spasms and pressure in the ureter, thereby leading to easier passage of the stone. One study reported a significant increase in patients passing the stone with tamsulosin (Flomax)—80.4% with tamsulosin versus 62.8% without.[11] Use of prednisone, trimethoprim-sulfamethoxazole, and nifedipine also led to increased rates of passage.[12] Analgesics with prednisone and nifedipine have also shown promise.[13]

V. COMPLICATIONS OF URETEROLITHIASIS

The general consensus is that stones less than 5mm have greater than 90% chance of passing. However, although ureteral peristalsis and pressures initially increase with ureterolithiasis, they decrease to 50% of pre-obstruction pressure within 5 hours, and continue to decrease thereafter. This can lead to the inability to pass even relatively small stones once they are impacted.

Most stones become impacted at the ureteral-vesicular junction, although the site varies with the size of the calculus. Other common sites for impaction include the ureteral-pelvic juncture, where the pelvis of the kidney significantly narrows into the ureter, and in the mid to distal ureter, where the ureters pass over the iliac vessels and pelvic brim.

A study in the radiology literature that examined the size, location, and outcome of stones detected on non-contrast CT found the chance of passing a stone was 87% for 1 mm diameter stones, 76% for stones 2–4 mm, 60% for stones 5–7 mm, 48% for stones 7–9 mm, and 25% for stones larger than 9 mm. Passage rates of stones were 48% in the proximal ureter (above the sacroiliac joints), 60% of mid ureteral stones (overlying the sacroiliac joints), 75% of distal stones (below the sacroiliac joints), and 79% at the ureterovesical junction.[14] In cases where the stone is proximal and greater than 5mm, consultation with a urologist may be warranted to ensure follow up. An additional indication for consultation is a return to the emergency department with persistent pain from a relatively small stone. The surgical management of obstructing renal calculi may include ureteroscopy with ureteral stent placement, extra-corporeal shock-wave lithotripsy for very proximal stones, or placement of a percutaneous nephrostomy tube.

It is important to note, especially with the findings in this case, that there are other causes of intrinsic ureteral obstruction, including ureteral strictures from previous urological or gynecological procedures, sloughed papilla in cases of papillary necrosis from analgesic overuse, tumors, and congenital abnormalities such as posterior urethral valves. Extrinsic causes of obstruction include uterine fibroids, tumors, and retroperitoneal fibrosis.

VI. OBSTRUCTION WITH INFECTION

In cases of complete obstruction, stasis of the urine leads to a higher risk of infection. This is made worse when a nidus for infection, the stone, is present. Decreased excretion of antibiotics into the urine resulting from decreased glomerular filtration in the affected kidney also complicates this situation. There is a very important difference between a non-obstructing renal calculus with a urinary tract infection and obstructing calculus with a urinary tract infection, as evidenced by hydronephrosis on the IVP, CT, or ultrasound. The evaluation of the patient's presenting symptoms should provide a clue as to the presence of an infection. Clear evidence of an infection would be the obvious signs of fever, hypotension, tachycardia, and altered mental status. In more subtle cases, the urinalysis should point to evidence of infection with the presence of pyuria, bacturia, and positive nitrite on the urine dip. However, it is difficult to always rely on the urinalysis in detecting infection proximal to the stone.

One complication of an obstructing calculus is rupture of the collecting system. This is relatively uncommon and usually involves conservative management with pain control, decompression and antibiotics.

VII. INDICATIONS FOR ADMISSION AND DISCHARGE INSTRUCTIONS

The major indications for admission in cases of ureterolithiasis are obstruction in a solitary native or transplanted kidney, large proximal stone, intractable pain, and obstructive stone with evidence of infection. Obstruction as evidenced by hydronephrosis, with adequate pain control, is not an indication for admission. Some larger emergency departments routinely admit uncomplicated renal colic patients to an emergency department observation unit for continued intravenous pain control.[15]

Patients with a UTI and a non-obstructing calculus may be discharged with appropriate antibiotics and follow-up. To be safe, I usually discuss any calculus with signs of infection with a urologist to ensure proper follow up.

If the patient meets discharge criteria, then specific discharge instructions should be given. This includes straining the urine; useful to confirm passage of the stone rather than to provide the stone for analysis. The patient is also instructed to return for worsening pain not controlled with prescribed medications, fever, and worsening dysuria, especially in patients with co-morbidities such as diabetes.

TEACHING POINTS ABOUT CASE 21:
- A urine negative for blood does not exclude stone.
- Once you have found a stone, ensure there is no infection. This patient had pyuria, leukocytosis and an elevated temperature. She also had a history of diabetes, placing her in a higher risk category. If there is obstruction and infection, then consult a urologist.
- Equivalent bioavailability is obtained with PO and IV levaquin.

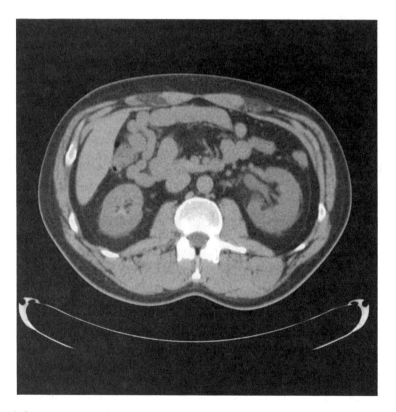

CT1. Axial noncontrast image at the level of the kidneys demonstrating left sided inflammatory changes including perinephric stranding. There is mild to moderate left hydronephrosis.

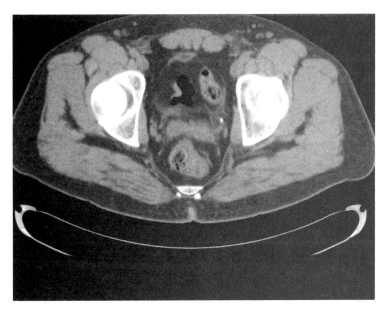

CT2. (Same patient) The offending calculus is seen at the distal left ureter a few centimeters proximal to the UVJ.

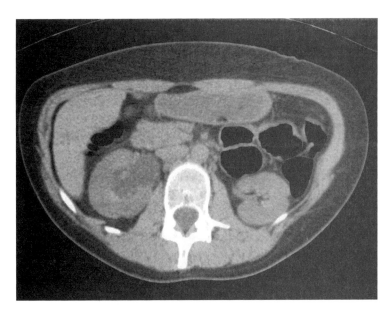

CT3. Axial noncontrast image at the level of the kidneys showing moderate to severe right sided hydronephrosis. The kidney appears enlarged and swollen.

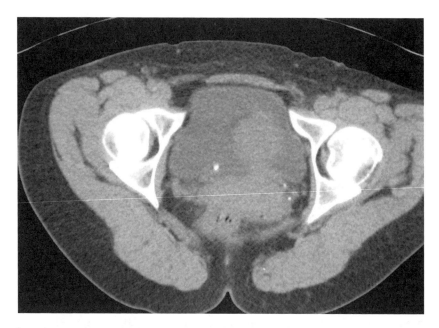

CT4. The obstructing calculus is seen at the right UVJ. At our institution, patients are scanned in the prone position if possible to ensure these types of calculi are not confused with a passed stone in the bladder.

Note: Thanks to Casey Rhodes, MD, for help with images.

REFERENCES

1. Bove P. Reexamining the value of hematuria testing in patients with acute flank pain. J Urol 1999;162: 685-7.
2. Stewart DP. Microscopic hematuria and calculus-related ureteral obstruction. J Emerg Med 1990;8: 693-5.
3. Cohen J, Powderly WG, eds. Infectious diseases, 2nd ed. London: Mosby, 2004: 764.
4. Menon M, Parulkar BG, Drach GW. Urinary lithiasis: etiology, diagnosis, and medical management. In Walsh PC, Retik AB, Vaughan ED, et al. (eds). Campbell's urology, 7th ed. Philadelphia:WB Saunders, 1998: 2661-705.
5. Escobar JI, Eastman ER, Harwood-Nuss AL. Selected urologic problems. In Marx J. Rosen's emergency medicine: concepts and clinical practice, 5th ed. St Louis:Mosby, 2002: 1414-31.
6. Ahmad NA. Incidental diagnosis of diseases on un-enhanced helical computed tomography performed for ureteric colic. BMC Urol 2003;3: 2.
7. Holdgate A. How accurate are emergency clinicians at interpreting noncontrast computed tomography for suspected renal colic? Acad Emerg Med 2003;10: 315-9.
8. Fowler KA. US for detecting renal calculi with nonenhanced CT as a reference standard. Radiology 2002;222: 109-13.
9. Larkin GL. Efficacy of ketorolac tromethamine versus meperidine in the ED treatment of acute renal colic. Am J Emerg 1999;17(1): 6-10.

10. Labrecque M, Dostaler LP, Rousselle R,et al. Efficacy of nonsteroidal anti-inflammatory drugs in the treatment of acute renal colic. A meta-analysis. Arch Intern Med 1994;154: 1381-7.
11. Cervenakov I, Fillo J, Mardiak J, et al. Speedy elimination of ureterolithiasis in lower part of ureters with the alpha 1-blocker—Tamsulosin. Int Urol Nephrol 2002;34:25-9.
12. Cooper JT, Stack GM, Cooper TP. Intensive medical management of ureteral calculi. Urology 2000;56: 575-8.
13. Saita A, Bonaccorsi A, Marchese F, et al. Our experience with nifedipine and prednisolone as expulsive therapy for ureteral stones. Urol Int 2004;72 Suppl 1: 43-5.
14. Coll DM. Relationship of spontaneous passage of ureteral calculi to stone size and location as revealed by unenhanced helical CT. AJR Am J Roentgenol 2002;178: 101-3.
15. Manthey DE. Nephrolithiasis. Emerg Med Clin North 2002;19: 633-54, viii.

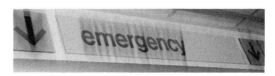

CASE 22

28 YEAR OLD PREGNANT FEMALE WITH SHORTNESS OF BREATH

Commentary:
Gregory L. Henry, MD, FACEP

CEO, Medical Practice Risk Assessment, Inc., Ann Arbor, Michigan
Clinical Professor, Department of Emergency Medicine
    University of Michigan Medical School, Ann Arbor, Michigan
Past President, American College of Emergency Physicians (ACEP)

Discussion:
Ryan Longstreth, MD, FACEP

Attending ED Physician
    Mt. Carmel St. Ann's Emergency Department, Westerville, Ohio
Assistant ED Director, St. Ann's Emergency Department

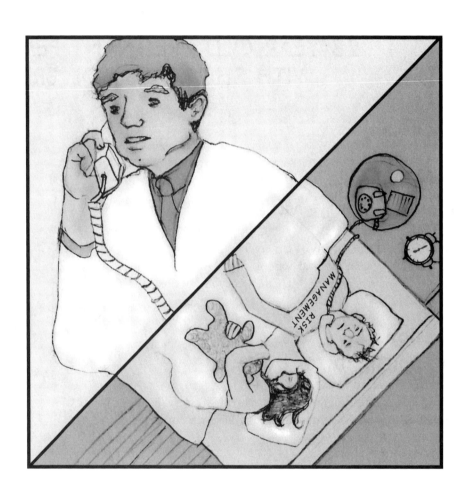

28 YEAR OLD PREGNANT FEMALE WITH SHORTNESS OF BREATH

—Initial Visit*—

*Authors' Note: The history, exam and notes are the actual documentation of the physicians and providers, including abbreviations (and spelling errors)

CHIEF COMPLAINT (at 02:52): Difficulty breathing

Time	Temp(F)	Rt.	Pulse	Resp	Syst	Diast	Pos.	O2 Sat	O2%
02:57	97.4	Oral	78	28	108	64	S	96	ra
03:30			100	30	110	70	S	88	ra
04:29			110	30	116	71	S	100	4lnc
04:51			116	30	114	64	S	100	4lnc

HISTORY OF PRESENT ILLNESS (at 03:33): This is a 28-year-old pregnant female, G1P0, approximately 38 weeks pregnant, who presents with 2 weeks of shortness of breath and dyspnea with exertion, orthopnea, and leg swelling. Also diffuse chest pain worse with exertion. Was seen by the family doctor and told that there was "no problem" (per husband). She denies fever or chills, cough, or chest pain. She has no other complaints today. She is non-English speaking and history is all from her husband and from a Somalian interpreter at the bedside. No fever, vomiting, rhinorrhea, headache, rash, blurred vision.

PAST MEDICAL HISTORY/TRIAGE:
No significant medical history.
No significant surgical history.
Allergies: Penicillin
Medications: Robitussin and Tylenol

EXAM (at 03:51):
General: Well-appearing; she is tachypnea with a resting respiratory rate of 26 on my exam
Head: Normocephalic; atraumatic
Eyes: PERRL
Nose: The nose is normal in appearance without rhinorrhea
Neck: No JVD or distended neck veins
Resp: Normal chest excursion with respiration; breath sounds clear and equal bilaterally; no wheezes, rhonchi, or rales
Card: Regular rhythm, without murmurs, rub or gallop
Abd: Gravid; non-tender, soft, without rigidity, rebound or guarding, no pulsatile mass
Chest: No pain with palpation

Skin: Normal for age and race; warm and dry without diaphoresis ; no apparent lesions
Extremities: Pulses are 2 plus and equal times 4 extremities, 2+ pitting edema of both LE

RESULTS (at 05:16):

Test	Flag	Value	Units	Ref. Range
WBC		9.3	K/uL	4.6-10.2
HGB	L	11.0	G/DL	12.0-16.0
PLT		318	K/uL	142-424
NA	L	130	MMOL/L	135-144
K		4.0	MMOL/L	3.5-5.1
CL		99	MMOL/L	98-107
AGAP		14.0	MMOL/L	6.0-18.0
CO2	L	21	MMOL/L	22-29
BUN		11	MG/DL	7-18
CREAT		1.1	MG/DL	0.6-1.3
ALB	L	2.5	G/DL	3.2-4.6
TP		7.0	GM/DL	6.4-8.2
BILT		.4	MG/DL	.0-1.0
BILD		0.1	MG/DL	0.0-0.3
BILI		.3	MG/DL	.0-1.0
ALT		42	U/L	22-65
ALP	H	189	U/L	42-144
AST	H	48	U/L	10-34
pH		7.428		7.350-7.450
PCO2	L	28.0		32.0-48.0
PO2	L	57.0		83.0-108.0
FI O2		21.00		
BNP	H	580	PG/ML	0-100

RADIOLOGY
CXR: Bilateral interstitial lung opacity, which is nonspecific and I suspect represents interstitial edema.

PROCEDURES (at 04:13):
FHT were ausculatated by doppler in the RUQ . The fetal heart rate was counted at 132beats per minute Fetal monitor: Pt. was placed on external fetal monitor at 0440. Fetal heart rate baseline felt to be 150's with accels to 170's with visible fetal motion noted. Two mild contractions that were not felt by pt noted during monitoring period and no decelerations in heart rate were noted. Fetal monitor was explained to husband and pt and informed that monitoring would cont after arriving to labor and delivery to insure fetal well being. OB resident was present and reviewed fetal monitor strip.

ORDERS (at 04:25): Chest CT angio R/O PE

PROGRESS NOTES:

Physician at 05:32: This patient is a 38 plus weeks pregnant and presents with shortness of breath. She is hypoxic. She needs to be admitted to the hospital and needs further workup to rule out blood clot. The patient wants to leave. I told her she does not have a choice because she is pregnant and is hypoxic. She's putting the fetus at risk if she wishes to leave and I'm not allowing her to leave at this point. Security has been called and they are at the bedside.

RN at 05:37: We got over to the elevator for the CT scan and pt refused to get on elevator to go to CT scan. Pt informed of risks to herself and her fetus and states "if I go home and die in my bed so be it". Informed of risk to unborn baby and pt keeps saying she is leaving. With much encouragement pt finally agreed to get back on cart and return to the ED but refuses to go to labor and delivery to monitor baby. Pt refuses to wear oxygen or be on cardiac monitor. OB resident called and informed of situation. Somalian interpreter called.

Physician at 05:52: I discussed with risk management patient's desire to leave - she is 38+ weeks pregnant and is hypoxic - my concern is that she is putting the unborn fetus at risk. He is looking into this and will call me back.

Social Work Consultation at 06:06: This clinician got involved in the case due to the pt wanting to leave.

According the ECC physician the pt is putting the life of the fetus in danger. This clinician paged the department manager, regarding the situation. She advised based on previous situations like this one, the physician has a right to hold the pt against her will provided 2 physicians concur that the pt is putting the fetus' life in danger then she can be hold long enough to pursue a probate court order to force treatment. The OB clinic social worker was also contacted.

Physician at 06:37: I had a long discussion with the patient and her husband regarding her critical illness at this time. The Somalian interpreter was present through the entire discussion. I told the patient that her oxygen level is too low to go home and she is at risk of dying. Her unborn baby is also at risk of dying. With the help of the interpreter, the patient repeated this back to me and states that she understands. Risk management concurs that she can leave AMA as long as she understands in the presence of an interpreter.

RN progress note at 06:57: The interpreter explained to the patient the risk of death for herself and her baby with the husband present as well as the OB doctor and the OB resident. She was strongly advised that her oxygen levels were too low and she was at great risk if she went home. She stated through interpreter that she understood. At one point, the husband requested treatment at another hospital and was given the option to transfer to facility of choice, but he ultimately refused that option. Pt. strongly advised to call 911 if chest pain or SOB worsened. Husband states they will follow up with their primary care doctor later today, but they will not give us the name of the doctor. The ED physician offered to call the PCP doctor to come to the ED to see the patient, but they refused. The patient signed the AMA form in the presence of her husband and the interpreter. The husband was also asked to sign since he was taking the patient home, but he refused to sign. Patient refused to allow fetal heart tones or repeat vital signs to be rechecked before discharge. Preliminary diagnosis was reviewed and the patient stated understanding. The proposed treatment was reviewed and the patient stated understanding. Alternative treatment was discussed and the patient stated understanding. The risks of refusing treatment (including the potential of death) was discussed and the patient stated understanding.

DIAGNOSIS (at 06:38):
1. Hypoxia
2. Dyspnea
3. Pregnant

DISPOSITION (at 06:42): The patient and her husband left against medical advice. The next day, there was a message left through interpretor for patient to return call or return immediately to the ED for admission. Mother is person who answered phone- states that patient doesn't live there and she will attempt to get in touch with her. Impressed upon her importance of her daughter returning to the emergency department.

Gregory L. Henry comments:

"Signing out AMA is a direct function of the patient's capacity. It might be argued that a 38 week pregnant woman, who may be going into an ecclamptic state with heart failure, is not in a competent position psychologically to sign an AMA form."

This particular case raises almost too many medical/legal issues to count. It is always problematic when the emergency physician feels a patient needs care and the patient refuses that. Much to the credit of the physicians involved in this case, most things were well documented.

The patient's disease entity was obvious. She is near-term pregnant, she has pedal edema, shortness of breath, and probably early congestive heart failure. This case required involvement of the OB/GYN service and the family; involvement of the husband at all times and use of a Somalian translator were both critical in this case. It was important to document that the degree of illness and recommendations for care were properly conveyed to the patient and her family.

The evaluation of this patient was excellent. The most important part was the documentation of the various people trying to convince the patient that she needed proper care. Involvement of social work and various other physicians is essential, but I am not sure I agree with the hospital's risk management personnel, allowing her to sign out against medical advice (AMA). Signing out AMA is a direct function of the patient's capacity. It might be argued that a 38 week pregnant woman, who may be going into an ecclamptic state with heart failure, is not in a competent position psychologically to sign an AMA form. Very little documentation was made about the interaction with the husband; perhaps a little more time could have been spent explaining what the husband thought and what he wanted done. I would have no problem with chemical sedation of the patient, with cardiology and OB/GYN at that time.

A second, and much more difficult, issue is that of the rights of the unborn child. Certain courts have ruled that pregnant women who are abusing drugs are actually harming their child and open to criminal prosecution. Although nothing as dramatic is taking place here, decisions are being made for the unborn child in clear contradiction to its best interests. Obtaining a court order for administration of medical care is not without precedent—the court system has an obligation to protect and defend children. Parents have guardianship, but not ownership of their children. This is a long and protracted, philosophical discussion, but the issue should not be overlooked.

Despite the excellent nature of the discussion on the chart, I am concerned that this physician may not have established the patient's capacity to competently give or withhold consent. If the patient or baby had died, the question remains whether the husband would have grounds for a lawsuit, claiming that he did not fully understand the gravity of the situation. The Somalian translator here is critical; his name should appear on the chart as well as some comment on his credentials, because he may be forced to testify on the family's understanding of what was honestly communicated.

Cultural differences aside, emergency physicians are obligated to protect both the mother and the child, and this case has no simple or correct answer... Cultural relativity be damned!

- Thoroughness of Documentation: 9 out of 10.

- Thoroughness of Patient Evaluation: 9 out of 10.

- Risk of Serious Illness Being Missed: Low

- Risk Management Legal Rating: High risk

28 YEAR OLD PREGNANT FEMALE WITH SHORTNESS OF BREATH

—Second Visit: 2 Days Later—

CHIEF COMPLAINT (at 02:29): Dyspnea

Time	Temp(F)	Rt.	Pulse	Resp	Syst	Diast	Pos.	O2 Sat	O2%
02:57	97.4	O	133	22	158	70	S	100	ra

HISTORY OF PRESENT ILLNESS (at 03:12): The patient is a 28 year old Somalian primip who is near term and presents with increased dyspnea over the last 3 weeks. She was in the ED 2 days ago and has gotten worse since then. She does have pain at the right scapular area. All systems negative including no significant cough. No fevers or chills.

PAST MEDICAL HISTORY/TRIAGE:
 Allergies: Penicillin

Medications: Sudafed
Past medical and surgical history: Negative
Social history: Alcohol. No tobacco or drugs.

EXAM (at 03:22):

General: Pregnant woman who is tachypnic, but not in severe distress
Head: Normocephalic; atraumatic
Oral: Membranes moist but lips are dry. Airway patent
Neck: Mild JVD. No thyromegaly
Resp: Decreased breath sounds bilaterally with distant breath sounds
Card: Increased rate, regular, no murmur or rub
Chest: Non tender to palpation
Abd: Gravid, no masses or tenderness. No HSM
Chest: No pain with palpation
Extremities: Marked edema which is pitting and bilateral up to the knees. She has 4+ pedal edema. Diffuse tenderness bilaterally

RESULTS (at 04:29)

Chest CT: Bilateral pleural effusions and increased heart size. No pulmonary embolic disease. Study most consistent with pulmonary edema. This may be secondary to peripartum cardiomyopathy.

Test	Flag	Value	Units	Ref.Range
WBC		8.2	K/uL	4.6-10.2
HGB	L	10.1	G/DL	12.0-16.0
PLT		288	K/uL	142-424
Test	Flag	Value	Units	Ref.Range
NA		137	MMOL/L	135-144
K		4.3	MMOL/L	3.5-5.1
CL		101	MMOL/L	98-107
CO2		22	MMOL/L	22-29
BUN		10	MG/DL	7-18

Urinalysis—Normal

ED COURSE: Lasix 40mg IV

DIAGNOSIS: Acute pulmonary edema associated with pregnancy

DISPOSITION (at 05:07): Admission

HOSPITAL COURSE:

Cardiology: She was admitted and an echocardiogram was performed the next day which showed moderate to severe left ventricular dilation and left atrial dilation secondary to severe mitral valve regurgitation from a rheumatic mitral valve. The EF was 55%.

OB: Two days after admission, in conjunction with cardiology, internal medicine, OB and anesthesia, it was decided to induce labor to decrease the fluid volume and workload on the heart.

Induction: She was placed on lasix drip and induction started. Pt. progressed to 7cm dilation, then began to have increased oxygen requirements.

Surgical intervention: It was decided that she could not tolerate labor further and her heart could not tolerate further pushing, so she was then taken for c-section. Delivery of a healthy infant. She was transferred to the ICU.

ICU course: Pt. transferred to ICU for vent management and CHF management. While in the ICU (5 days after admission), she had a TEE which showed a severely dilated left atrium with 4+ mitral regurgitation. EF 40-45%. She also had a thorocentesis which was normal. She remained intubated for 7 days. Transferred to the floor 3 days after extubation. Repeat ECHO showed EF 50-55%. She developed a fever and was diagnosed with UTI and treated with levaquin. Her recovery was also complicated by hypotension. She was discharged on cozaar, lasix, potassium, and toprol.

SUBSEQUENT ED PRESENTATION: Returned to the ED 2 weeks later with SOB and cough. Exam showed heart rate of 110, respirations 28 and pulse ox 91% on room air. The Lung exam revealed bibasilar rales and decreased breath sounds. Heart exam found 2/6 systolic murmur. Labs were normal with Hb 12.3, normal lytes and cardiac enzymes. No ECG changes compared to previous ECG. Oxygen saturation was 98% on 2L nasal canula. CXR showed acute pulmonary edema. She was treated with lasix. A repeat ECHO showed 4+ MR and EF 55-60%. She was admitted.

Hospital course: Admitted to medicine with a cardio consult. Repeat TEE and this showed that MV repair was feasible, so cardiothoracic surgeon was consulted and they agreed to do the surgery. Family wanted to help make the decision, so patient went home to follow up as an outpatient.

FINAL DIAGNOSIS: Cardiomyopathy secondary to severe mitral valve regurgitation and pregnancy.

No further information is available about this patient.

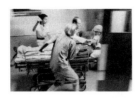

EVALUATION OF SHORTNESS OF BREATH IN PREGNANCY. HYPERTENSIVE DISORDERS AND CARDIOMYOPATHY OF PREGNANCY

Ryan Longstreth, MD, FACEP

I. INTRODUCTION

Talk about a nightmare! Could the creators of "ER" come up with a scenario as bizarre as this? A non-English speaking, pregnant female presents to the ED with her non-English speaking spouse, complaining of trouble breathing. She was found to be hypoxic and tachypneic. For an unknown reason, she refused hospitalization. The treating physician was clearly unsure of the potential legal ramifications involved. Given the fact she was hypoxic and pregnant with a full term infant, is the physician allowed to let her leave, or is he legally obligated to do everything in his power (including chemical paralysis and intubation) to hospitalize the patient? He went so far as to keep security at the bedside to prevent patient from leaving while he discussed the case with the hospital's legal consultants.

Despite multiple attempts by the emergency physician to convince the patient and her husband that she was extremely ill and did require hospitalization, the patient left against medical advice. One may argue that the patient was not competent to sign out against medical advice, given her hypoxia. There was no documentation of her mental status and when considering the choices she made, one wonders if she was, in fact, disoriented. There was also an attempt to have a husband sign the AMA form, but he refused.

Two days later, she returned to the ED hypertensive and in acute pulmonary edema. At this point, she met criteria of severe preeclampsia. Was there any consideration given to administration of magnesium? She subsequently spent five days in the ICU, was on a ventilator for a week, and ultimately diagnosed with severe mitral regurgitation secondary to presumed rheumatic heart disease. Thankfully she gave birth to a healthy infant by cesarean.

II. PHYSIOLOGICAL CHANGES SEEN IN PREGNANCY

A woman's normal physiology goes through various changes during pregnancy. Cardiovascular alterations include increased heart rate, increased heart size, and increased stroke volume, resulting in increased cardiac output by 30 to 50%.[1] The patient in this case was tachycardic on both visits, although I doubt that it was due to normal physiological changes. Pulmonary changes include elevation of the diaphragm as pregnancy progresses, resulting in increased minute ventilation. The normal CO_2 in a pregnant female ranges from 27 to 32, resulting in a mild respiratory alkalosis.[2] Up to 70% of healthy women complain of dyspnea or a "sense of breathlessness" during pregnancy.[1] The blood volume of a pregnant woman increases by 33%, resulting in a dilutional anemia; our patient did have a hemoglobin ranging from 10 to 11.

III. DYSPNEA IN PREGNANCY

The evaluation of shortness of breath in pregnancy is challenging. More often than not, dyspnea during pregnancy may be attributed to a normal increase in minute ventilation. However, several potentially life-threatening emergencies must be ruled out, including asthma, pneumonia, pulmonary embolism, or pulmonary edema due to preeclampsia or dilated cardiomyopathy of pregnancy. Pulmonary embolism has been thoroughly discussed elsewhere in this text.

Asthma, the most common respiratory disorder complicating pregnancy, affects 1 in 100 pregnant women.[3] The effect of pregnancy on pre-existing asthma is unpredictable; approximately one-third of patients improve during pregnancy, one-third worsen, and one-third remain unchanged.[4] Management of asthma during pregnancy is not much different than in nonpregnant patients. Guidelines published in 2004 from the National Asthma Education and Prevention Program (NAEPP) make recommendions based on the severity of the exacerbation. Management of pregnant patients with a mild asthma exacerbation (Peak expiratory flow—PEF $\geq$ 50%) include a beta-2 agonist up to 3 doses in the first hour, oxygen to achieve oxygen saturation $\geq$ 95%, and oral systemic steroids if there is not an immediate response or if the patient had recently been on steroids. Management of a severe exacerbation (PEF $\leq$ 50%) is the same with the exception that oral systemic steroids are always given. Patients with impending or actual arrest are managed with intubation, nebulized beta-2 agonist and ipratropium bromide, and IV steroids[5].

Pneumonia is the most common non-obstetrical infectious cause of maternal death during pregnancy.[6] The alteration in a pregnant woman's thorax makes clearing of respiratory secretions more difficult. Also, decreased lymphocyte proliferation and decreased helper T cells may make viral pneumonias more virulent. The most common cause of bacterial pneumonia is S. pneumonia, as in non-pregnant patients.[7] The recommended inpatient treatment is a third-generation cephalosporin, such as ceftriaxone, in combination with a macrolide, such as azithromycin. Quinolones are contraindicated during pregnancy. Many authors do recommend hospitalization for all pregnant women with radiographically confirmed pneumonia.

IV. DIAGNOSTIC IMAGING IN PREGNANCY

When considering radiological investigations in the pregnant patient, one must weigh the potential risks of radiation to the developing fetus against the risk to both the mother and the fetus of misdiagnosis. The 2 main concerns are teratogenic and oncogenic. Teratogenic risks include congenital malformations or embryonic death, of greatest concern during the first seven weeks, when organogenesis is occurring. In addition, several studies have shown a small but statistically significant increase in the relative risk of developing childhood cancer after the unborn fetus is exposed to radiation.[10]

Significant risk is unlikely when the fetus is exposed to less than 10 rads (10,000 mrad).[8] However, with exposure to 15 rads or greater, there is a 6% chance of severe mental retardation and 15% chance of microsomia.[9] Interestingly enough, the fetus will be exposed to an average of 50–100 mrad of naturally occurring radiation during nine months of pregnancy.[9] Table 1 lists estimated radiation dose to the fetus by imaging modality. For example, between 3,000 and 10,000 chest x-rays can be safely done during pregnancy.

Traditional teaching suggested that a nuclear ventilation-perfusion (V/Q) scan was the test of choice to rule out PE, providing a safe radiation exposure to the unborn fetus. More than 200 V/Q scans can be done with a total rad exposure would be less than 10 (Table 1). However, a 2002 study suggests that helical CT may be better.[22] This study compared fetal radiation dose between nuclear scan and CT and concluded that the average fetal radiation dose with CT was substantially less during all 3 trimesters. The authors stated "pregnancy should not preclude use of helical CT for the diagnosis of PE."

Table 1. Estimated Radiation Dose to Fetus

- C-SPINE (< 1 mrad)
- CHEST XRAY (1–3 mrad)
- KUB (200-500 mrad)
- PELVIS XRAY (200–500 mrad)
- L-SPINE (600-1000 mrad)
- CT HEAD/CHEST WITH ABDOMINAL SHIELDING (<1000 mrad)
- CT ABDOMEN (3000 mrad)
- CT PELVIS (3000–9000 mrad)
- V/Q SCAN (<55 mrad)
- CT PULMONARY ANGIOGRAM (405 mrad via Femoral, <50 mrad via brachial with abdominal shielding)

Adapted from Harwood-Nuss AL, ed. The clinical practice of emergency medicine. 3rd ed. Philadelphia: Lippincott Williams & Wilkins, 2001:621; Rosen P, ed. Emergency medicine concepts and clinical practice. 4th ed. St. Louis: Mosby-Year Book, 1998:2335.

V. HYPERTENSIVE DISORDERS OF PREGNANCY

Gestational hypertension is a blood pressure of greater than 140/90, without proteinuria, which returns to normal after delivery of the fetus (as opposed to chronic hypertension), and is not associated with other features of preeclampsia.[11] The simple diagnosis of gestational hypertension does not apply to this patient's second visit. She did have a blood pressure greater than 140/90, but she had other signs of preeclampsia, including pulmonary edema. Preeclampsia is defined as a blood pressure greater than 140/90 with associated proteinuria. Preeclampsia is often subdivided into a mild and severe. Mild preeclampsia includes elevated blood pressure, but the diastolic is less than 110 and there are no associated features of severe preeclampsia. Severe preeclampsia includes a diastolic pressure of greater than 110 and/or any of the following features: oliguria, pulmonary edema, thrombocytopenia, right upper quadrant abdominal pain, headache, and visual changes (blurry vision or seeing spots).[12] Our patient would be considered to have severe preeclampsia, with a systolic blood pressure greater than 140 and evidence of pulmonary edema. The HELLP syndrome is a subset of severe preeclampsia defined by **H**emolysis, **E**levated **L**iver enzymes, and a **L**ow **P**latelet count. Eclampsia is seen in pre-eclamptic patients that subsequently develop changes in mental status, such as generalized seizures or coma.

For unclear reasons, the incidence of preeclampsia is decreasing, with a threefold decline from the early 1970's to the late 1990's.[13] Nearly 1 in 4 first-time pregnancies will be complicated by hypertension, and approximately 5–10% of these will ultimately develop preeclampsia.[8] Approximately 1 in 1000 pregnancies result in eclampsia.[2]

Preeclampsia consists of an initial "placental phase" followed by a "systemic phase" affecting multiple organ systems. In normal pregnancy, a change occurs in the uterine vascular system, resulting in decreased vascular resistance. In preeclampsia, these vessels retain their normal vascular resistance, with subsequent placental ischemia. This ischemia triggers the release of chemicals, such as prostaglandins, leading to necrosis, platelet aggregation, and vasospasm.[14] A series of events follow: 1) proteinuria from renal necrosis; 2) right upper quadrant pain and increased LFT's due to hepatocellular necrosis; 3) decreased intravascular volume leading to increased peripheral resistance, hypertension, and increased cardiac output; 4) microangiopathic hemolysis with anemia and thrombocytopenia; and 5) thrombus formation or hemorrhage resulting in headaches and eventually seizures. Risk factors for developing preeclampsia are listed in Table 2.

Table 2. Risk Factors for Developing Preeclampsia

- Nulliparity
- Extremes of age
- Preexisting hypertension, diabetes, renal disease, or autoimmune disease
- Family history of preeclampsia
- Multiple (twin, triplet) pregnancy
- Molar pregnancy
- Obesity
- Prior history of preeclampsia

Is there any way to predict which patients with preeclampsia will develop eclampsia? One retrospective study showed that the presence of oliguria or anuria is predictive of eclampsia.[15] Another prospective study showed that preeclamptic patients with headache or greater than 3+ DTR's on physical exam are more likely to develop eclampsia.[16] Low dose (81 mg) daily aspirin in patients with risk factors was associated with a decreased risk of preeclampsia, preterm deliveries, and fetal demise.[2]

VI. EVALUATION OF PREECLAMPSIA

The initial history should focus on potential warning signs such as visual changes, headache, chest pain, shortness of breath, right upper quadrant abdominal pain, and decreased urine output, in addition to risk factors listed above. On physical exam, a persistent elevated blood pressure reading greater than 140/90 is consistent with mild preeclampsia, and greater than 160/110, along with signs of end-organ damage, is consistent with severe preeclampsia. Tachypnea and distant or adventitious lung sounds may be present due to underlying pulmonary edema. In our case, the patient was hypertensive and tachypneic with evidence of pulmonary edema (distant lung sounds) on physical exam. A detailed neurological exam should also be performed; hyperreflexia is a high-risk exam finding. It is interesting to note that no neurological exam was performed on either of our patient's visits. A seizure in the third trimester should be attributed to eclampsia until proven otherwise, and focal neurological deficits should heighten suspicion for intracranial hemorrhage.

Lab evaluation includes a CBC, BUN/creatinine, uric acid, and liver function tests. Anemia may be due to pregnancy itself, or secondary to underlying HELLP syndrome (along with thrombocytopenia and elevated transaminases). Elevation of creatinine and/or uric acid is also a high-risk feature of preeclampsia.

Chest x-ray is indicated if the patient is complaining of dyspnea. This patient's chest x-ray was consistent with acute pulmonary edema.

VII. MANAGEMENT OF PREECLAMPSIA AND ECLAMPSIA
The definitive treatment of preeclampsia and eclampsia is prompt delivery of the fetus; it is indicated for all pregnancies beyond 36 weeks, and is usually considered the treatment of choice for pregnancies past 32 weeks. Management prior to 32 weeks is controversial and beyond the realm of this discussion.

Magnesium is considered the drug of choice for eclamptic seizures. Other options include diazepam and phenytoin. One large multicenter randomized trial found the most effective anticonvulsant (compared to diazepam and phenytoin) was magnesium sulfate, with a lower risk of recurrent seizures, ICU admission, maternal and neonatal intubation, and pneumonia. However, it did not show any statistically significant difference in overall maternal outcome.[17] Magnesium is also indicated in both mild and severe preeclampsia for seizure prophylaxis, although no good evidence exists to support its efficacy in mild preeclampsia. The loading dose is 4-6 g IV, followed by an infusion of 2–3 g/hr, with a goal of maintaining a serum magnesium level of 5-8 mg/dL.[20] I would argue that the treating physician in this case should have administered magnesium for seizure prophylaxis, since the patient displayed signs and symptoms of severe preeclampsia.

What about managing the hypertension? Hydralazine is the initial drug of choice, with a target blood pressure below 160/100. Decreasing blood pressure too rapidly may cause uterine hypoperfusion and fetal distress.

Steroids are recommended for all preeclamptic patients less than 34 weeks gestation to promote lung maturity of the developing fetus; they may also have a direct positive impact in treating preeclampsia[18]. One low power study did demonstrate better blood pressure control and increased urine output with the administration of IV dexamethasone versus IM betamethasone.[19]

VIII. CARDIOMYOPATHY OF PREGNANCY
The term cardiomyopathy refers to a broad spectrum of disorders, both acute and chronic, that affect the myocardium. Cardiomyopathies are divided into three categories: dilated, hypertrophic, and restrictive. Cardiomyopathy of pregnancy is a dilated, high output form of cardiac failure which is often transient. It can occur during the last month of pregnancy, but most cases are encountered in the first 3 months postpartum.[20] Risk factors for developing cardiomyopathy of pregnancy include advanced age, African-American multips, and preeclampsia. Complications include development of a mural thrombus and subsequent pulmonary embolism. The chest x-ray may show cardiomegaly, with signs of pulmonary edema such as Kerley B lines or interstitial infiltrates. The 2D echo will reveal dilated chambers and thin cardiac walls, consistent with a dilated cardiomyopathy. In this case, there was suspicion for cardiomyopathy of pregnancy, but the 2-D echo demonstrated underlying valvular disease as the likely precipitant of pulmonary edema.

IX. VALVULAR HEART DISEASE AND PREGNANCY

Mitral stenosis caused by rheumatic heart disease is the most common valvular disease in pregnancy. Almost three-fourths of patients have clinical deterioration in their condition during pregnancy, including the development of heart failure and arrhythmias, but maternal mortality is uncommon. There is an increase in preterm delivery and intrauterine growth retardation, more pronounced in patients with severe disease.[21]

X. CASE SUMMARY

During our patient's initial presentation, she was hypoxic—she left AMA, possibly for cultural reasons, although she may have not understood the true implications of her illness, given her degree of hypoxia. She returned with a BP of 158/70, pulmonary edema, and 4+ pitting edema of her extremities. She was ultimately found to have severe mitral regurgitation as the cause of her pulmonary edema. One of the most difficult patients to manage is the one who doesn't understand you (or one that you don't understand)—this case illustrates that point beautifully.

TEACHING POINTS ABOUT CASE 22:
- One must have a normal sensorium to make an informed decision regarding medical decisions.
- When a patient leaves against medical advice, document ability to make this decision as well as the understanding of its implications.
- Mild preeclampsia is defined by BP greater than 140/90 without evidence of end organ failure. (i.e., pulmonary edema, renal failure, etc.), whereas the severe preeclamptic does show evidence of end organ damage.
- One must weigh the benefit of any particular radiographic study against the potential risk to the patient/unborn fetus—if there is any doubt, consult the obstetrician and/or radiologist.

REFERENCES
1. Lain KY, Roberts JM. Contemporary concepts of the pathogenesis and management of preeclampsia and eclampsia. JAMA 2002;287: 3183-5.
2. Brooks MB. Pregnancy, Eclampsia. 2004; http://www.emedicine.com/emerg/topic796.htm
3. Alexander S, Dodds L, Armson BA.Perinatal outcomes in women with asthma during pregnancy. Obstet Gynecology 1998;92:435-40.
4. Juniper EF, Newhouse MT. Effect of pregnancy on asthma: a systematic review and meta-analysis. In: Schatz M, Zeiger RS, Claman HC, eds. Asthma and immunological diseases in pregnancy and early infancy. New York:Marcel Dekker; 1993:401-27.
5. Asthma and pregnancy – update 2004. NAEPP Working Group Report on Managing Asthma During Pregnancy: Recommendations for Pharmacologic Treatment—Update 2004. NIH Publication No. 05-3279. Bethesda, MD. U.S. Department of Health and Human Services; National Institutes of Health; National Heart. Lung, and Blood Institute, 2004. http://www.nhlbi.nih.gov/health/prof/lung/asthma/astpreg/astpreg_full.pdf
6. Kaunitz AM, Hughes JM, Grimes DA, et al. Causes of maternal mortality in the United States. Obstet Gynecol 1985;65:605-612.
7. Martinez FG. Pulmonary disorders during pregnancy. Emergency care of the woman. New York:McGraw-Hill, 1998:191-227.
8. Trauma during pregnancy: ACOG technical bulletin. American College of Obstetricians and Gynecologists. November 1991.

9. Wagner LK, Lester RG, Saldana LR. Exposure of the pregnant patient to diagnostic radiations: a guide to medical management. Philadelphia:Lippincott, 1985.

10. Ginsberg JS, Hirsh J, Rainbow AJ, et al. Risks to the fetus of radiological procedures used in the diagnosis of maternal venous thromboembolic disease. J Thromb Haemost 61:189,1989.

11. National High Blood Pressure Education Program Working Group on High Blood Pressure in Pregnancy. Am J Obstet Gynecol 2000;183:1-22.

12. Selvidge R, Dart R. Emergencies in the second and third trimesters: hypertensive disorders and antepartum hemorrhage. Emerg Med Prac 2004;6 :1-19.

13. Ventura SJ, Martin JA, Curtin SC, et al. Births: Final data for 1998. Natl Vital Stat Rep 2000;28:1-100.

14. Granger JP, Alexander BT, Llinas MT, et al. Pathophysiology of hypertension during preeclampsia linking placental ischemia with endothelial dysfunction. Hypertension 2001;38:718-22.

15. Small M, Valsaint P, Copel J, et al. The utility of common clinical and laboratory parameters to distinguish eclamptic from preeclamptic women in a developing country. Am J Obstet Gynecol 2001;185 (Dec. suppl): S176.

16. Witlin AG, Saade GR, Mattar F, et al. Risk factors for abruptio placentae and eclampsia: analysis of 445 consecutively managed women with severe preeclampsia and eclampsia. Am J Obstet Gynecol 1999;180:1322-9.

17. Group TETC. Which anticonvulsant for women with eclampsia? Evidence from the Collaborative Eclampsia trial. Lancet 1995;345:1455-62.

18. Crowley P. Prophylactic corticosteroids for preterm birth. Cochrane Database Syst Rev 2000;(2): CD000065.

19. Isler CM, Barrilleaux PS, Magann EF, et al. A prospective randomized trial comparing the efficacy of dexamethasone and betamethasone treatment of antepartum HELLP syndrome. Am J Obstet Gynecol 2001;184:1332-9.

20. Harwood-Nuss AL, ed. The clinical practice of emergency medicine. 3rd ed. Philadelphia: Lippincott Williams & Wilkins, 2001.

21. Elkayam U, Bitar F. Valvular heart disease and pregnancy. Part I: native valves. J Am Coll Cardiol 2005;46:223-30.

22. Winer-Muram HT, et al. Pulmonary embolism in pregnant patients: fetal radiation dose with Helical CT. Radiology 2002;224:487-92.

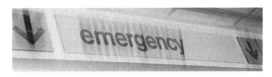

CASE23
51 YEAR OLD MALE WITH BACK PAIN

Commentary:
Gregory L. Henry, MD, FACEP

CEO, Medical Practice Risk Assessment, Inc., Ann Arbor, Michigan
Clinical Professor, Department of Emergency Medicine
  University of Michigan Medical School, Ann Arbor, Michigan
Past President, American College of Emergency Physicians (ACEP)

Discussion:
Michael B. Weinstock, MD

Clinical Assistant Professor, Division of Emergency Medicine
  The Ohio State University, College of Medicine
  Columbus, Ohio
Attending ED physician, Director of Medical Education
  Mt. Carmel St. Ann's Emergency Department
  Westerville, Ohio

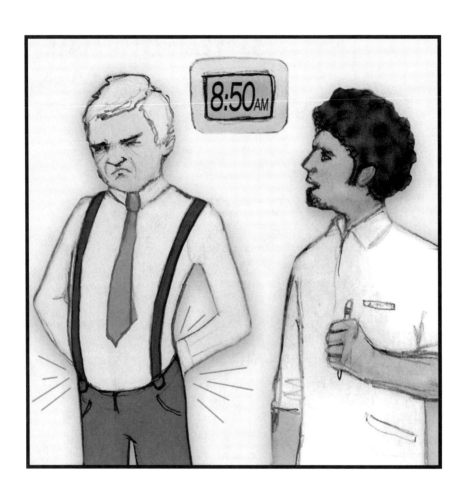

51 YEAR OLD MALE WITH
BACK PAIN

—Initial Visit*—

*Authors' Note: The history, exam and notes are the actual documentation of the physicians and providers, including abbreviations (and spelling errors)

CHIEF COMPLAINT: Back pain

```
VITAL SIGNS                                              Pain
Time  Temp(F)  Rt.   Pulse  Resp  Syst  Diast  Pos.  Scale
08:25  96.8   Tym.    88     18    164   107    S      8
```

HISTORY OF PRESENT ILLNESS (at 08:50): This is an otherwise healthy 51 y/o male who presents with a three to four week history of waxing and waning lower back pain. He denies any definite injury prior to symptom onset. He denies saddle paresthesias, bowel or bladder incontinence, weakness or numbness in the arms or legs. No fever or IV drug abuse. No prior back surgery. No meds prior to arrival. No fever, vomiting, chest pain, dysuria, urinary frequency, paresthesias.

PAST MEDICAL HISTORY/TRIAGE:
No private physician
No known allergies.
Meds: The patient is not taking medications at this time
No significant medical history.
No significant surgical history.

EXAM (at 08:52):
General: Well-appearing; well-nourished; A&O X 3, in no apparent distress
Head: Normocephalic; atraumatic.
Nose: The nose is normal in appearance without rhinorrhea
Abd: Non-distended, non-tender, soft, without rigidity, rebound or guarding
Back: There is pain with palpation musculature low back. No midline cervical/thoracic/lumbar sacral tenderness to palpation = + lipoma on lower T-spine
Neuro: Strength 5/5 for flexion and extension bilateral lower extremities, patellar DTR's normal X2, straight leg raise negative X2, sensation grossly intact bilateral lower extremities. No evidence of urinary incontinence

PROGRESS NOTES(at 09:05): His blood pressure remained 160/100 on recheck. He has no chest pain, shortness of breath, or lateralizing weakness or paresthesias. I suspect this blood pressure elevation is due to acute pain. I have given him instructions on blood pressure and he is to follow-up with his physician in the next few days for a recheck of his blood pressure. He received ibuprofen 600mg in the ED at 09:04.

PROCEDURES: Urine dip stick: WNL except: Trace protein

DIAGNOSIS: LBP (Low back pain)

DISPOSITION: Aftercare Instructions for LS strain and elevated blood pressure, prescriptions for ibuprofen and vicodin. Patient left the ED at 09:14.

Gregory L. Henry comments:

"Middle-aged men do not seek healthcare unless they have specific problems"

A 51 year old male with a new onset of back pain is always troubling. Areas of concern include the urinary tract and aneurysm of the aorta. Middle-aged men do not seek healthcare unless they have specific problems. This patient has no doctor, is on no medication, and has no significant medical history; this indicates a significant problem may be occurring.

The history in this case is important; the pain is recent onset, has had a waxing and waning nature, and is seemingly unrelated to activity or a previous injury. He has no neurological symptoms at this time.

The evaluation in the emergency department shows a reasonable history with an excellent review of systems. Examination of the back seems normal, but it should be noted that there is no cervical, thoracic, or lumbar tenderness to palpation. No specific motor activity, such as lifting the legs, or movement, causes pain. This is not the typical physical examination of a patient with musculoskeletal back pain.

A urinalysis is ordered on the patient; what is this for? Patient symptomatology would not defend evaluation for urinary tract infection. If we are looking for blood in the urine, lack of hematuria does not rule out a kidney stone or other urinary tract problems.

The documentation on this case is adequate, but fails to complete the thought process. The question remains: "Is there a lesion in the back that may be causing this discomfort?"

Additional comments and risk management rankings follow Second Visit

—Second Visit: 14 Days Later—

CHIEF COMPLAINT: Back pain

```
VITAL SIGNS                                            Pain
Time   Temp(F)  Pulse   Resp   Syst   Diast  Pos.  scale
06:55    98       84     16     170    107     S     10
08:10             74     18     152    100     S      6
08:53                                                4-5
```

HISTORY OF PRESENT ILLNESS (at 07:21): 51yo BM comes to the ED with c/o having persistent low back pain and now radiating down his right leg into his knee. Patient reports that the pain has moved down his leg for about a week. Was seen here a while ago with the same low back pain and did not get any relief with the ibuprofen and vicodin. Patient reports that he just wants to the pain to go away. No urinary/bowel problems. No saddle paresthesias. Patient denies any back problems prior to this last month or so. Patient reports that he's a security guard and walking around on his feet a lot, but no heavy lifting. No h/o trauma. No fever, chills, n/v/d, abd. pain, chest pain, palpitations, SOB, cough, dysuria, hematuria, urinary frequency or incontinence of urine.

PAST MEDICAL HISTORY/TRIAGE:
No private physician
No known allergies.
Meds: The patient is not taking medications at this time
No significant medical history.
No significant surgical history.
Social history: Patient denies alcohol use. Patient denies drug use.

EXAM (at 07:27):
General: Alert, well-appearing BM in no acute distress; appropriate with exam
Head: Normocephalic; atraumatic.
Eyes: PERRL
Oropharynx: MMM
Nose: The nose is normal in appearance without rhinorrhea
Resp.: Normal chest excursion with respiration; breath sounds clear and equal bilaterally; no wheezes, rhonchi, or rales
Cardio: Regular rhythm, without murmurs, rub or gallop
Abd: Non-distended; non-tender, soft, without rigidity, rebound or guarding
Back: No cervical/thoracic/lumbar tenderness to palpation; FROM of back without much difficulty; 5/5 strength bilaterally DF/PF, HS/quads/IS; 2+ DP/PT pulses bilaterally; normal sensation to light touch bilaterally; normal gait; neg. SLR bilaterally

Ext: no calf tenderness
Skin: Normal for age and race; warm and dry

ORDERS (at 07:28): Prednsione 60mg po, Percocet 5mg po x2

PROGRESS NOTES (at 08:11): Patient aware of blood pressure and needs to f/u with PCP. At 08:53 he said he was feeling better.

PROCEDURES: Urine dip stick: WNL except: Protein 30 mg/dl

DIAGNOSIS: Sciatica

DISPOSITION: Discharged to home. Prescriptions for naprosyn, percocet, prednisone. Aftercare instructions for sciatica. He released from the ED at 08:54.

Additional comments by Gregory L. Henry:

On the second visit, some 14 days later, the patient again has a reasonable examination and history performed. Again a urine dipstick is positive for protein suggesting a potential problem in the kidneys. Again the patient is considered to have sciatica, and yet the physical examination shows no actual discomfort in the area of the sciatic notch. The diagnosis of sciatica does not fit from a physical exam/anatomic standpoint. A study, such as a helical CT, which involves the bone structures, kidneys, and aorta, would be appropriate.

- Thoroughness of Documentation: 8 out of 10.

- Thoroughness of Patient Evaluation: 5 out of 10.

- Risk of Illness Being Missed: Low risk.

- Risk Management Legal Rating: Low risk.

51 YEAR OLD MALE WITH BACK PAIN

—Third Visit: 2 Days Later—

CHIEF COMPLAINT: Back pain

```
VITAL SIGNS                                          Pain
Time    Temp(F)  Pulse  Resp  Syst  Diast  Pos.  scale
07:33    98.5     90     18    153    103    S
14:30             88     18    160     80    S     10
```

HISTORY OF PRESENT ILLNESS (at 08:32): This is a 51-year-old male who complains of persistent right-sided back pain radiating down the right leg for the past seven weeks. Today, he has also developed upper abdominal pain and dizziness. He has been seen here twice since symptoms started and was diagnosed with sciatica. He denies urinary symptoms, chest pain, headache, or shortness of breath. He has taken Vicodin, Percocet, and Prednisone with some temporary resolution of symptoms. He has been given referrals to private care physicians, but has not gone to see them. No fevers, vomiting, dysuria, hematuria, HA.

PAST MEDICAL HISTORY/TRIAGE:
No private physician
No known allergies.
Meds: The patient is not taking medications at this time
No significant medical history.
No significant surgical history.
Social history: Patient denies alcohol use. Patient denies drug use.

EXAM (at 08:33):
General: Well-appearing; well-nourished; A&O X 3, in no apparent distress
Head: Normocephalic; atraumatic.
Eye: Pupils are equal and reactive to light. Extraocular muscles are intact.
Nose: The nose is normal in appearance without rhinorrhea
Resp: Respiratory rate and effort appear normal. The lungs are clear to auscultation bilaterally. No retractions noted.
Cardio: The heart has a regular rate and rhythm; normal S1, S2; no S3 or S4; no murmurs, rubs, or gallops. The pulses are equal bilaterally. There is no peripheral edema of the extremities.
Abd: Non-distended, minimal epigastric tenderness - no RUQ tenderness; soft, without rigidity, rebound or guarding
Back: There is pain with palpation musculature low back. No midline cervical/thoracic/lumbar sacral tenderness to palpation

Neuro: Strength 5/5 for flexion and extension bilateral lower extremities, patellar DTR's normal X2, straight leg raise negative X2, sensation grossly intact bilateral lower extremities. No evidence of urinary incontinence

ORDERS:

Meds: Vicodin 5mg, give 2 PO, dilaudid 1mg IVP, phenergan 12.5mg IVP

IV: .9NS-1L bolus then to 125 cc/hour

RESULTS (at 09:35):

Test	Flag	Value	Units	Ref. Range
WBC		4.9	K/uL	4.6-10.2
HGB	L	8.7	G/DL	13.5-17.5
PLT		326	K/uL	142-424
NA		137	MMOL/L	135-144
K		4.1	MMOL/L	3.5-5.1
CL		103	MMOL/L	98-107
CO2		26	MMOL/L	22-29
BUN		16	MG/DL	7-18
CREAT		1.2	MG/DL	0.6-1.3
GLUC		93	MG/DL	70-110
AMY		77	U/L	25-115
LIP	H	438	U/L	114-286
ION CAL		1.30	MMOL/L	1.15-1.37
LACTIC		0.7	MMOL/L	0.4-2.0
LDH	H	403	U/L	100-190
IRON	L	10	UG/DL	59-158
TIBC		269	UG/DL	228-428
FERRITIN		97	NG/ML	3-244
ABS RETIC	H	23.5	X 10 3	23.5-140.3

LFT's and coagulation studies: WNL

Urine dip stick: WNL except: Protein—100 mg/dL
  Blood—trace

RADIOLOGY

Unenhanced helical CT abdomen and pelvis, r/o stone: There is some diaphragmatic elevation on the right. The left kidney is visualized and appears unremarkable. No normal right kidney is identified but rather there is a large, heterogeneous mass occupying the right renal fossa, very suspicious for a huge right renal neoplasm. The study also demonstrates a destructive lesion of the vertebral body and right pedicle of, I believe, the L2 vertebra. Additional information will be found in the associated post-contrast dictation.

Enhanced CT abdomen and pelvis - Impression: There is a huge 15.6 x 13.0-cm mass likely representing a renal cell carcinoma of the right kidney with evidence for multiple intrahepatic metastasis and bony metastasis to the lumbar spine, I believe L2. These findings were communicated to the clinical service at the time of dictation.

DIAGNOSIS (at 11:55): Cancer—urinary system

DISPOSITION: Admitted to medical/surgical bed and went to the floor at 14:52.

HOSPITAL COURSE AND FOLLOW UP:

He was subsequently prescribed dilaudid and referred to a cancer center where he was scheduled for kidney surgery. His appointment was 8 days after discharge, but he returned to the ED 6 days later with continued pain and received a refill of the dilaudid.

FINAL DIAGNOSIS: Renal cell cancer with metastases.

Additional Greg Henry comments:

By the third visit, 16 days after the initial visit, a helical CT scan is performed and a proper diagnosis is obtained. In this case, diagnostic delay of a few days probably had no long-term effect on the patient or the outcome. However, earlier use of the CT scan would have at least provided an earlier diagnosis, regardless of the outcome.

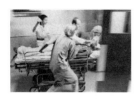

DIAGNOSIS AND MANAGEMENT OF NON-TRAUMATIC LOW BACK PAIN AND RENAL CELL CANCER

Michael B. Weinstock, MD

I. INTRODUCTION, DIFFERENTIAL DIAGNOSIS, AND RED FLAGS

Back pain is a common complaint in the ED as well as primary care. Between 70 and 85% of adults will have back pain at some point in their lives; the annual prevalence ranges from 15–45%.[2] Back pain is one of the great deceivers; since it is commonly due to a benign etiology, one can be lulled into complacency. Much to the credit of the physician on the first ED visit, the diagnosis was general: "low back pain." No attempt was made to attribute the pain to a lumbosacral strain or other mechanical problem. It is common that we are not able to arrive at an exact diagnosis in the ED. The progress note is well thought out regarding the incidental finding of elevated blood pressure (though it would have been nice to have a repeat blood pressure prior to discharge), but the presenting complaint is not mentioned. When a definitive diagnosis cannot be established in the ED, there should be a plan for further evaluation.

Back pain can be divided into 2 groups; mechanical/discogenic and non-mechanical. Mechanical etiologies include idiopathic or nonspecific (strain/sprain) low back pain, discogenic pain, spinal stenosis, and chronic low back pain. Non-mechanical etiologies include malignancy, infection, inflammation (rheumatoid arthritis, ankylosing spondylitis), gynecologic, renal (UTI/pyelonephritis, renal colic, renal artery occlusion), gastrointestinal (peptic ulcer disease, pancreatitis), and vascular (ruptured AAA). (Table 1). Red flags for more serious disease include age > 65, history of malignancy, unexplained weight loss, recent trauma, fever, failure to improve after 1 month of therapy, nocturnal pain, injection drug use, morning stiffness, and history of peripheral vascular disease.[1] We do not know if this patient had weight loss, as is typical with malignancy—this question was not asked on any of his 3 visits.

Table 1. Differential Diagnosis of Low Back Pain

MECHANICAL LOW BACK OR LEG PAIN (97%)↑	NONMECHANICAL SPINAL CONDITIONS (ABOUT 1%)‡	VISCERAL DISEASE (2%)
Lumbar strain, sprain(70%)§	Neoplasia (0.7%)	Disease of pelvic organs
Degenerative processes of disks and	Multiple myeloma	Prostatitis
facets, usually age-related (10%)	Metastatic carcinoma	Endometriosis
Herniated disk (4%)	Lymphoma and leukemia	Chronic pelvic inflammatory
Spinal stenosis (3%)	Spinal cord tumors	disease
Osteoporotic compression fracture (4%)	Retroperitoneal tumors	Renal disease
Spondylolisthesis (2%)	Primary vertebral tumors	Nephrolithiasis
Traumatic fracture (<1%)	Infection (0.01%)	Pyelonephritis
Congenital disease (<1%)	Osteomyelitis	Perinephric abscess
Severe kyphosis	Septic diskitis	Aortic aneurysm
Severe scoliosis	Paraspinous abscess	Gastrointestinal disease
Transitional vertebrae	Epidural abscess	Pancreatitis
Spondylolysis¶	Shingles	Cholecystitis
Internal disk disruption or diskogenic	Inflammatory arthritis (often associated with	Penetrating ulcer
low back pain‖	HLA-B27) (0.3%)	
Presumed instability **	Ankylosing spondylitis	
	Psoriatic spondylitis	
	Reiter's syndrome	
	Inflammatory bowel disease	
	Scheuermann's disease (osteochondrosis)	
	Paget's disease of bone	

Note: references omitted.

Source: Deyo RA, Weinstein JN. Low back pain. N Engl J Med 2001; 344:365. Used with permission. Copyright 2001. Massachusetts Medical Society. All rights reserved.

II. HISTORY AND PHYSICAL EXAM

A directed history should exclude serious causes of back pain. Inquire about mechanism of injury, onset, exacerbating factors, successful treatments, past history of back pain, and "red flags" as listed above. Include questions for common causes of non-mechanical back pain, looking for diagnoses such as pyelonephritis, ureterolithiasis, pancreatitis, cholecystisis, and varicella zoster. Certain causes of mechanical back pain which require more timely diagnosis and management include spinal stenosis, herniated disc and traumatic back pain. The history documented on the first 2 visits is brief. On the first visit, there is an excellent review of symptoms, but we only learn 3 things from the "history of the present illness:" duration is 3–4 weeks, pain is "waxing and waning,"and there was not a definite injury prior to symptom onset. It may have been helpful to know if the pain was worse with motion, if there was a history of similar pain, if this pain was positional or otherwise worsened by motion (as would be expected with mechanical back pain). If the answers to these final questions were negative, our suspicion of more serious illness may be heightened.

The physical exam begins with a visual inspection of the back (zoster) and proceeds with palpation, range of motion, percussion (for CVA tenderness), and neurologic testing (sensation, strength, reflexes, and straight leg raise testing). Nonmechanical causes of back pain may be sought with an abdominal, pelvic, or rectal exam. The straight leg raise (SLR) test is performed by using one hand to lift the heel while using the other hand to keep the knee extended. A positive test is the reproduction of sciatica with leg elevation between 30 and 60%. The "crossed straight leg raise sign" is performed by lifting the well leg in a similar fashion and is positive with reproduction of sciatica in the affected leg.[15]

In 1999, Vroomen, et al., studied the value of the history and physical exam in the diagnosis of sciatica due to disc herniation. They found 37 studies which met their selection criteria. These studies were pooled, and they found that the only test consistently sensitive was the straight leg raise test, with a sensitivity of 85% and specificity of 52%, using testing such as CT, MRI or myelography as the gold standard. When operative findings were used as the gold standard, the pooled sensitivity and specificity were 91% and 32%, respectively. One study used an angle > 60% to produce pain as a positive SLR test, while others used different findings. The crossed SLR test had a sensitivity and specificity of 32% and 98% in the nonsurgical population.

These findings suggest that standard SLR testing is sensitive, and crossed SLR testing is specific. Paresis was not sensitive, but one study found that when present, the probability of nerve root involvement from disc herniation was > 90%. Sensory deficits were insensitive and nonspecific. Depressed reflexes of the knee were not sensitive, and there was disagreement of the specificity of the knee and ankle deep tendon reflexes.[14]

A thorough neurologic exam was performed on all visits. The physical exam on the first and third visits documents reproducible pain with palpation of the low back. A complete history and physical examination will often lead to a diagnosis, or exclude serious causes of back pain; when it does not, then further testing should be considered.

III. TESTING

Nonmechanical causes of back pain may be evaluated with urinalysis, bedside ultrasound, and imaging. The following discussion will focus on evaluation of mechanical back pain.

Imaging studies are controversial in evaluating back pain. Previously, plain films were recommended in those patients with fever, history of cancer, history of IVDU, age greater than 50, trauma, neurological deficits, or unexplained weight loss.[17] These criteria were established 11 years ago based on earlier data, before MRI was widely available. The sensitivity of a plain film is low for most of these conditions (spinal infection, cancer, etc.). If these diagnoses are being entertained, a more sensitive test such as MRI or CT should be considered.

A high incidence of disc pathology is found in asymptomatic patients, making interpretation of a positive MRI difficult (Table 2). Therefore, these tests should be reserved for patients with suspicion of cancer, ureterolithiasis, vascular disease, infection, or those patients with persistent neurologic deficits in whom surgery would be considered.

Incidental findings such as herniated/bulging/degenerative discs may be asymptomatic positives and may lead to unnecessary interventions, patient anxiety, lifestyle modification to accommodate the disease, and assumption of the sick role. Findings which are unusual in an asymptomatic population include extruded disc herniation, displacement of the nerve root, and interruption of the annulo-ligamentus complex.[21]

Table 2. Representative Results of Magnetic Resonance Imaging Studies in Asymptomatic Adults

STUDY	SUBJECTS	ANATOMICAL FINDINGS				
		HERNIATED DISK	BULGING DISK	DEGENERATIVE DISK	STENOSIS	ANNULAR TEAR
		prevalence (%)				
Boden et al.	Volunteers <60 yr old	22	54	46	1	NR
	Volunteers =60 yr old	36	79	93	21	NR
Jensen et al.	Volunteers (mean age, 42 yr)	28	52	NR	7	14
Weishaupt et al.	Volunteers (mean age, 35 yr)	40	24	72	NR	33
Stadnik et al.	Patients referred for head or neck imaging (median age, 42 yr)	33	81	72	NR	56

*NR denotes not reported.
References omitted.

Source: Deyo RA, Weinstein JN. Low back pain. N Engl J Med 2001;344:366. Used with permission. Copyright 2001. Massachusetts Medical Society. All rights reserved.

IV. PROGNOSIS AND MANAGEMENT OF ACUTE BACK PAIN—IDIOPATHIC, HERNIATED DISC, AND SURGICAL EMERGENCIES

About 60–70% of patients recover from an acute episode of back pain by 6 weeks, and by 12 weeks 80–90% have recovered. Recurrences of low back pain occur in up to 40% of patients by 6 weeks.[3] Interestingly, less than 50% of patients disabled for 6 months will return to work, and at 2 years this rate is close to zero.[2] Return to work is influenced by social and economic factors.[1] A high correlation with psychological factors exists, but 94–95% of patients with concomitant substance abuse and anxiety had these syndromes before they developed back pain. Depression may develop before or after the onset of back pain.[18] Operative treatment improves satisfaction and pain relief in patients with herniated nucleus propulsus (HNP), but does not lead to earlier return to work at 1 and 4 years.[20]

Management of acute idiopathic (sprain, strain) back pain is controversial, but effective methods include NSAIDS, muscle relaxants, pain medications, and rapid return to normal activities. Spinal manipulation and physical therapy have a limited effectiveness, and should be delayed until pain has persisted for at least 3 weeks, since 50% of patients will improve in this time. Massage has shown promise in early studies. Therapies shown to be ineffective include bed rest, back exercises in the acute phase, lumbar supports, facet joint injections, and acupuncture.[1]

In the acute phase, management of HNP is similar to management of nonspecific back pain. The natural history of HNP is improvement; at 6 weeks, only 10% have pain severe enough to consider surgery. At 6 months, sequential MRI's show partial or complete regression of the herniated disc in two-thirds of patients. Surgical management (discectomy) has been shown to provide superior pain relief at 4 years, but may not have an advantage at 10 years.[1]

Surgical emergencies causing acute low back pain include ruptured abdominal aortic aneurysm and epidural compression syndromes such as caudina equina syndrome and conus medullaris syndrome. These may be caused by massive midline disc herniation, spinal canal hemorrhage, infection or tumors. Cauda equina syndrome is a rare finding. Symptoms include "saddle" anesthesia (a sensory deficit over the buttocks, posterior-superior thighs and perineal regions), urinary retention, sciatica, sensory and motor deficits, diminished anal sphincter tone, and abnormal SLR's. Sensitivity of urinary retention is 90% and the predictive value of *not* having urinary retention is 95%.[15] Cauda equina syndrome is a surgical emergency and should be treated with dexamethasone 10mg IV before confirmatory MRI is ordered, to minimize progression of the compression and subsequent neurologic damage.[22]

V. CHRONIC BACK PAIN

Chronic back pain has been defined as pain lasting longer than 7–12 weeks, or pain which lasts beyond the expected period of healing.[2] These are not patients that most of us enjoy treating. The reasons are simple; they want relief from their pain, usually with a request for pain medications, and we want to ensure there is not a serious cause for their pain. The patient in this case had only 4 weeks of pain on his initial presentation, and by his second visit had almost 6 weeks of pain.

Management of chronic back pain can be complicated; select patients may benefit from referral to a multidisciplinary pain center. A recent meta-analysis of 9 randomized, controlled trials, including 504 patients with an average of 10 years of back pain, found that antidepressants had a small but significant effect in reducing back pain but not in improving activities of daily living. Only 2 of these studies excluded people with depression, so it is questionable if antidepressants would benefit patients without depression.[4] Therapeutic massage seems to be effective when compared to acupuncture and self education, but traditional Chinese acupuncture was relatively ineffective.[5] Another proven strategy is intensive exercise, which reduces pain and improves function, but adherence is difficult.[6,7] Cyclobenzaprine is modestly more effective than placebo, but the effect occurs mostly during the first 4 days after the onset of back pain, and there are significant side effects including drowsiness.[8] Long term opioid therapy is common, but many patients have side effects such as drowsiness, headache, and constipation, as well as tolerance to medications and addiction.[9] Calcitonin has been shown to have an analgesic effect in patients with osteoporosis-related vertebral fracture.[13]

Is it possible to separate those patients who have organic disease from those seeking narcotics? In 1980, Waddell devised a set of physical signs to differentiate these patients.[12] Three or more physical signs on exam strongly suggest a non-organic component to back pain.

Waddell's signs:

1. Overreaction to the physical exam
2. Widespread superficial tenderness that does not correspond to an anatomical distribution
3. Pain on axial loading of the skull or simultaneous rotation of the shoulders and pelvis
4. Severe limitation on straight leg raise in patients able to sit forward with legs extended
5. Weakness or sensory loss that does not correspond to a nerve root distribution

In a small study in 2002, Blom, et al., described the "heel-tap" test, which seemed to correlate with Waddell's signs but was easier to perform. The examiner tells the patient that the test may cause low back pain, and then gently taps on the patient's heels while seated with hips and knees flexed to 90°. A sudden onset of low back pain is a positive test.[18]

VI. INDICATIONS FOR SURGERY
Indications for surgery from Deyo and Weinstein (reference 1) are listed below.

Table 3. Indications for Surgical Referral among Patients with Low Back Pain

SCIATICA AND PROBABLE HERNIATED DISKS
The cauda equina syndrome (surgical emergency): characterized by bowel or bladder dysfunction (usually urinary retention), numbness in the perineum and medial thighs (i.e., in a saddle distribution), bilateral leg pain, weakness, and numbness Progressive or severe neurologic deficit Persistent neuromotor deficit after 4-6 weeks of nonoperative therapy Persistent sciatica (not low back pain alone) for 4-6 weeks, with consistent clinical and neurologic findings (in this circumstance, and for persistent neuromotor deficit, surgery is elective, and patients should be involved in decision making)
SPINAL STENOSIS
Progressive or severe neurologic deficit, as for herniated disks Back and leg pain that is persistent and disabling, improves with spine flexion, and is associated with spinal stenosis on imaging tests; surgery is elective, and patients should be involved in decision making
SPONDYLOLISTHESIS
Progressive or severe neurologic deficit, as for herniated disks Spinal stenosis with referral indications as above Severe back pain or sciatica with severe functional impairment that persists for a year or longer

Source: Deyo RA, Weinstein JN. Low back pain. N Engl J Med 2001;344:368. Used with permission. Copyright 2001. Massachusetts Medical Society. All rights reserved.

VII. RENAL CELL CANCER
About 31,000 cases of renal cancer are diagnosed per year in the US, with a mortality of almost 40%. At the time of diagnosis, 25–30% of patients have metastatic disease, with 95% having multiple metastases,[11] as occurred in our patient. Renal cell carcinoma occurs in 2% of patients diagnosed with cancer.[16] The classic triad of flank pain, hematuria, and flank mass only occurs about 10% of the time; 25–39% of patients are asymptomatic at the time of the diagnosis. As in our patient, the diagnosis is often found incidentally during unrelated testing.[11]

Initial symptoms of renal cell carcinoma may be from metastatic lesions or paraneoplastic syndromes. Findings may include hematuria, flank or back pain, hypercalcemia, erythrocytosis, elevation of liver function tests, weight loss, cachexia, anemia, fever, polyneuromyopathy, amyloidosis, dermatomyositis or hypertension.[11]

One oft-quoted study of 1,975 walk-in patients with back pain found no cancer if all of the following were true: age less than 50 years without a history of cancer, no unexplained weight loss, absence of conservative therapy failure.[10] This study found that only 0.66% of primary care patients with back pain have a malignant neoplasm, primary or metastatic, as the cause of their pain. The study found 13 patients with tumors which were thought to be causing their back pain, so this should not be interpreted to mean that if a patient meets the above criteria, there is no chance they have cancer. This was also an indigent population at a public hospital in the early 1980's, so the results are not applicable to all populations.

Surgery is the treatment of choice for renal cell cancer, even if the patient has metastatic disease. Radiation and chemotherapy are useful for palliation, but have not proven effective as adjuvant therapy. Interferon alpha or interleukin-2 are occasionally effective in inducing remission.[11]

VIII. CONCLUSION

Our patient had no history of back pain, and an onset of pain which occurred without a definite mechanism of injury. The physical exam was not particularly convincing for a musculoskeletal etiology. He did not have much pain with range of motion, and only the first exam documented any pain with palpation, though the amount or location of pain is not defined; both are clues that a diagnosis other than mechanical back pain may exist. A CT scan was done to exclude renal stone, and metastatic renal cancer was found.

In the ED, the first step in back pain evaluation is exclusion of life-threatening or reversible causes of back pain, specifically abdominal aortic aneurysm, epidural compression syndromes, infection, and tumor. A reasonable approach to a patient with low back pain without acute surgical symptoms may be initial conservative therapy, such as anti-inflammatory, muscle relaxant, and pain medications. Discuss potential etiologies of pain and the importance of follow up.

TEACHING POINTS ABOUT CASE 23:

- If the mechanism of injury and exam are inconsistent with the diagnosis, an alternate diagnosis should be considered and definite follow up arranged.
- 80% of patients with back pain eventually diagnosed with a malignancy are greater than 50. The prevalence of cancer is <1% in all patients with back pain.
- If a tumor has caused an epidural compression syndrome, the entire spine should be imaged since 10% will have other epidural metastases which may change the management.[22]
- There is a high percentage of asymptomatic people with herniated and degenerative lumbar disc disease evident on MRI.
- Red flags for more serious disease include age > 65, history of malignancy, unexplained weight loss, recent trauma, fever, failure to improve after 1 month of therapy, nocturnal pain, injection drug use, morning stiffness, and history of peripheral vascular disease.[1]

REFERENCES

1. Deyo RA, Weinstein JN. Low back pain. N Engl J Med 2001;344: 363-70.
2. Anderson GBJ. Epidemiologic features of chronic low back pain. Lancet 1999;354: 581-5.
3. Carey TS, Garrett JM, Jackman A, et al. Recurrence and care seeking after acute back pain: results of a long-term follow-up study. BMJ 1998;37: 157-64.
4. Salerno SM, Browning R, Jackson JL. The effect of antidepressant treatment on chronic back pain. Arch Intern Med 2002;162: 19-24.

5. Cherkin DC, Eisenberg D, Sherman KJ, et al. Randomized trial comparing traditional Chinese medical acupuncture, therapeutic massage, and self-care education for chronic low back pain. Arch Intern Med 2001;161:1081-8.

6. van Tulder MW, Koes BW, Bouter LM. Conservative treatment of acute and chronic nonspecific low back pain: a systematic review of randomized controlled trials of the most common interventions. Spine 1997;22: 2128-56.

7. Frost H, Lamb SE, Klaber-Moffett JA, et al. A fitness programme for patients with chronic low back pain: 2 year follow up of a randomized controlled trial. Pain 1998;75: 273-9.

8. Browning R et al. Cyclobenzaprine and back pain. Arch Intern Med 2001;161: 1613-20.

9. Jamison RN Jackson JL, O'Malley PG. Opioid therapy for chronic noncancer back pain: a randomized prospective study. Spine 1998;23: 2591-600.

10. Deyo RA, Diehl AK. Cancer as a cause of back pain: frequency, clinical presentation, and diagnostic strategies. J Gen Intern Med 1988;3: 230-8.

11. Curti BD. Renal cell carcinoma. JAMA 2004;292: 97-100.

12. Waddell G, McCulloch JA, Kummel E, et al. Non-organic physical signs in low back pain. Spine 1980;5: 117-25.

13. Blau LA, Hoehns JD. Analgesic efficacy of calcitonin for vertebral fracture pain. Ann Pharmacother 2003;37: 564-70.

14. Vroomen PC, de Krom MC, Knottnerus JA. Diagnostic value of history and physical examination in patients suspected of sciatica due to disc herniation: a systematic review. J Neurology. 1999;246: 899-906.

15. Deyo RA, Rainville J, Kent DL. What can the history and physical examination tell us about low back pain? JAMA. 1992;268: 760-5.

16. Motzer RJ, Bander NH, Nanus DM. Renal cell carcinoma. N Engl J Med 1996;335:865-75.

17. Bigos S, Bowyer O, Braen G, et al. Acute low back problems in adults. Clinical practice guideline no. 14. Rockville, Md.: Agency for Health Care Policy and Research, Dec. 1994. (AHCPR Pub. No. 95-0642).

18. Blom A, Taylor A, Whitehouse S, et al. A new sign of inappropriate lower back pain. Ann R Coll Surg Engl 2002;84: 342-3.

19. Polatin PB, Kinney RK, Gatchel RJ, et al. Psychiatric illness and chronic back pain. The mid and the spine—which goes first? Spine 1993;18: 66-71.

20. Atlas SJ, Chang Y, Kammann E, et al. Long term disability and return to work among patients who have a herniated lumbar disc: the effect of disability compensation. J Bone Joint Surg Am 2000;82-A: 4-15.

21. Stadnik TW, Lee RR, Coen HI, et al. Annular tears and disk herniation: prevalence and contrast enhancement on MR images in the absence of low back pain or sciatica. Neuroradiology 1998;206: 49-55.

22. Tintinalli JE, ed. Emergency medicine. A comprehensive study guide. 6th ed. New York: McGraw-Hill, 2004: 1773-9.

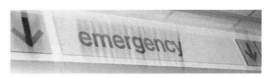

CASE24
48 YEAR OLD MALE WITH BACK PAIN & FEVERS

Commentary:
Gregory L. Henry, MD, FACEP
CEO, Medical Practice Risk Assessment, Inc., Ann Arbor, Michigan
Clinical Professor, Department of Emergency Medicine,
   University of Michigan Medical School, Ann Arbor, Michigan
Past President, American College of Emergency Physicians (ACEP)

Discussion:
Frank Orth, DO, FACEP
Past Physician Facilitator for Performance Improvement of the Emergency Care Center
President of Medical Staff at Mount Carmel St. Ann's Hospital
Past President, Immediate Health Associates
Attending ED physician
   Mt. Carmel St. Ann's Emergency Department, Westerville, Ohio

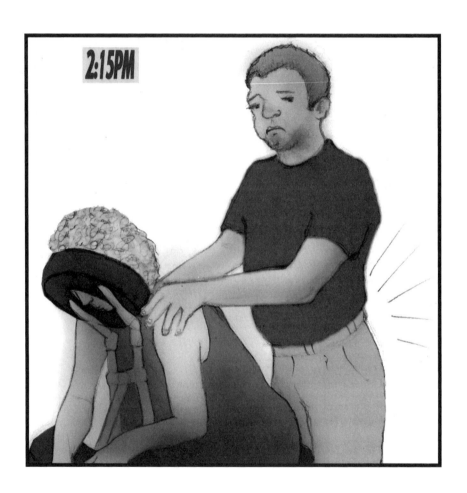

48 YEAR OLD MALE WITH

BACK PAIN & FEVERS

—Initial Visit—

*Authors' Note: The history, exam and notes are the actual documentation of the physicians and providers, including abbreviations (and spelling errors)

CHIEF COMPLAINT (at 09:22): Back pain/spasms

VITAL SIGNS						
Time	Temp(F)	Pulse	Resp	Syst	Diast	Pain
09:28	96.0	80	16	114	60	9
10:56		88	17	108	58	9
12:00		80	18	101	57	0-1
13:50		83	16	102	59	0

HISTORY OF CHIEF COMPLAINT: This 48-year-old white male presents by private auto with friend. He states he has had significant spasms in his left sacroiliac area since last evening. Presents here because of spasms being so severe that he is unable to control the pain anymore. He also gives history of having intermittent fevers throughout the past week. He has had a significant work up by his PCP four days prior with all the test results being normal. He denies any trauma to his back. The patient denies any sensation as far as fever or chills at this time. He denies any bowel or bladder dysfunction. He points to the left sacroiliac area as the area of discomfort. He denies any significant pain down in his buttocks or into his leg. He has never had this type of symptoms before. The patient denies any abdominal pain. All other systems were reviewed and were negative.

PAST MEDICAL HISTORY/TRIAGE (at 09:40):
   Allergies: No known drug allergies.
   Medications: Advil as needed.
   Past medical history: Mitral valve prolapse.
   Past surgical history: Inguinal hernia.
   Social history: Nonsmoker, nondrinker. He is a massage therapist.

PHYSICAL EXAMINATION:
   General: In no acute respiratory distress, alert and cooperative with exam.
   Lungs: Clear to auscultation with good breath sounds bilaterally, no accessory muscle use is noted, or areas of consolidation are heard.
   Cardiovascular: Heart is regular rate and rhythm. He does have a systolic murmur heard.
   Abdomen: Positive bowel sounds, soft, nontender, no masses.

Extremities: Show no signs of trauma or deformity, seemed to move all extremities well. Neurocirculatory status appears intact of the lower extremities

Back: His back examination is limited initially because any movement seems to cause him increase pain in the above noted area

EMERGENCY DEPARTMENT COURSE: The patient was having such severe spasms that it limited my physical exam initially. Therefore, (at 10:30) he was given IV Toradol 30mg and IV Robaxin 1gm, then (at 11:30) requiring IV Demerol 50mg and IV Valium 5mg as well to help calm down his symptoms. He did improve, but did have intermittent exacerbations in the emergency department. He was eventually given (at 12:51) further Valium 2.5mg and Decadron 10mg intravenously. I did review all his lab work that was done by his PCP earlier in the week for his intermittent fevers, all of which did appeared normal. [These labs included CBC, chemistry, glucose, LFT's and urinalysis. All were normal. The WBC count was 6.5 and hemoglobin was 12.6.]

I did not feel with him being afebrile at this time that any further work up from this standpoint is warranted. I really doubted it was related to the problems he is presenting with today. The patient was able to stand, but any significant flexion or extension of his back did cause spasms in his left sacroiliac area. I did not feel there is any further emergency department course or work up necessary. X-rays were not warranted because he has had no trauma. He is agreeable with symptomatic treatment at this time and requesting discharge.

DIAGNOSIS (at 13:01): Acute left lumbosacral spasm/pain.

DISPOSITION: The patient is discharged to home with friend in improved condition. He is given prescription for Percocet, #30; prednisone 40 mg a day for the next five days; and also Valium 5 mg tablets #20. Told to follow up with his PCP beginning next week. Otherwise return to the emergency department for any worsening or concerning symptoms. He was discharged from the ED at 13:58.

Gregory L. Henry comments:

"A social history specifically inquiring about a history of IV drug use should have been taken; a drug abuser with back pain is an abscess until proven otherwise"

A chief complaint of back pain is common in the emergency department. We are so often focused on musculoskeletal pain that an abscess or other infection can be extremely difficult to diagnose. This is an extremely subtle case in a healthy appearing patient with normal vital signs. However, it is important to note that this patient had a history of fever and was worked up 4 days earlier by his family practitioner. With a history of intermittent fever, an attempt to find a potential relationship to his presenting complaint should be made. Fever and back pain are commonly, but not exclusively, associated with urinary tract infections. A social history specifically inquiring about a history of IV drug use should have been taken; a drug abuser with back pain is an abscess until proven otherwise.

The evaluation of this patient seems reasonable—an adequate history and physical examination were performed. However, in the cardiovascular exam, a systolic murmur was heard, but no further delineation of this murmur is noted. With his history of mitral valve prolapse, the murmur might have prompted further investigation. In addition, a skin exam is not performed. In a patient with potentially infectious disease, skin examination for exanthem or petechiae is advisable.

Importantly, there was no specific time given for re-evaluation; this is always a mistake. A patient needs to know when to return, and why.

- Thoroughness of Documentation: 8 out of 10.

- Thoroughness of Patient Evaluation: 8 out of 10.

- Risk of Serious Illness Being Missed: Medium risk.

- Risk Management Medical legal Rating: Medium risk.

48 YEAR OLD MALE WITH
BACK PAIN AND FEVERS

—Second Visit: 5 Days Later—

CHIEF COMPLAINT (at 10:48): Back pain.

VITAL SIGNS								
Time	Temp(F)	Rt.	Pulse	Resp	Syst	Diast	Pulse ox	Pain
10:47	96.3	Tym.	80	20	102	62		
12:45			83	16	90	62		0
14:45			91	16	115	53		0
15:55			94	16	106	65	98%	0

HISTORY OF PRESENT ILLNESS (at 11:15): This is a 48-year-old male who states prodrome, started having fevers about three weeks ago. The fevers have been getting up to about 103. A little over a week ago he noted some small vesicular lesions on his skin that have now completely resolved, however he continues to have fevers at night. He states when he woke up this morning his fever was 101, took a couple of Advil for it. But, the main reason why the patient is here is he is having significant pain and he points to the left SI joint. He has been having this tremendous back pain and spasm on the left side. It started about four or five days ago and has just gradually gotten worse. He describes it as pain in the SI joint and into the gluteal area where he has just tremendous spasms mostly with movement. The pain is worse when he coughs, but he has had no chest pain or sputum. He denies any radicular pain, denies any numbness or tingling, denies any bowel or bladder dysfunction. He is able to get into a position where he is laying on his back with his knees crouched up. That does seem to cause no pain. However, he denies any pain with range of motion in the hip, knee, or foot. He was seen here in the emergency department on Friday, five days ago, was placed on Valium, Percocet and prednisone, states he had no pain relief with that and it only made him groggy, thus he called his primary care doctor on Monday, 2 days ago, and had an x-ray of his lumbar spine done that day, which just showed some chronic changes in the lumbar region, but he returns today for the significant pain. [Radiologist reading of XR per PCP: There is a spondylosis within the arch of L5 without slipping of L5 on S1. There is mild degenerative spondylosis involving the L5-S1 disk. The disks are satisfactory as are the vertebral bodies. No destructive process is apparent.]

Denies ear pain, rhinorrhea, or sore throat. No chest pain, dyspnea, sputum. Complains of no abdominal pain. He has had a little bit of nausea, but no vomiting, diarrhea, constipation, or melena. Denies any flank pain, denies dysuria, hematuria, frequency, or urgency. With the fevers he has been having some headaches. They were worse a week ago, but have significantly improved this week. He states he has no headache at this time. He denies any neck pain or neck stiffness. He has had fevers for over three weeks, ranging from 103 to last night 101.

PAST MEDICAL HISTORY/TRIAGE:

(Per RN): Patient presents per medic with complaint of back pain

Allergies: No known drug allergies.

Medications: Valium, Percocet, last dose of prednisone was to be taken this morning, however he did not take it.

Past medical history: Mitral valve prolapse. He has had no history of any back injuries, no history of any recent injury that he can recall.

Past surgical history: None

Social history: Denies alcohol, tobacco, and drug use.

PHYSICAL EXAMINATION (AT 11:18):

Vital signs: Blood pressure 102/64, pulse 80, respirations 20, temperature 96.3.

General: Alert and oriented times three.

HEENT: Within normal limits. Neck is supple, negative Kernig's, negative Brudzinski, no lymphadenopathy.

Lungs: Lungs are completely clear to auscultation bilaterally, no wheeze, rales, or rhonchi, good aeration throughout.

Cardiovascular: Heart regular rate and rhythm without murmur.

Abdomen: Abdomen is nondistended, bowel sounds are heard in all four quadrants, very soft, no voluntary, involuntary guarding, no rebound, no referred tenderness, no hepatosplenomegaly or masses, nontender to all four quadrants, no flank tenderness.

Musculoskeletal: He is nontender to the thoracic or the lumbar vertebra midline, but as I palpate in the left SI joint he has some mild tenderness there and some mild tenderness in the paraspinal muscles just above the SI joint, very tender in the gluteal muscles. This caused significant spasm and pain for him when I palpated the gluteal area. With range of motion of the waist this does cause pain into the gluteal area, but he actually has a straight leg raise with no radicular pain, thus caused some pain again in the low back region, on the left side. He has full range of motion of the left hip without any tenderness, full flexion, extension, internal and external rotation does cause some mild pain with flexion however. Full range of motion of the knee and ankle.

Extremities: Pedal pulses are good, capillary refill is brisk, has sensation distally.

Neuro: Deep tendon reflexes are 2/4 bilaterally of the lower extremities.

EMERGENCY DEPARTMENT COURSE: We did obtain a CBC (results below). Urinalysis was completely negative for leukocyte esterase, no blood, no nitrite. It was sent for culture and sensitivity. We did obtain a CT of his pelvis in the gluteal area. (Results at 14:15). It did show a little bit of free fluid in the cul-de-sac, however there was no abscess and the muscle and the gluteal area all appears to be fine, so it is a negative CT. We did give him an IV of 0.9 normal saline KVO, and (at 12:08) Dilaudid 1 mg IV, and Phenergan 12.5 mg IV. This did sedate him and he was able to get somewhat comfortable. We will go ahead and release him to home, still off work for the rest of the week. I gave him a referral to the orthopedist on-call, or follow up with his PCP. We continued the Percocet. I gave him 10 mg Percocet, one by mouth every four hours. We continued him on the Valium, 5 mg one q.8. As the prednisone seemed to be not effective, we switched him to Vioxx 50 mg one daily and off work for the next few days.

RESULTS (at 11:55):

Test	Flag	Value	Units	Ref. Range
WBC		7.4	K/uL	4.6-10.2
HGB	L	10.6	G/DL	12.0-16.0
PLT	L	132	K/uL	142-424

Urinalysis: WNL

CT PELVIS WITH PO AND IV CONTRAST: Impression (per radiologist at 14:15): The urinary bladder appears somewhat distended, but, otherwise, unremarkable. I believe that there is a small amount of free fluid in the cul-de-sac of uncertain etiology. No pelvic mass, lymphadenopathy or abscess is identified. No obvious abnormality of the gluteal muscles are noted.

IMPRESSION: (1) Acute left gluteal spasms. (2) Fever, unknown origin.

Disposition: He was released from the ED, ambulatory, with family at 14:15.

48 YEAR OLD MALE WITH BACK PAIN AND FEVERS

—Third Visit: 6 Days Later—

CHIEF COMPLAINT (at 22:33): Fever and fatigue

VITAL SIGNS						
Time	Temp(F)	Rt.	Pulse	Resp	Syst	Dias
22:42	98.1	Tym.	93	20	126	76

HISTORY OF PRESENT ILLNESS (at 23:43): 48 year old male with one month history of intermittent fevers, fatigue who had been seen by his family doctor who thought he possibly had bacterial endocarditis. Several days ago he did have some visual loss and saw an ophthalmologist who recommended ECHO to rule out endocarditis. He did have a cardiac ECHO today and there was a thick mitral valve leaflet and a question of vegetation. He is scheduled for a transesophageal ECHO tomorrow. He has had some headaches. Vomited once in the last month. Did have some rash on his face and trunk which were red and then a scab appeared and then they resolved. No rashes now. Intermittent nonproductive cough.

PAST MEDICAL HISTORY/TRIAGE (at 22:37):
PMH: Mitral valve prolapse
PSH: Hernia surgery. Heart catheterization in the 1960's to evaluate for rheumatic heart disease and it was normal.

FH: Heart disease and cancer
SH: No tobacco, occ. Alcohol
Meds: Valium, vioxx, percocet

PHYSICAL EXAMINATION (at 23:47):

General: Awake and alert.
HEENT: Unremarkable
Eyes: Funduscopic exam normal. No macular edema appreciated.
Neck: Supple without JVD, bruits, LAN
Chest: Diminished aeration but clear. No rales or rhonchi, no wheezing or stridor
CV: Regular with apical rate of 90, no gallops. Has grade II/VI systolic murmur
Abdomen: Soft, nontender, BS active
Extremities: A lot of pain with movement of the left hip. Good distal function and sensation in all of the extremities and good pulses in all extremities.
Skin: No splinter hemorrhages under the nails. No cyanosis or clubbing.
Neuro: No focal deficits. Cranial nerves intact.

TESTING:

ECG with NSR and a rate of 97 (actual ECG not available)

RESULTS (at 00:52):

Test	Flag	Value	Units	Ref. Range
WBC		8.1	K/uL	4.6-10.2
HGB	L	10.2	G/DL	12.0-16.0
PLT		242	K/uL	142-424

Chemistry and LFT's - WNL

Test	Flag	Value	Units	Ref. Range
CK		272	NG/ML	
TROPI	H	1.06	NG/ML	.00-.27
WSR	H	77	MM/HR	0-15

ED COURSE: IV with normal saline, IV vancomycin and gentamicin.

DIAGNOSIS (at 01:21):

1. Febrile illness of unknown etiology
2. Mitral regurgitation, rule out endocarditis
3. Anemia
4. Left hip pain, rule out septic arthritis

DISPOSITION: Admission to tele bed. He was discharged from the ED to the floor at 03:31.

HOSPITAL COURSE:

He was admitted, continued on IV antibiotics and underwent cardiac evaluation:

Transthoracic ECHO: EF 60%. Mitral valve with thickening and prolapse of anterior leaflet with probable vegetation.

Transesophageal ECHO: There is 0.5-.075cm vegetation on the tip of the anterior leaflet of the mitral valve which prolapses into the left atrium with coaptation of the valve. There is 3+ to 4+ mitral regurgitation. Left atrium is dilated. No atrial thrombus or patent foramen ovale.

MRI left hip 3 days after admission: Enhancement of the inferior endplate of L5 and superior endplate of S1 with mild enhancement within the L5-S1 disc. Mild disc bulge. Consistent with osteomyelitis/diskitis L5-S1

Blood cultures X 2 on day of admission and then X 2 one week later were all negative

FINAL DIAGNOSIS: Culture negative endocarditis

OUTPATIENT FOLLOW UP AND "SUBSEQUENT EVENTS"

Four months later he underwent mitral valve repair, ligation of the left atrial appendage, and closure of patent foramen ovale. He was released after 4 days. He was left with permanently diminished vision in his left eye.

Subsequent events: The patient later sued the first two ED physicians and the primary care physicians with a failure to diagnose. The main allegation against the ED physicians is that blood cultures were not obtained as this may have helped with the diagnosis. It was subsequently revealed in the deposition that the patient had a history of mitral valve prolapse with regurgitation and underwent a dental procedure 3 weeks prior to onset of symptoms. He had been prescribed antibiotics, but had not taken then. The case was dropped by the plaintiff before trial.

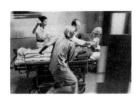

EVALUATION OF FEVER IN ADULTS AND INFECTIOUS ENDOCARDITIS

Frank Orth, DO, FACEP

I. CASE SUMMARY

Despite several visits to the ED and his primary care physician, our patient continued to experience symptoms of fever and severe back pain. When he developed visual loss he saw an ophthalmologist, who may have seen Roth spots on his retina and recommended an ECHO to rule out endocarditis. He was sent back to the ED for admission and workup for endocarditis. Transthoracic and transesophageal ECHO showed mitral valve vegetations. Blood cultures were negative on admission and again one week later. He eventually underwent valve repair, but unfortunately had residual visual loss.

II. DEFINITION AND DIFFERENTIAL DIAGNOSIS OF FEVER

Fever is the chief complaint in 6% of adult and 40% of pediatric ED visits. Pediatric fevers are usually secondary to an infectious source, while adults are more likely to have either an infectious or non infectious etiology. Fever is generally considered a temperature above 100.4° F (38° C). Hyperthermia is defined as a temperature above 106.7° F (41.5° C). The differential diagnosis of fever is separated below into non infectious and infectious etiologies (Table 1).[1]

Table 1. Differential Diagnosis of Fever in Adults

INFECTIOUS	NON-INFECTIOUS
1. Bacterial	1. Collagen vascular/autoimmune/vasculitides
2. Viral (including HIV)	2. Neoplasms
3. Fungal	3. Granulomatous diseases
4. Parasitic	4. Thromboembolic diseases
	5. Drug fever
(Opportunistic pathogens of any of	6. Inherited diseases (e.g., Familial Mediterranean fever)
the above categories predominantly	7. Endocrine (Hyperthyroidism, adrenal insufficiency)
seen in immunosuppressed hosts)	8. Factitious fever
	Other: Neuroleptic malignant syndrome, malignant hyperthermia, transfusion reactions, etc.

III. EVALUATION OF FEVER—HISTORY

The bedside evaluation of the adult with fever begins with the history, which helps to establish a differential diagnosis to guide the physical examination and diagnostic testing. The history and physical examination will establish a diagnosis 70–85% of the time.[2,3]

The onset, duration, and magnitude of the fever, as well as associated symptoms, should be documented. The history should include any recent travel, medications including antipyretics, surgery, chronic illnesses, or orthopedic implants. History should also seek to elicit whether the patient has sick contacts in the home or workplace, as well as pet and insect exposures. Risk factors for HIV should be explored, including IV drug abuse; patients without risk factors but concerning symptoms should be tested.

In this case the initial physician documented an intermittent fever and the use of an antipyretic (Advil), but it is unclear if the patient used the Advil prior to the visit. Mitral valve prolapse is also mentioned in the history, but his symptoms seem to point to a musculoskeletal etiology for his pain with an unrelated elevated temperature. There is no rash or mention of recent procedures. The visit to the primary care physician seemed to be primarily for fever, and the ED physician documented review of labs obtained by the family physician, but did not specify results.

The history obtained on the second visit 5 days later was more extensive. The fever and its pattern were explored in greater depth and documented that the patient used Advil before coming to the ED. The outpatient lumbar spine film results were reviewed, but did not add to the case. Because the patient's primary complaints were fever and gluteal pain, a CT was performed to search for an abscess. The results were negative and the patient was discharged with adjustments to his medications.

The history on the final visit is straight forward; the patient now has a presumptive diagnosis established by the ophthalmologist, and he was admitted for further workup and treatment.

IV. EVALUATION OF FEVER—PHYSICAL EXAM

Oral or rectal temperature are considered the most accurate methods of measuring temperature. The presence of a tachycardia can be related to the fever; the pulse rate may increase 10 beats per minute for every one degree celsius of temperature elevation. Tachypnea can reflect sepsis or pulmonary infection, pulse oximetry may reveal hypoxemia, and septic patients may have altered mental status. Diffuse adenopathy occurs with the acute antiretroviral syndrome as well as other processes. Rigors are present in less than 50% of bacteremic patients.[4]

Funduscopic exam may reveal Roth spots, suggesting endocarditis. This may have been the case in our patient, but findings of the ophthalmologist are not included. Examination of the mouth may reveal dental caries, pharyngitis, or abscesses. Sinus tenderness could indicate sinusitis which is often a source of unexplained fever. The neck may exhibit lymphadenopathy, nuchal rigidity, masses, or an enlarged, tender thyroid gland. Lymphadenopathy is often tender and bilateral if associated with infections; non infectious causes include malignancies and medications, such as phenytoin, methyldopa, and procainamide.

Auscultation of the lungs may reveal the typical sounds of pneumonia or decreased breath sounds from a parapneumonic effusion. Patients with pericarditis may have a friction rub. A new heart murmur can stem from endocarditis, particularly in intravenous drug users, patients with history of indwelling lines and catheters, or elderly patients. The abdomen should be evaluated for peritoneal signs and distension; also patients with ascites and fever should be presumed to have spontaneous bacterial peritonitis (SBP). A tender, boggy prostate, due to prostatitis, can cause fever, and a tender mass around the rectum could suggest an abscess.

Pelvic examination may reveal cervical motion tenderness or vaginal discharge present in pelvic inflammatory disease or tuboovarian abscess. The testicular exam may reveal the enlarged painful testicle of orchiitis, epidydimitis, or possibly Fournier's gangrene.

Skin may exhibit clues to cellulitis, abscesses, or particular findings of systemic infections such as a maculopapular exanthem of viral etiology. The finding of petechial or purpuric rashes may indicate meningitis/meningococcemia. Splinter hemorrhages under the fingernails may be present in patients with endocarditis. The back exam, a system often missed in evaluation of the febrile adult, can reveal localized pain due to diskitis, osteomyelitis, or epidural abscess.

During our patient's initial visit, the physical examination did not uncover an etiology of the fever. The exami-nation was reasonable; a murmur was heard on the cardiac examination but not explored further. The physical examination on visit #2 did not reveal an objective fever, but the patient had taken ibuprofen prior to arrival. Here, the cardiac examination documented absence of a murmur, in contradiction to the initial visit. This discrepancy was not commented upon—it seems that the initial chart was not reviewed during the second visit.

V. LABORATORY EVALUATION OF FEVER

WBC Count

An elevated WBC count does increase the likelihood of a bacterial infection, but is neither sensitive nor specific for the presence or severity of infection. An absolute neutrophilia with left shift is also non-specific, and can be seen in a wide variety of clinical presentations, from an acute emotional event to strenuous exercise to overwhelming sepsis.[1,2] The WBC count should be used in conjunction with the history, examination, and other testing.

Urine

Young females with typical symptoms and a positive dipstick do not need a urine culture. Males with dysuria need a prostate examination and urine culture. Pyuria on urinalysis has a sensitivity of 95% and specificity of 71%; bacteriuria is 40–70% sensitive and 85–96% specific. Presence of nitrite or leukocyte esterase on dipstick has sensitivity of 75% and specificity of 82%.[3] There are several non-infectious causes of false positive dipsticks, including interstitial nephritis, nephrolithiasis, or leukocytes which are vaginal in origin. A positive urine culture is considered the gold standard for the diagnosis of UTI, but some controversy exists about what determines a positive culture. Traditionally, a colony count of greater than 100,000 was required for the diagnosis; however, infections exist below this colony count threshold. Associated bacteremia can occur at colony counts < 100,000.

Blood cultures

Bacteremia does not have well-defined clinical signs. In the elderly, mental status change may indicate bacteremia, but false positive and negative results are common.[8,9] Blood cultures may identify the infectious agent in pneumonia, meningitis, pyelonephritis, occult abscess, endovascular infections, or patients with signs of sepsis. If endocarditis is suspected, then 3 sets of blood cultures should be obtained at least 1 hour apart prior to administering antibiotics.

Blood cultures should be considered in patients with sickle-cell disease, steroid-dependency, immunocompromised state, or in patients with signs of sepsis or meningitis. The American Thoracic Society and the Infectious Diseases Society of America recommend blood cultures in patients admitted with pneumonia. Blood cultures should not be obtained in patients with uncomplicated cholecystitis, appendicitis, or bowel perforation.[2,4]

Cerebral spinal fluid (CSF)
The evaluation of CSF should include cell count, glucose, protein, gram stain and culture. CSF gram stain has a sensitivity of about 75% in identifying the infectious agent; the CSF culture is positive in 70–85% of patients with meningitis.[8] The classic signs of meningitis are often blunted or absent in the elderly and immunocompromised patients, and a low threshold for lumbar puncture and CSF examination should be used in these high-risk patients.

Let's return to our patient. He was seen in the ED twice and by his family physician twice, then developed visual changes which suggested endocarditis. The use of the Duke criteria for diagnosis of endocarditis is based on blood cultures and echocardiographic findings, information rarely available in the initial ED evaluation. In addition, blood cultures at the last ED visit and again 1 week later (a total of 4 cultures) were all negative. His final diagnosis was culture-negative endocarditis.

VI. INFECTIOUS ENDOCARDITIS—EPIDEMIOLOGY, ORGANISMS, MORTALITY
The incidence of infectious endocarditis (IE) is about 1–6.2/100,000, or 10,000–20,000 cases per year.[9,10,11,12] IE is the fourth leading cause of life-threatening infectious disease following urosepsis, pneumonia, and intra abdominal sepsis.

There are 3 subgroups of endocarditis: native valve IE, prosthetic valve IE, and IV drug use IE. Native valve IE, which can be acute or sub-acute, comprises about 59–70% of cases.[13] Prosthetic valve IE, which comprises about 14–30% of cases, can occur in the early post-operative period or years later. IE associated with IV drug use has an incidence of 11–16% of cases. Risk in IV drug users is 2–5% per year, mean age is 30 years, and infection usually occurs in the tricuspid valve.[25]

The most common valve affected in native valve IE is the aortic valve, followed by the mitral and tricuspid valves.[26] In the past, IE was often related to valvular disease secondary to rheumatic fever; with the advent of antibiotics, rheumatic fever is rarely encountered in industrialized countries, but remains the most frequent cardiac condition predisposing patients to IE in developing countries.

The most common bacteria responsible for native valve IE has historically been *Streptococcus viridans*, but has recently been replaced by *Staphylococcus aureus*.[25] Blood cultures are ultimately positive in 95% of cases of IE;[14] however, the incidence of culture-negative IE is increasing, likely due to poor culture technique, fastidious organisms, and prior antibiotic use.[15,16]

The overall mortality rate for IE approaches 40%;[17] each sub-group has its own level of mortality. Native valve mortality ranges from 16–27%, and the development of CHF predicts a poor outcome.[18] Those who develop prosthetic valve IE in the early post-op period (less than 60 days) have a mortality of 30-80%, whereas those greater than 60 days post-op have a mortality of 20-40%.[19] IVDA-associated endocarditis has a mortality of about 8%.[20]

VII. INFECTIOUS ENDOCARDITIS—PREDISPOSING FACTORS

The most common cardiovascular diagnosis predisposing patients to IE is mitral valve prolapse, particularily if associated with mitral regurgitation or thickened mitral leaflets.[25] (Table 2)

Table 2. Predisposing Conditions to the Development of IE

A. Cardiac conditions
• High risk
Prosthetic cardiac valves
Previous bacterial endocarditis
Complex cyanotic congenital disease
Prosthetic shunts or conduits
• Moderate risk
Other congenital cardiac malformations
Acquired valvular dysfunction
Hypertrophic cardiomyopathy
Mitral valve prolapse (High risk with cardiac dysfunction)
B. Recurrent Bacteremic States
Intravenous drug use
Intravascular prosthesis
Hemodialysis shunts
Infected central line catheters
Extensive burn injury
Significant dental infection

Source: Tilden F, Woolridge D. Infectious endocarditis: A comprehensive review for emergency physicians. Emerg Med Rep 1999; 20(26): 263.

VIII. INFECTIOUS ENDOCARDITIS—CLINICAL PRESENTATION AND DIAGNOSIS

Fever (T>38° C) is present in > 90% of patients overall, and in > 98% of IV drug users. Fever is less likely to occur in the elderly, or patients with heart failure or renal failure.[26] A heart murmur may be present in 24–95% of cases, but is not sensitive or specific for the diagnosis.[21, 22, 23]

Clinical evidence of heart failure (such as pulmonary edema, JVD, or peripheral edema), may be present due to valvular dysfunction. Various vascular findings, such as Janeway lesions (painless red lesions on palms and soles), conjunctival hemorrhages, Roth spots (retinal exudative lesions), Osler's nodes (painful raised lesion on fingers, toes, or feet which are violet colored), splinter hemorrhages (subungual hemorrhages), arterial emboli, septic pulmonary infarctions and mycotic aneurysms may also be seen. These are more commonly encountered in the subacute form of IE and are each present in less than 10% of patients. The presentation of IE ranges from extremely vague, non-specific, chronic complaints to immediate life threatening cardiac events. (Table 3)

Table 3. Clinical Features of IE

Symptoms	Laboratory findings
Fever	Persistently positive blood cultures
Chills	Positive serologic studies
Arthralgia/myalgia	Anemia (Hb ≤ 10 g/dL)
Back pain	Elevated ESR (> 30 mm/hr)
Pleuritic chest pain	Elevated WBC (> 10,000 cells/mm3)
Malaise/weight loss	Positive rheumatoid factor
Mental confusion	Hematuria (gross or microscopic)
Symptoms of CHF	Pyuria
Signs	Proteinuria
Temperature > 38°C	Renal insufficiency
New or changing murmur	Chest x-ray:
Pneumonia	congestive heart failure
Vascular phenomena:	septic emboli
Janeway lesions	pneumonia
conjunctival hemorrhage	**Echocardiography**
Immunologic phenomena:	Vegetation
Osler's nodes	Valvular thickening
Roth's spots	Endocardial abscess
Petechiae	Valvular dehiscence
Hepatomegaly	Cardiac dysfunction
Splenomegaly	**CNS abnormalities**
Clubbing	Intracranial hemorrhage
Splinter hemorrhages	Arterial embolism
CNS manifestations	Aseptic meningitis
	Mycotic aneurysm

Adapted from Tilden F, Woolridge D. Infectious endocarditis: A comprehensive review for emergency physicians. Emerg Med Rep 1999; 20(26): 265.

Endocarditis is a difficult diagnosis to make in the ED, given its wide array of clinical presentations. Often, the patient is admitted for blood cultures and an echocardiogram. A high index of suspicion should be maintained for patients at risk. The diagnostic criteria for IE are classically based on those originally proposed by a group at Duke University[27] and have been subsequently modified[28] (Table 4). These criteria are considered the "gold standard" for the clinical diagnosis of IE.

Table 4. Modified Duke Diagnostic Criteria for Infective Endocarditis

Major criteria

Microbiologic

Typical microorganism isolated from two separate blood
cultures: viridans streptococci, *Streptococcus bovis,* HACEK
group, *Staphylococcus aureus,* or community-acquired
enterococcal bacteremia without a primary focus

or

Microorganism consistent with infective endocarditis isolated
from persistently positive blood cultures

or

Single positive blood culture for *Coxiella burnetii* or phase I
IgG antibody titer to *C. burnetii* >1:800

Evidence of endocardial involvement

New valvular regurgitation (increase or change in preexisting
murmur not sufficient)

or

Positive echocardiogram (transesophageal echocardiogram
recommended in patients who have a prosthetic valve,
who are rated as having at least possible infective endocarditis
by clinical criteria, or who have complicated
infective endocarditis)

Minor criteria

Predisposition to infective endocarditis that includes
certain cardiac conditions and injection-drug use

Fever Temperature >38°C (100.4°F)

Vascular phenomena

Immunologic phenomena

Microbiologic findings

Table modified from ref 29 and criteria are those from Li et al 28. IE is *definite* if fulfillment of two major criteria, one major criterion plus three minor criteria or five minor criteria; they are defined as *possible* if they fulfill one major and one minor criterion, or three minor criteria. HACEK (haemophilus species (*Haemophilus parainfluenzae, H. aphrophilus,* and *H. paraphrophilus*), *Actinobacillus actinomycetemcomitans, Cardiobacterium hominis, Eikenella corrodens,* and *Kingella kingae.*

Modified from: Mylonakis E, Calderwood SB. Infective endocarditis in adults. N Engl J Med 2001; 345(18):1318-30.N Engl J Med 2001;344:368. Used with permission. Copyright 2001. Massachusetts Medical Society. All rights reserved.

Our patient did fulfill one major criteria (positive ECHO) and 3 minor criteria (predisposition to IE with the hx of MVP, fever per history, and vascular phenomena with the positive funduscopic findings per the ophthalmologist).

IX. CULTURE-NEGATIVE ENDOCARDITIS

This patient had culture-negative endocarditis, which occurs in 5–7% of patients who have not received antibiotics prior to blood cultures, and can be due to infections by fungus, fastidious organisms, or intracellular pathogens that are not easily culturable. These include the HACEK group of bacteria (see Table 4), *Brucella species*, *Coxiella* (the agent of Q fever), *Bartonella spp*, (agent of Cat Scratch disease), *Legionella*, *Chlamydia*, and *Tropheryma* (the agent of Whipple's disease). These diagnoses are based on specialized culture techniques, serological testing, PCR identification of the organism, or histopathology of the infected valve.[30]

X. MANAGEMENT

Because the definitive diagnosis requires culture results and echocardiogram, therapy is usually not started in the ED. For true culture-negative endocarditis, antibiotics include β-lactams such as ampicillin in combination with an aminoglycoside, ceftriaxone, or doxycycline and TMP/SMX usually in combination with an aminoglycoside depending on the organism. Anticoagulation should not be used, as it has not been shown to decrease embolic events, but does increase the risk of intracerebral hemorrhage.[25]

XI. SUMMARY

I find it interesting that despite 3 evaluations in the emergency department, an objective fever wasn't found; analgesics may have been the reason. The presenting complaint of back pain was confusing; the physical examination points to a very localized type of pain, concerning to the second physician, but the CT scan was negative for abscess. The astute ophthalmologist discovered Roth spots on funduscopic examination after the patient developed visual changes. As it turned out, the patient was found to have osteomyelitis/diskitis of L5-S1 when admitted. These conditions are related to the embolic nature of IE.

Though IE has a wide array of clinical presentations with multiple organ system involvement and non-specific complaints, several clues were present that could have led to a presumptive diagnosis. A history of several weeks of fever in a patient with a past history of mitral valve prolapse does increase the risk of IE. Anemia was noted on the CBC, a nonspecific finding, but one found to occur in patients with IE. This was a difficult case, but these clues could have provoked a suspicion of endocarditis.

TEACHING POINTS FROM CASE 24:
- Fever is present in about 90% of patients with IE, but may be absent if the patient has recently used antipyretics.
- The most common cardiovascular diagnosis predisposing patients to IE is mitral valve prolapse, particularly if associated with mitral regurgitation or thickened mitral leaflets.
- Reviewing charts of previous visits will often assist in the workup. In this case, documentation of a mitral valve prolapse with a murmur occurred during the initial visit.
- When IE is in the differential, the patient should be questioned about history of IV drug use.

REFERENCES

1. Shah SM., Searls, L. The febrile adult: part 1, a systemic approach to diagnosis and evaluation. Emerg Med Rep 1998;19: 173-81.
2. Stapczynski JS. Evaluation of the febrile adult in the emergency department. Ann Emerg Med 1990;19: 481.
3. Keating HJ, Klimek JJ, Levine DS, et al. Effects of aging on the clinical significance of fever in ambulatory adult patients. J AM Geriatr Soc 1984;32: 282-7.
4. Fontanarosa PB, Kaeverlein SJ, Gerson LW, et al. Difficulty in predicting bacteremia in elderly emergency patients. Ann Emerg Med 1992;21: 842-8.
5. Gelfand JA, Dinarello CA.Alterations in body temperature. In: Fauci AS, Martin JB, Braunwald E, et al., eds. Harrison's principles of internal medicine. New York:McGraw-Hill 1998:84-90.
6. Young GP. CBC or not CBC? That is the question. Ann Emerg Med 1986;15: 367-71. A study revealed that only 2 out of 860 WBC's had a clear benefit for the outcome of the patient.
7. Fihn SD. Acute uncomplicated urinary tract infection in women. N Engl J Med 2003;349: 259-66.
8. Scheld MW. Bacterial meningitis, brain abscess, and other suppurative intracranial infections. In: Fauci AS, Martin JB Braunqald E, et al., eds. Harrison's principles of internal medicine. New York:McGraw-Hill; 1998: 2419-26.
9. Watanakunakorn C, Burkert T. Infective endocarditis at a large community teaching hospital,1980-1990: A review of 210 episodes. Medicine 1993;72: 90-102.
10. Hogevik H, Olaison L, Andersson R, et al. Epidemiologic aspects of infective endocarditis in an urban population: a 5-year prospective study. Medicine 1995;74: 324-39.
11. Bayer AS, Bolger AF, Taubert KA, et al. Diagnosis and management of infective endocarditis and its complications. Circulation 1998;98: 2936-48.
12. Durack DT, Prevention of infective endocarditis. N Engl J Med 1995;332: 38-44.
13. Sandre RM, Shafran SD. Infective endocarditis: review of 135 cases over 9 years. Clin Infect Dis 1996;22: 276-86.
14. Werner AS, Cobbs CG, Kaye D, et al. Studies on the bacteremia of bacterial endocarditis. JAMA 1967;202: 199-203.
15. Hoen B, Selton-Suty C, Lacassin R, et al. Infective endocarditis in patients with negative blood cultures: analysis of 88 cases from a one year nationwide survey in France. Clin Infect Dis 1995; 20: 501-6.
16. Pazin GJ, Saul S, Thompson ME. Blood culture positivity: suppression by outpatient antibiotic therapy in patients with bacterial endocarditis. Arch Intern Med 1982;142: 263-8.
17. Dwyer DE, Chen SC, Wright EJ, et al. Hospital practices influence the pattern of infective endocarditis. Med J Aust 1994;160:709-18.
18. Sandre RM, Shafran SD. Infective endocarditis: review of 135 cases over 9 years. Clin Infect Dis 1996;22: 276-86.
19. Vongpatanasin W, Willis L, Lange R. Prosthetic heart valves. N Engl J Med 1996;335: 407-16.
20. Pulvirenti J, Kerns E, Benson C, et al. Infective endocarditis in injection drug users: importance of human immunodeficiency virus serostatus and degree of immunosupression. Clin Infect Dis 1996; 22:40-5.
21. Del Pont JM, De Cicco LT, Vartalitis C, et al. Infective endocarditis in children: clinical analysis and evaluation of two diagnostic criteria. Pediat Inf Dis J 1995;14: 1079-86.

22. Stockheim JA, Chadwick EG, Kessler S, et al. Are the Duke Criteria superior to the Beth Israel Criteria for the diagnosis of infective endocarditis in children? Clin Infect Dis1998;27: 1451-6.

23. Matthew J, Addai T, Anand A, et al. Clinical features, site of involvement, bacteriologic findings and outcome of infective endocarditis in intravenous drug users. Arch Int Med 1995;155: 1941-8.

24. Gernsheimer J, Hlibczuk V, Bartniczuk D, et al. Antibiotics in the ED: how to avoid the common mistake of treating not wisely, but too well. Emerg Med Prac 2005;7: 1-32.

25. Mylonakis E, Calderwood SB. Infective endocarditis in adults. N Engl J Med 2001;345: 1318-30.

26. Rothman R, et al. Infectious endocarditis. In: Tintinalli JE, ed. Emergency medicine: a comprehensive study guide. 6th ed. New York:McGraw-Hill;2004: 937-43.

27. Durack DT, Lukes AS, Bright DK. New criteria for diagnosis of infective endocarditis: utilization of specific echocardiographic findings. Duke Endocarditis Service. Am J Med 1994;96: 200-9.

28. Li JS, Sexton DJ, Mick N, et al. Proposed modifications to the Duke criteria for the diagnosis of infective endocarditis. Clin Infect Dis 2000;30: 633-8.

29. Mylonakis E, Calderwood SB. Infective endocarditis in adults.N Engl J Med 2001;345: 1318-30.

30. Brouqui P, Raoult D. Endocarditis due to rare and fastidious bacteria. Clin Microbiol Rev 2001;14: 177-207.

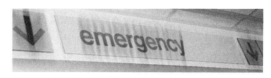

CASE25

6 YEAR OLD MALE WITH ABDOMINAL PAIN

Commentary:
Gregory L. Henry, MD, FACEP

CEO, Medical Practice Risk Assessment, Inc., Ann Arbor, Michigan

Clinical Professor, Department of Emergency Medicine
  University of Michigan Medical School, Ann Arbor, Michigan

Past President, American College of Emergency Physicians (ACEP)

Discussion:
Ann Dietrich, MD, FAAP, FACEP

Attending ED physician, Columbus Children's Hospital

Associate Professor, The Ohio State University College of Medicine
  Columbus, Ohio

Editor-in-chief, Pediatric Emergency Medicine Reports

Editor-in-chief, Trauma Reports

ACEP, Section Affairs Emergency Medicine Committee

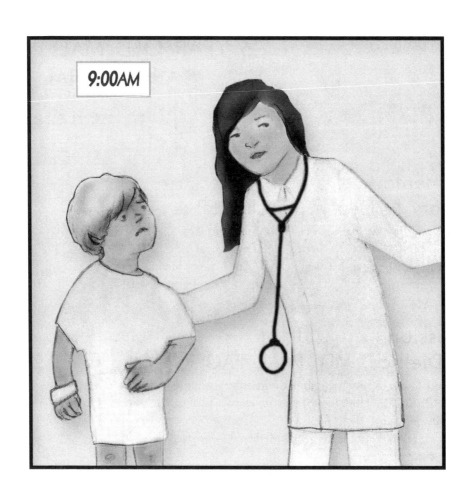

6 YEAR OLD MALE WITH ABDOMINAL PAIN

—Initial Visit*—

*Authors' Note: The history, exam and notes are the actual documentation of the physicians and providers, including abbreviations (and spelling errors)

CHIEF COMPLAINT (at 14:04): Abdominal pain

```
VITAL SIGNS
Time   Temp(F)   Rt.    Pulse   Resp   Syst   Diast   O2 sat
14:04  98.8      Oral   144     36     127    91      98%(room air)
                        120     28     127    92
```

HISTORY OF PRESENT ILLNESS (at 14:35): Diffuse abd. pain which is constant and beg. 5 days ago gradually and the pain is severe. They were at the Children's hospital emergency department one morning last week and were diagnosed with constipation and prescribed miralax which he tried but vomited up. They did use prune juice which resulted in some loose stool. Did have temp 103-104 degrees last week and then 2 days ago awoke at 5AM after feeling a "pop" in the abdomen. No blood in stool or urine. Not able to describe the character of the pain.

PAST MEDICAL HISTORY/TRIAGE:
  Allergies: NKDA
  Current meds: Zyrtec
  PMH/PSH: No significant past medical or surgical history

EXAM (at 14:36):
  General: Tired-appearing; quiet, alert, in no apparent distress.
  Eyes: PERRL
  Ears: TM's normal, no bulging or signs of otitis media, canals normal
  Oral: Posterior pharynx is pink without exudates, erythema, or any oral lesions
  Nose: The nose is normal in appearance without rhinorrhea
  Resp: Breath sounds clear and equal bilaterally; no wheezes, retractions, rhonchi, or rales.
  Card: Regular rhythm, without murmurs, rub or gallop
  Abd.: Minimally-distended; diffusely tender with some voluntary guarding, without rigidity or rebound
  Skin: Warm and dry; no apparent lesions

RESULTS (labs received and reviewed at 16:01):

Test	Flag	Value	Units	Ref. Range
WBC		11.4	K/uL	5.0-14.5
HGB		12.3	G/DL	11.5-15.5
PLT		306	K/uL	142-424

Test	Flag	Value	Units	Ref. Range
NA	L	129	MMOL/L	135-144
K		4.1	MMOL/L	3.5-5.1
CL	L	89	MMOL/L	98-107
CO2		26	MMOL/L	22-29
BUN		12	MG/DL	7-18
CREAT		0.6	MG/DL	0.5-1.0

Urinalysis—WNL except ketones 50mg/dl and protein 30mg/dl.

Acute abdominal series (as read by the radiologist): The chest demonstrates normal cardiothymic silhouette and clear lungs. There is no free subdiaphragmatic air. There are distended large and small bowel loops with multiple air-fluid levels. The degree of dilatation appears to be slightly more prominent in the small bowel. Overall appearance is most consistent with an adynamic ileus, although with the small bowel dilatation and prominence an early mechanical obstruction cannot be excluded. If symptoms persist, follow up radiographs would probably be necessary to determine the exact etiology.

PROGRESS NOTES (at 16:38): He does have an acute abdomen and no stool on XR and even if CT here was neg., he would still need pediatric evaluation so I will send him for evaluation at Children's hospital emergency department.

DIAGNOSIS (at 16:39): 1. Abdominal pain, 2. Vomiting - and nausea

DISPOSITION: He left at 18:54 en route to Children's hospital.

FOLLOW UP: He was seen at Children's hospital and found to have a ruptured appendix and taken to the OR.

FINAL DIAGNOSIS: Ruptured appendix

Gregory L. Henry comments:

"If the patient has an appendix, whether age 6 or 86, it could be appendicitis"

A six-year-old with abdominal pain tests the knowledge base of all physicians. Early on, serious intra-abdominal pathology is very difficult to diagnose. This child was at another hospital five days earlier, and now has decidedly different exam findings, which makes the diagnosis much simpler at the second ER visit.

Although appendicitis is classically described as having an 18–36 hour time course, a 5-day course is certainly not without precedence. The area of inflammation can wax and wane in intensity, and only with actual rupture will the pain increase. A history of a popping sensation in the abdomen is rarely obtained; most abscess ruptures are more subtle.

The evaluation and the decision-making in this case are perfectly reasonable. However, no documentation of amount of fluid or antibiotics is found. In a patient like this, I believe preoperative antibiotics would be perfectly appropriate, assuming time to hang the medication prior to transfer.

Appendicitis is still the most common intra-abdominal catastrophe leading to litigation in emergency medicine. If the patient has an appendix, whether age 6 or 86, it could be appendicitis. The first hospital was not negligent in their diagnosis, but the follow-up program on such children is extremely important. The diagnosis of constipation should always be made tentatively; most children are not constipated, and another cause for their abdominal discomfort can usually be found.

- Thoroughness of Documentation: 9 out of 10.

- Thoroughness of Patient Evaluation: 9 out of 10.

- Risk of Serious Illness Being Missed: On this visit, low risk.

- Risk Management Legal Rating: Medium risk.

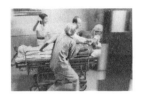

EVALUATION OF ABDOMINAL PAIN IN CHILDREN AND DIAGNOSIS OF APPENDICITIS

Ann Dietrich, MD, FAAP, FACEP

I. INTRODUCTION

It is common for children to present to the emergency department with abdominal and gastrointestinal complaints. In the majority, the symptoms are the result of a simple, limited condition, such as a viral gastroenteritis or constipation, and will resolve spontaneously. On our patient's initial visit he was diagnosed with constipation. Unfortunately, we do not have access to the chart from this encounter. On the current visit it is documented that he was at "Children's Hospital" last week and that he had a temperature of 103–104° last week; it would be interesting to know which occurred first. Diagnosing constipation in a child with a temperature of 103–104° would be hard to imagine, so probably the constipation occurred first, then the temperature elevation occurred. Did they receive instructions to return with a fever or continued pain? Were these instructions verbal or written? Were they understood? We do not have access to this information, but these issues highlight the importance of timely follow up in patients with abdominal pain. If the pain continues longer than 8–12 hours or if the symptoms change or worsen, the patient should be rechecked.

II. EVALUATION OF ABDOMINAL PAIN—HISTORY AND PHYSICAL EXAM

Abdominal pain in children is often benign, but it may also be the harbinger of an underlying serious condition, for which the diagnosis should not be delayed. Frequently parents and children are poor historians. Although they may be able to relate that their child is in pain, the location of the pain may be elusive. In children, the history should focus on the onset of pain, the pattern of pain (crampy, intermittent pain is associated with intussusception), other gastrointestinal complaints such as emesis (projectile, non-bilious emesis in an infant is associated with pyloric stenosis and bilious emesis may be associated with malrotations and volvulus), a history of cough and fever (pneumonia may cause abdominal pain) or altered mentation (associated with intussusception).

The physical exam may also be challenging, especially in the younger child. Careful observation of the child, prior to physical contact, may reveal very helpful information, such as the child's overall appearance, vital signs, respiratory status, perfusion, pain level, and degree of mobility. A 2-year-old lying still on a cot should raise suspicion of significant pathology. Gently approach the child and warm your hands if they are cold. In older children, ask them to identify the area of most pain and then start away from that area and gently examine the abdomen. Always examine the entire child, noting any bruises, distention of the abdomen, or abnormalities in the area of the genitalia (hernias may be painful if incarcerated, and testicular pain may be difficult to elicit from a scared preteen boy).

III. SPECIFIC DIAGNOSES PRESENTING WITH ABDOMINAL PAIN

Certain combinations of historical and physical exam findings suggest certain disease processes.

- Hypertrophic pyloric stenosis (HPS) usually presents in the third to fifth week of life with projectile, non-bilious emesis. Typically the children are very hungry, and on physical examination peristaltic waves or a palpable olive may be present. In the child with HPS who has prolonged vomiting, the laboratory studies may show a hypochloremic, hypokalemic metabolic alkalosis.
- Infants with congenital malrotation of the intestines and a volvulus peak in presentation during the first month of life, but may present at any time. Characteristically these infants present in one of three ways: sudden onset of abdominal pain and bilious emesis, bilious emesis that appears to be a bowel obstruction, or failure to thrive with a feeding intolerance.[24] Bilious emesis is always worrisome in an infant and should be considered a surgical emergency until proven otherwise.
- Intussusception should be suspected in a child, particularly at < 1 year old, who presents with intermittent colicky abdominal pain, vomiting, and bloody mucous stools. Although this classic triad is encountered only 20–40% of the time, the presence of two of these characteristics occurs in 60% of patients. This diagnosis should also be considered in a child < 2 years old with an altered mental status. A palpable mass in the right upper or lower quadrant may help with the diagnosis, but is uncommonly present.
- Incarcerated hernias occur in 1–3% of all children, more frequently in males, and most frequently on the right side. More than two-thirds of incarcerated hernias occur during the first year of life. The key to diagnosis is evaluation of the genitalia and identification of any bulges.

IV. APPENDICITIS IN CHILDREN—GENERAL

Appendicitis is the most common surgical emergency in childhood and affects approximately 4 of every 1,000 children. It is estimated that appendicitis is the cause of abdominal pain in 2.3% of children seen in ambulatory clinics or EDs.[9] It typically occurs in older children and young adults, with the highest incidence in males between 10–14 years and females 15–19 years old.[7] The diagnosis of appendicitis, especially in younger children, is frequently delayed, and reported perforation rates of 23–73% are present, significantly higher than in adults. Neonatal appendicitis, a very uncommon diagnosis, has been reported to have an 82% perforation rate and 28% mortality rate.[21] Nance ML et al., found that in children < 1 year old, there was a 100% perforation rate, and for children aged 1–2 years old, the perforation rate was 93%.[22] Nelson DS found that in their series, 100% of children < 4 years old, 55% of the 4–5 year olds, 42% of the preteen age group and 13% of the 14–16 year olds had a perforated appendicitis at the time of presentation.[23] Consequences of delayed diagnosis of appendicitis include perforation, peritonitis, abscess formation, sepsis, adhesions and bowel obstruction. Up to one-half of children with a perforation will experience a complication.[14]

V. PRESENTATIONS OF APPENDICITIS

The "classic" presentation of appendicitis—generalized abdominal pain migrating to the right lower quadrant, with anorexia followed by vomiting and fever—is seen less often in the pediatric patient.[10] Approximately one-third of children with acute appendicitis have atypical clinical findings.[13] In addition, some literature suggests that children present earlier in their clinical course than adults, with only mild or nonspecific symptoms. A history of vomiting preceded by abdominal pain may be helpful in distinguishing appendicitis from a viral illness (gastroenteritis). Diarrhea, especially in younger children, does not exclude the diagnosis of appendicitis.[12] The most common findings in children with appendicitis include right lower quadrant pain, abdominal tenderness, and guarding.[11]

It should be noted that rebound tenderness and Rovsing's sign both have a high sensitivity and specificity in children.[11]

VI. DIAGNOSIS OF APPENDICITIS

A. Laboratory evaluation

No laboratory test is 100% sensitive or specific for appendicitis. The WBC count is neither sensitive nor specific, but may be helpful to categorize children with abdominal pain. If the child's history and physical arouse a low suspicion for appendicitis and the child has a normal WBC, then the likelihood of appendicitis is low. If the child's WBC is elevated, then further tests or observation may be indicated. A urinalysis should be completed, but the clinician should remember that an inflamed appendix, next to a ureter, may result in mild pyuria, hematuria, or bacteriuria. A urine pregnancy test should be completed in any patient of the appropriate age to exclude ectopic pregnancy. C-reactive protein has been studied as a marker for appendicitis, but has not been found to be more sensitive or specific than the WBC count.[15,16]

B. Diagnostic radiology

1. Plain radiographs

A plain film abdominal series will typically have nonspecific findings and is of low yield in cases of appendicitis. It has been shown to be relatively insensitive and adds unnecessary costs and radiation exposure.[8] In patients with non-perforated appendicitis, abdominal radiography is usually normal with diffuse air-fluid levels or mild bowel dilatation. Radiographic findings that may be associated with appendicitis include a focally dilated loop in the right lower quadrant (sentinel loop), psoas sign, an appendicolith (unusual and present in only about 10% of true appendicitis cases), small bowel obstruction, and a soft tissue mass or extraluminal air following perforation and abscess formation.[18]

2. Ultrasound

Graded-compression sonography has been used for the diagnosis of appendicitis for over 15 years (Picture 1). Operator skill is important with this diagnostic modality, with wide ranges of sensitivities and specificities reported. An overall sensitivity of 85% and specificity of 92% has been reported using meta-analysis of pediatric and adult studies published between 1986 and 1994.[19] For many clinicians, ultrasound is the imaging test of choice for children because it is noninvasive, rapid, doesn't require oral or IV contrast, and limits exposure to radiation. Graded compression is used to determine the presence or absence of inflammation. An inflamed appendix will typically be aperistaltic, noncompressible and larger than 6mm in diameter. It is important to image the entire appendix to avoid a false-negative reading (appendiceal tip inflammation). The mucosal lining of the appendix may be intact or poorly defined and a fecalith may or may not be visualized. Color-flow doppler may be added to increase the accuracy of the sonographic evaluation, and typically demonstrates an increase in blood flow to the area of an inflamed appendix.[17] Ultrasound has also been found to be useful in establishing an alternative diagnosis. One study found that only 22% of children referred for ultrasonography for suspected appendicitis had the diagnosis, while another 29% had other specific diagnoses detected by ultrasonography.[5] Most false-negative diagnoses result from failure to visualize the appendix. This may be secondary to operator dependency, retrocecal position of the appendix, or appendiceal perforation.[20] False-positive results have also been reported. A study by

Roosevelt and Reynolds did not show any significant differences in the perforation rate or the cost of care in children who underwent ultrasound compared with those who did not.[6]

Picture 1—Appendicitis Demonstrated on Ultrasound

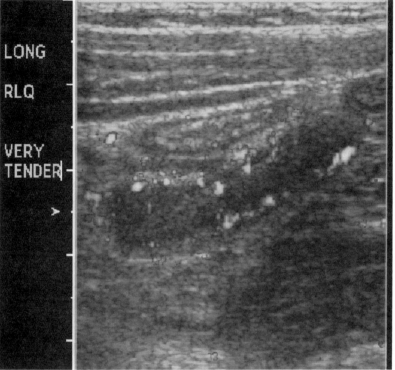

3. CT scan

In recent years, CT has become the diagnostic procedure of choice when ultrasound is unable to provide a definitive diagnosis. Numerous studies advocate different techniques, including triple-contrast, rectal contrast, or non-contrast unenhanced CT.[2] CT has greater accuracy, the ability to identify alternative diagnosis, and lower negative laparotomy rates.[4] A normal appendix is identified at CT in approximately one-half of children. Computed tomography signs of acute appendicitis include a distended appendix greater than 7 mm in maximal diameter, appendiceal wall thickening and enhancement, an appendicolith, circumferential or focal apical cecal thickening, pericecal fat stranding, adjacent bowel wall thickening, focal or free peritoneal fluid, mesenteric lymphadenopathy, or intraperitoneal phlegmon or abscess. The reported sensitivity of CT for the diagnosis of acute appendicitis ranges from 87–100% and the specificity ranges from 89–98%. CT has also been found to be better than ultrasonography for evaluating the complications of acute appendicitis. There is evidence that supports improved patient outcomes with the use of CT, by significantly decreasing the negative laparotomy rate.[4] CT is also useful in establishing an alternative diagnosis. In one series in 37% of children with a true-negative diagnosis for appendicitis at CT, an alternative diagnosis was established. False negative CT scans may occur, especially in patients with an atypical location of the appendix, tip appendicitis, and stump appendicitis. False positives have also been reported and may be secondary to Crohn's disease, cecal diverticulitis, or gynecologic abnormalities.[1]

VII. MANAGEMENT OF APPENDICITIS
The initial management of a child with appendicitis focuses on stabilization of the ABCs, most commonly correction of shock from sepsis or dehydration. The patient should not be allowed to eat or drink, and any electrolyte abnormalities should be corrected. If there are any clinical or radiographic signs of perforation, then antibiotics should be initiated in the ED and should include coverage for gram-negative and anaerobic bacteria.

VIII. SUMMARY
Since the early diagnosis of appendicitis will lead to a better outcome, a high degree of suspicion should be maintained. If the clinical suspicion for appendicitis is high, consultation with a surgeon prior to diagnostic imaging is appropriate. However, many surgeons will request a diagnostic study to decrease the likelihood of a negative laparotomy. Any child who is evaluated in the ED, with a chief complaint of abdominal pain, and determined to be well enough to go home, should have a very specific and thorough discharge plan. All children with abdominal pain should be evaluated within 8–12 hours of leaving the ED.

TEACHING POINTS ABOUT CASE 25:
- There are no laboratory tests which definitely exclude appendicitis. In this case, the WBC count was only minimally elevated at 11.4.
- Abdominal pain is difficult to assess in children; frequent reassessments are valuable. Any child with abdominal pain that is discharged from the ED should have follow-up in 8–12 hours.
- Appendicitis is the cause of abdominal pain in 2.3% of children seen in ambulatory clinics or EDs.

REFERENCES
1. Levine CD, Aizenstein O, Wachsberg RH. Pitfalls in the CT Diagnosis of Appendicitis. The Br J Radiol 2004;77: 792-9.
2. Garcia Pena BM, Mandl KD, Kraus SJ, et al. Ultrasonography and limited computed tomography in the diagnosis and management of appendicitis in children. JAMA 1999;282: 1041-6.
3. Pena BM, Taylor GA, Lund DP, et al. Effect of computed tomography on patient management and costs in children with suspected appendicitis. Pediatrics 1999;104: 440-6.
4. Rao PM, Rhea JT, Rattner DW. Introduction of appendiceal CT: impact on negative appendectomy and appendiceal perforation rates. Ann Surg 1999;229: 344-9.
5. Siegel MG, Carel C, Surratt S. Ultrasonography of acute abdominal pain in children. JAMA 1991;266: 1987-9.
6. Roosevelt GE, Reynolds SL. Does the use of ultrasonography improve the outcome of children with appendicitis? Acad Emerg Med 1998;5: 1071-5.
7. Addiss DG, Shaffer N, Fowler BS, et al. The epidemiology of appendicitis and appendectomy in the United States. Am J Epidemiol 1990;132: 910-25.
8. Eisenberg RL, Heinekien P, Hedgcock MW, et al. Evaluation of plain abdominal radiographs in the diagnosis of abdominal pain. Ann Intern Med 1982;97: 257-61.

9. Wagner JM, McKinner WP, Carpenter JL. Does this patient have appendicitis? JAMA 1996;276: 1589-94.

10. Williams N, Bello M. Perforation rates relates to delayed presentation in childhood acute appendicitis. J Royal College Surg Edinburgh 1998;43: 101-2.

11. Saidi RF, Ghasemi M. Role of Alvarado score in diagnosis and treatment of suspected acute appendicitis. Amer J Emerg Med 2000;18: 230-1.

12. Horwitz JR, Gursoy M, Jaksic T, et al. Importance of diarrhea as a presenting symptom of appendicitis in very young children. Amer J Surg 1997;173: 80-2.

13. Sivit CJ, Newman KD, Boenning DA, et al. Appendicitis: usefulness of ultrasound in a pediatric population. Radiology 1992;185: 549-52.

14. Pieper R, Kager L, Nasman P. Acute appendicitis: a clinical study of 1,018 cases of emergency appendectomy. Acta Chir Scand 1982;148: 51-62.

15. Chung JL, Kong MS, Lin SL, et al. Diagnostic value of C-reactive protein in children with perforated appendicitis. European J Peds 1996;155: 529-31.

16. Paajanen H, Mansikka A, Laato M, et al. Are serum inflammatory markers age-dependent in acute appendicitis? Amer College Surgeons J 1997;184: 303-8.

17. Quillan SP, Siegel MJ. Diagnosis of appendiceal abscess in children with acute appendicitis: value of color doppler sonography. AJR Am J Roentgenol 1995;164: 1251-4.

18. Sivit CJ. Imaging the child with right lower quadrant pain and suspected appendicitis: current concepts. Pediatr Radiol 2004;34: 447-53.

19. Orr RK, Porter D, Hartman D. Ultrasonography to evaluate adults for appendicitis: decision-making based on meta-analysis and probabilistic reasoning. Acad Emerg Med 1995;2: 644-650.

20. Sivit CJ, Applegate KE, Stallion A, et al. Imaging evaluation of suspected appendicitis in a pediatric population: effectiveness of sonography versus CT. AJR Am J Roentgenol 2000;175: 977-80.

21. Karaman A, Cavusoglu YH, Karaman I, et al. Seven cases of neonatal appendicitis with a review of the English language literature of the last century. Pediatr Surg Int 2003;19: 707-9.

22. Nance ML, Adamson WT, Hedrick HL. Appendicitis in the young child: a continuing diagnostic challenge. Pediatr Emerg Care 2000;16: 160-2.

23. Nelson DS, Bateman B, Bolte RG. Appendiceal perforation in children diagnosed in a pediatric emergency department. Pediatr Emerg Care 2000;16: 233-7.

24. Lin JN, Lou CC, Wang KL. Intestinal malrotation and midgut volvulus: a 15-year review. J Formos Med Assoc 1995;94: 178-81.

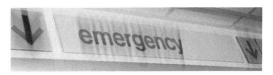

CASE26

53 YEAR OLD FEMALE WITH HEADACHE & EYE PAIN

Commentary:
Gregory L. Henry, MD, FACEP

CEO, Medical Practice Risk Assessment, Inc., Ann Arbor, Michigan
Clinical Professor, Department of Emergency Medicine
    University of Michigan Medical School, Ann Arbor, Michigan
Past President, American College of Emergency Physicians (ACEP)

Discussion:
Frank J. Weinstock, MD, FACS

Professor of Ophthalmology, Northeastern Ohio University College of Medicine
Past President, Society of Geriatric Ophthalmology
Recipient Lifetime Achievement Award 2000, American Academy of Ophthalmology
Editorial Board, Geriatric Ophthalmology, Journal of Refraction, Review of
    Ophthalmology, and the Ohio State Medical Journal
Ophthalmologist, Canton Ophthalmology Associates, Canton, Ohio

Michael B. Weinstock, MD

Clinical Assistant Professor, Division of Emergency Medicine
    The Ohio State University, College of Medicine
    Columbus, Ohio
Attending ED physician, Director of Medical Education
    Mt. Carmel St. Ann's Emergency Department

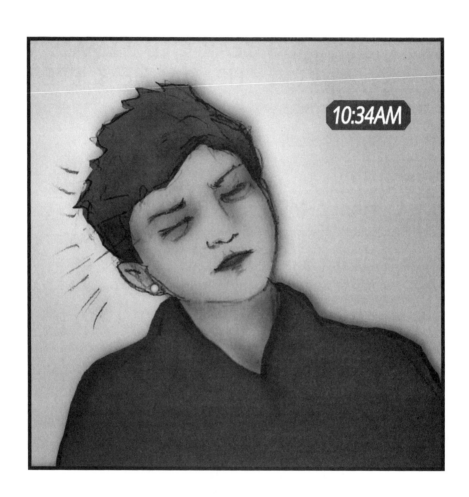

53 YEAR OLD FEMALE WITH HEADACHE & EYE PAIN

—Initial Visit*—

*Authors' Note: The history, exam and notes are the actual documentation of the physicians and providers, including abbreviations (and spelling errors)

CHIEF COMPLAINT (at 19:50): Headache

VITAL SIGNS									Pain
Time	Temp(F)	Rt.	Pulse	Resp	Syst	Diast	Pos.	02%	Scale
19:53	98.2	Tym.	74	16	155	79	S		10
22:27			58	18	148	72	L	100	3

HISTORY OF PRESENT ILLNESS (at 20:27): Pt has hx severe HA's in past but none for 10 years until 4 days ago. This HA is no worse than previous HAs and was gradual onset. The patient presents with a severe right frontal headache that began gradually 4 day(s) ago. The symptoms are constant, The discomfort is currently 10/10. The pain began while at rest. She does have photophobia. The patient describes the headache as dull, aching, and throbbing. She has had identical HA's in the past, but has never seen a neurologist. She was at an urgent care last night and given an injection, but doesn't know the name of the medicine. She was at her family doctor's office today and given imitrex. Neither of these therapies significantly improved her pain. She also used vicodin which was minimally effective. She denies fever, rash, paresthesias, weakness of extremities, slurred speech, diplopia, blurred vision, aura, cough, SOB, rhinorrhea, neck stiffness, diaphoresis, abd. pain, or nausea/vomiting.

PAST MEDICAL HISTORY/TRIAGE:

Allergies: No known allergies
Meds: Synthroid, Vicodin, Maxalt, and Fioricet
PMH: Thyroid problem, headaches.
PSH: Ovarian cyst removal
SOCIAL HISTORY: The patient is a smoker, but denies alcohol or drug use. She is married.

EXAM:

General: Well-appearing; well nourished; A&O X 3, in no apparent distress.
Head: Normocephalic; atraumatic.
Eyes: PERRL, EOMs grossly intact. Funduscopic no hemm/exud./papilledema
Ears: TM's normal;
Nose: Normal nose; no rhinorrhea;
Throat: Normal pharynx with no tonsillar hypertrophy.
Neck: Supple; non-tender; no cervical lymphadenopathy.

Card: Regular rate and rhythm, no murmurs, rubs or gallops

Resp: Normal chest excursion with respiration; breath sounds clear and equal bilaterally; no wheezes, rhonchi, or rales.

Skin: Normal for age and race; warm and dry; no apparent lesions

Neuro: Alert and oriented to person, place and time. Cranial nerves II-XII intact, normal gait. Motor strength and sensation intact

ORDERS (at 20:34): Dilaudid 1mg IVP, Phenergan 12.5mg IVP, Torodal 30mg IVP, .9NS-500cc bolus then to 125cc/hour

RESULTS: CT; Exam: brain w/o contrast: Tiny punctate area of high attenuation seen in the right basal ganglia, possibly a small calcification. I doubt that this is hemorrhage. Ventricles and cisternal spaces are normal. No evidence of hemorrhage or mass. No extracerebral or subdural collections.

PROGRESS NOTES (at 21:55): Patient is feeling better. Patient is ready to go home

DIAGNOSIS: Cephalgia

DISPOSITION: The patient was discharged to Home ambulatory. F/u PCP in 5 days if not better. Aftercare instructions for headache. Patient released from the ED at 22:32.

Gregory L. Henry comments:

"She had seen her own physician, as well as an urgent care, and was not improving. The thought of a more aggressive work up should come to mind"

Headache evaluation in the emergency department is always directed at deadly disease entities or those we can fix. The patient had 4 days of headache, but no headaches in the previous 10 years; this should raise the possibility that the usual migraine or tension headache is not the most likely diagnoses. The steady, dull, aching pain she describes is inconsistent with most migraine headaches. This was her third visit to a medical facility; she had seen her own physician, an urgent care physician, and was not improving. The thought of a more aggressive work up should come to mind.

The evaluation of this patient is reasonable, except the head exam which was noted "normocephalic," atraumatic." Palpation of the head was not done to assess for tender temporal arteries. Temporal arteritis in a patient of this age would not be out of the question. The eye examination seems to be rather complete and no lesions were found. Neurological examination was adequate. The patient did receive a CT scan without evidence of mass effect. However, for a complete work up of one of the life threatening causes of headache, a spinal tap would be in order. If this patient's spinal tap had been clear and the rest of the examination normal, I believe she could have been followed up as an outpatient.

The discharge instructions for follow up in 5 days is inappropriate; most headaches should be resolving within 12 to 24 hours. This is a more appropriate time frame for follow up care.

- Thoroughness of Documentation: 8 out of 10.

- Thoroughness of Patient Evaluation: 6 out of 10.

- Risk of Serious Illness Being Missed: Medium risk.

- Risk Management Legal Rating: Medium risk.

53 YEAR OLD FEMALE WITH HEADACHE AND EYE PAIN

—Second Visit: 1 Day Later—

CHIEF COMPLAINT (at 09:48): Headache

```
VITAL SIGNS
Time      Temp(F)  Pulse  Resp   Syst  Diast  Pos.  Pain
09:58      99.9      64     18     128    75     S     10
21:59                72     16     108    60     L      6
```

HISTORY OF PRESENT ILLNESS (at 10:06): 53-year-old with a remote history of headaches 10 years ago and has had no problems until 5 days ago when she had gradual onset of right frontal headache behind the right eye. She was seen by her doctor and treated with several medications which have not helped her. She was seen here last night and received 1 mg of dilaudid which helped her pain significantly, she had a negative CAT scan and was sent home. She had interrupted sleep secondary to her pain last night and returns today with identical pain over the right eye but now has some swelling of the eyelid. She states the right eye vision is normal, the pain is achy, constant, 9/10, and nonradiating. She denies any neck pain or stiffness. This headache is similar to headaches she's had a past and not the worst headache of her life. She has had nausea and vomiting but denies any diarrhea. No paresthesias or weakness in her extremities, abd. pain, chest pain, SOB, and denies hearing changes. She denies any fever, stiff neck, rhinorrhea, sore throat or cough, or rash. No dizziness, facial droop or dysuria. She has not had pain medicine today.

PAST MEDICAL HISTORY/TRIAGE:
   Medication, common allergies: No known allergies
   Meds: Synthroid, Vicodin, Maxalt, and Fioricet
   SH: Nonsmoker, no alcohol
   PAST HISTORY: No change

EXAM:

General: Well-appearing; well nourished; A&O X 3, in no apparent distress.

Head: Normocephalic; atraumatic. There is swelling about the upper and lower right lid and the orbit. There is no erythema, she is nontender over the right temple area. No evidence of temporal arteritis.

Eyes: PERRL, EOMs grossly intact, no pain with EOM motion. Visual acuity: Right eye: uncorrected 20/70. Left eye: uncorrected 20/50. Tonometry - Using Tonopen: L EYE= 29, R EYE = 33 and 35

Ears: TM's normal; No blood

Nose: Normal nose; no rhinorrhea;

Throat: Normal pharynx with no tonsillar hypertrophy.

Neck: Supple; no nuchal rigidity. non-tender; no cervical lymphadenopathy.

Card: Regular rate and rhythm, no murmurs, rubs or gallops

Resp: Normal chest excursion with respiration; breath sounds clear and equal bilaterally; no wheezes, rhonchi, or rales.

Abd: Non-distended; non-tender , without rigidity, rebound or guarding

Skin: Normal for age and race; warm and dry; no apparent lesions

ORDERS:

At 10:12: Benadryl 25mg IVP, reglan 10mg IVP, dilaudid 0.5mg IVP

At 12:55: Decadron 10mg IVP, imitrex 6mg SQ

At 13:22: Demerol 25mg IVP

RESULTS:

Test	Flag	Value	Units	Ref. Range
WBC		6.5	K/uL	4.6-10.2
HGB		12.8	G/DL	12.0-16.0
PLT		247	K/uL	142-424

PROGRESS NOTES (at 14:50): I spoke with the primary care physician and she requests an LP. Pt. never complains of pain and has 2 ED visits, one to the PCP and one to an UC in the last 3-4 days.

RESULTS LUMBAR PUNCTURE:

Test	Flag	Value	Units	Ref. Range
CSFTUBE		3	ML	
CSF COLOR		COLORLESS		
CSF APPEAR		CLEAR		CLEAR
CSF WBC CT		1	CMM	0-8
CSF RBC CT		0	CMM	0-8
CSFGLUC		58	MG/DL	40-75
CSFPROT		42.8	MMOL/L	15.0-45.0

RESULTS LAB:

Test	Flag	Value	Units	Ref. Range
WSR		9	MM/HR	0-30
ANA ROUT		NEGATIVE		NEGATIVE

PROGRESS NOTES (at 20:32): We were prepared to discharge this patient however pain returned and appeared to be intractable. In addition , Tonopen IO pressures were somewhat elevated so we felt that admission was the best course. (At 20:49) we ordered Dilaudid 0.5mg IVP, and nafcillin 1.5grams IVPB

DIAGNOSIS (at 20:48): Orbital cellulitis, Cephalgia, intractable pain

DISPOSITION: Admitted. Pt. was transported to the floor at 23:05.

53 YEAR OLD FEMALE WITH HEADACHE AND EYE PAIN

—Hospital Course—

INITIAL HISTORY PER ADMITTING PHYSICIAN:
I discussed this case at length with the physician assistant last night. Eye examination was unremarkable. Funduscopic exam demonstrated no papilledema. The patient underwent a CT scan of the head, which demonstrated no significant abnormalities on initial report. The patient was treated with Dilaudid with improvement of her pain, as well as some Demerol. After my evaluation of the patient, I discussed this case with the ophthalmologist by phone. It was agreed that the symptomatology was more consistent with an orbital cellulitis. I placed the patient on some IV antibiotics, continued IV fluid resuscitation therapy, as well as ophthalmic eye drop solution.

Differential diagnosis and plan: Differential diagnosis does include orbital cellulitis, herpes ophthalmicus, herpes zoster ophthalmicus, and acute angle glaucoma. Given this fact and her persistent deterioration, recommend that ophthalmology be consulted emergently. At this point, she is on intravenous Nafcillin, intravenous Solu-Medrol, and Levaquin eye drops. I have not seen a typical vesicular lesion at this point.

INPATIENT COURSE: Over the next 24-48 hours she developed vesicles on the right side of the nose and face and a diagnosis of herpes zoster ophthalmicus was established. She was placed on IV acyclovir and was in the hospital a total of 5 days. CSF culture was negative for growth at 48 hours.

FINAL DIAGNOSIS: Herpes zoster ophthalmicus

When the patient returned, the diagnosis still was not clear. Lumbar puncture was completely appropriate. The eye examination, at least initially, was not terribly impressive except for the mildly elevated increased intraocular pressure. During the hospital course, the diagnosis of herpes zoster ophthalmicus was established, which could not have been predicted from the initial examination. The diagnosis of herpes zoster ophthalmicus requires at least some lesions, conjunctival injection, or a definite localization of the pain. Sometimes it is only with the passage of time that we are able to identify the disease entity.

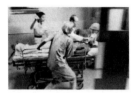

EVALUATION OF NONTRAUMATIC EYE PAIN, DISCUSSION OF VARICELLA ZOSTER VIRUS AND ZOSTER OPHTHALMICUS

Frank J. Weinstock, MD, FACS
Michael B. Weinstock, MD

I. INTRODUCTION AND SUMMARY OF THE CASE

The patient is a 53 year old woman presenting with severe headaches and photophobia. The pain was severe enough to cause her to seek help earlier in the day at her primary care physician's office, at which time she received medication without alleviation of her pain.

Headaches are extremely common, but rarely severe enough for a patient to seek medical attention twice in the same day. During the initial visit, the evaluation in the Emergency Department ruled out the presence of a significant tumor, but did not delve into ocular causes for headache. The patient felt better and was discharged. However, the relief of pain was somewhat misleading since the narcotic may have masked her symptoms.

The history on the second visit is essentially the same with a few questions directed to the eye, but no information that might lead to a diagnosis of zoster or other eye disease. The intraocular pressure (IOP) was elevated and was one of the reasons for admission, but there was no clinical evidence of acute glaucoma. With isolated elevated IOP, the patient can be referred for ophthalmology follow up within 24 hours.[1]

In the following section, we will discuss the evaluation of patients with eye pain, the evaluation and management of varicella zoster virus (shingles), and zoster ophthalmicus.

II. HISTORY OF PATIENTS WITH NONTRAUMATIC EYE PAIN

During evaluation of headaches, the eyes should be evaluated since they may be the primary etiology of the headache, or may reveal a non-ophthalmologic source. Patients often interpret ocular discomfort as a headache. Concerning symptoms include redness of the eye, decreased vision, photophobia, double vision, or eye pain. Obtaining history of onset acuity and the activity when symptoms began may yield a diagnosis. However, in the case presented, no ocular history or significant eye exam findings provided a diagnosis.[2]

It is important to determine if ocular complaints are new and if they coincide with the headache; for example, a patient may have amblyopia or long-standing poor vision, with no recent changes and of no significance in the current evaluation. A medication list may provide information not offered by the patient.

III. PHYSICAL EXAMINATION OF PATIENTS WITH NONTRAUMATIC EYE PAIN

The history helps direct the physical examination. The visual acuity should be measured with a chart, if possible.[5] If no chart is available, ask the patient to compare the corrected vision in each eye and note any difference and determine if the difference is acute or chronic.

Most of the eye exam requires only an ophthalmoscope.[3] In addition to allowing evaluation of the retinal and optic disc, the ophthalmoscope serves as a flashlight and a source of magnification to allow visualization of corneal or conjunctival foreign bodies. The fluorescein staining of corneal abrasions is seen clearly with the green (red-free) lens. Conjunctival redness, corneal clarity, pupillary size, and muscle function require no special instrumentation. Evaluation of the eye should include inspection of the lids and periorbital areas.

If the pupils are not equal, check with the patient, or family, to find out if this is a new occurrence or chronic; for example, congenital, from a prior injury, eye trauma, eye surgery, or eye drops.[7]

Emergency physicians should attain a certain proficiency in the use of the slit lamp,[4] a magnifying microscope used to diagnose conditions such as iritis, and corneal or conjunctival foreign bodies.[5,6,7] There are various techniques to evaluate IOP. Normal pressure is less than 20 mmHg.

Confrontation visual fields may reveal a field defect, aiding in the diagnosis of stroke or tumor. Stand in front of the patient and first cover the patient's left eye and your right eye. Ask the patient to look at your eyes. With testing of the right eye, bring your left hand (showing 1, 2 or 3 fingers) from the left, right, up and down. Ask the patient to tell you when he or she can see your fingers and tell you the correct number. Assuming that you have a full visual field, you and the patient should see and count the fingers at roughly the same time. If the examiner can see the fingers as they are brought in and the patient cannot, assume there is a visual field defect. Confirmation and more detail are obtained by formal visual field testing in the ophthalmologist's office. Hemianopias, due to CVA's or tumors, are relatively easy to demonstrate, but smaller defects are more difficult to find.

IV. SPECIFIC OCULAR CONDITIONS WHICH MAY CAUSE EYE PAIN

Acute angle closure glaucoma usually causes significant eye pain which may be referred to the head. The condition may be confused with abdominal problems if there is associated nausea and vomiting.[1]

Vision may be decreased, and the patient may reveal a history of rainbow colored halos with past headaches. Inquire about a family history of acute angle-closure glaucoma.

On exam, patients with acute angle closure glaucoma will have a red eye, semi-dilated or dilated pupil, cloudy cornea, decreased vision, a shallow anterior chamber (as seen with the slit lamp or with a flashlight directed across the anterior chamber), and an elevated IOP. In the case presented, acute angle closure glaucoma was in the differential diagnosis, but the elevated intraocular pressure turned out to be an incidental finding.

If angle closure glaucoma is suspected, consult an ophthalmologist to decide on the next course of action. Ophthalmologists usually prefer that patients be sent to their offices since most hospitals do not have the specialized equipment necessary for diagnosis and management of elevated IOP. Acute angle closure glaucoma can usually be treated with medications or a laser.

Chronic simple open angle glaucoma rarely causes any pain or headache. Although elevated, an isolated IOP of 33 mmHg does not warrant hospitalization. Our patient had elevated pressure in both eyes, but only had pain in one eye—further evidence that the elevated pressure was not the etiology of the pain. The eyes were not red, with normal pupillary reactions. If the patient was questioned regarding a history of increased IOP, the patient may have reported this finding or that treatment for elevated IOP had been given. We would normally see this type of patient the next day in the office.

Appropriately, orbital cellulitis was considered in the differential diagnosis.[8] Orbital cellulitis involves the orbit posterior to the lids and is most commonly caused by Staph aureus.[16] Signs include swelling of the lids, with redness of the conjunctiva, as well as proptosis of the eye and double vision due to involvement of the extra ocular muscles. It is usually painful and may be accompanied by a fever. Except for radiographic studies, special equipment is not necessary for making the diagnosis. A CAT scan often shows sinus involvement, since the most common bacterial source is orbital extension from ethmoid sinusitis.[16] Vision may be reduced with more advanced infections. Orbital cellulitis is a life-threatening emergency requiring hospitalization and systemic antibiotics.

Iritis or other inflammatory eye diseases may present with photophobia and pain, usually with some blurred vision and a varying degree of headache. The pupil of the affected eye may be small. An ocular injury, recent ocular surgery, or history of an eye infection may progress to iritis or endophthalmitis.

A foreign body or corneal abrasion may evoke sufficient pain and redness to cause a patient to initially complain of headache. Inquire if the patient has been in a windy environment or if the onset of pain was sudden, as occurs with a foreign body.

A hyphema or globe disruption/rupture may occur following trauma and is discussed at length in another chapter.

Double vision, which is present when both eyes are open and which disappears when one eye is covered or closed, may be caused by involvement of the intraocular nuclei from aneurysm, diabetes, tumor, or stroke. Diabetes may be responsible for acute third or other cranial nerve palsies and usually resolves in 2–4 months without any special treatment. If double vision is present, it is very uncomfortable for the patient, and may be eliminated completely by patching either eye while awaiting resolution or definitive diagnosis.

Herpes simplex primarily involves the cornea with characteristic dendritic appearing lesions, but may also cause uveitis and severe scarring of the cornea.[11]

When considering these conditions, an ophthalmologist should be consulted, follow up arranged, and the communication documented.

V. VARICELLA ZOSTER VIRUS (VZV)

Varicella Zoster virus causes varicella (chickenpox) and its reactivation causes herpes zoster (shingles). The primary risk factor for shingles is increased age. The overall incidence is 2 cases per 1,000 person years, which increases to 10 cases per 1,000 person years in patients older than 75 years.[14] Other risk factors include history of neoplastic diseases, patients on immunosuppressive medications, organ transplant recipients and human immunodeficiency virus (HIV). Healthy patients with a new diagnosis of zoster do not need a work up for underlying cancer.[15] While usually a minor infection, zoster can be devastating, involving the skin, eyes and central nervous system.[12]

Prodrome of zoster include mild tingling of the skin to severe pain, headache, photophobia and malaise.[15] Pain is more common in older and immunocompromised patients.[13] The patient may offer a history of discomfort when combing hair.

Skin involvement (classically a maculopapular rash with clusters of clear vesicles) occurs in a unilateral, dermatomal distribution and is visible between 1 and 7 days after the prodromal symptoms.

VI. ZOSTER OPHTHALMICUS

Ocular involvement, zoster ophthalmicus, occurs with involvement of the first division of the trigeminal nerve. Symptoms include pain and tension around the eye and the forehead and nose. CNS involvement may be responsible for double vision by affecting the third, fourth or sixth cranial nerves.[11] Usually the infection is localized to the lids, scalp, and face. However, when the lesions occur on the tip of the nose (Hutchinson sign), it is an indication of corneal involvement, with possible corneal scarring and visual loss.

VII. ANTIVIRAL THERAPY FOR ZOSTER OPHTHALMICUS

Oral antiviral therapy may reduce the incidence of ocular complications (keratitis, episcleritis, iritis) of zoster ophthalmicus from 50% (untreated) to 20–30%.[15] Antivirals (acyclovir, famciclovir, valacyclovir) should be started in the Emergency Department and continued for 10 days. The Sanford Guide To Antimicrobial Therapy recommends oral therapy for varicella-zoster ophthalmicus with a suggested primary regimen of famciclovir (500mg TID) or valacyclovir (1g TID) and alternative regimen of acyclovir (800mg, 5 times per day).[22] Antiviral therapy for admission is usually not necessary, but timely follow up should be arranged.

VIII. POSTHERPETIC NEURALGIA (PHN), ANTIVIRALS, AND STEROIDS

By definition, PHN occurs when pain persists for 1 month after the acute rash. It occurs more commonly in the elderly. One study of 421 patients with a first episode of zoster found that 94% of patients aged 0–49 years, and 50% of patients over 70 years, were pain-free at 1 month. At 12 months, 100% of patients in the first group were pain free and 96% of patients in the second group were pain free. Only 4% of these patients were treated with antiviral medications at the time of the rash.[17]

Treatment with antivirals have been shown to decrease the interval to scabbing and complete healing. They decrease the duration and pain of PHN, but not the incidence.[18,19] Famciclovir and valacyclovir have have better dosing profiles, but acyclovir is less expensive; the efficacy is comparable.[15]

Prednisone, when combined with antivirals, decreases healing time, interrupted sleep, and use of analgesics during the first month in some patients, but does not decrease the incidence or duration of PHN.[19,20]

IX. INVESTIGATIONAL VACCINE
An investigational live vaccine given to 38,546 adult, asymptomatic patients over 60 years of age was found to decrease the incidence of zoster by 51.3% (315 among vaccine recipients and 642 among placebo recipients) and to decrease the incidence of PHN by 66.1% (27 vs. 80).[21]

X. FINAL DISCUSSION
Could the eventual diagnosis of herpes zoster have been made earlier? If the patient were specifically questioned about the presence of tenderness of the skin or scalp, suspicion of zoster may have increased, but without a rash, diagnosis would have been difficult to confirm. Before the onset of rash, zoster is difficult to diagnose due to its nonspecific prodrome and ability to affect different portions of the central nervous system and the skin; that was the situation in our patient.

TEACHING POINTS ABOUT CASE 26:
- An elevated IOP, without other symptoms or signs of acute angle closure glaucoma, does not warrant admission.
- Prodrome of zoster includes mild tingling of the skin to severe pain, headache, photophobia, and malaise. The patient may complain of discomfort when combing the hair.
- Antiviral medications decrease the interval to scabbing and complete healing, but do not decrease the incidence of PHN. Prednisone, when used with antivirals, decreases symptoms during the first month, but does not decrease the incidence or duration of PHN.

REFERENCES
1. Caprioli J, Bateman JB, Gaasterland DE, et al. Primary angle closure. Preferred practice pattern. American Academy of Ophthalmology Sept. 2000 (Clinical practice guideline). Available at: http://www.aao.org/education/library/ppp/loader.cfm?url=/commonspot/security/getfile.cfm&PageID=1286
2. Caprioli J, Bateman JB, Gaasterland DE, et al. Comprehensive adult medical eye evaluation. Preferred practice pattern. American Academy of Ophthalmology Sept. 2000 (Clinical practice guideline). Available at: http://www.aao.org/education/library/ppp/loader.cfm?url=/commonspot/security/getfile.cfm&PageID=1275
4. Anderson DP, Sullivan PM, Luff AJ, et al. Direct ophthalmoscopy versus slit lamp biomicroscopy in diagnosis of the acute red eye. R Soc Med 1998; 91:127-8. (Prospective, controlled clinical trial; 98 patients)

5. Roberts JR, Hedges JR, eds. Clinical procedures in emergency medicine. 3rd ed. Philadelphia: W.B. Saunders;1998: 127.

6. Roberts JR, Hedges JR, eds. Clinical procedures in emergency medicine. 3rd ed. Philadelphia:W.B. Saunders;1998: 1241.

7. Talbot EM. A simple test to diagnose iritis. Br Med J (Clin Res Ed) 1987;295(6602): 812-13. (Consecutive series)

8. Rose GE, Pearson RV. Unequal pupil size in patients with unilateral red eye. BMJ 1991;302(6776): 571-2. (Consecutive series)

9. Donahue SP, Khoury JM, Kowalski RP. Common ocular infections. A preserver's guide. Drugs 1996;52: 526-40. (Review)

10. Cooper M. The epidemiology of herpes zoster. Eye 1987;1: 413-21.

11. Rogozzino MW, Melton LJ, Kurland LT, et al. Population-based study of herpes zoster and its sequelae. Medicine 61:310-6, 1982.

12. Shapiro DW, Miedziak AM. Contemporary approaches to varicella-zoster virus eye infections. Contemporary Ophthalmology 2003;2: 13.

13. Rockley PF, Tyring SK. Pathophysiology and clinical manifestations of varicella zoster virus infections. Int J Dermatol 1994;33: 227.

14. Marsh, RJ, Cooper M. Ophthalmic herpes zoster. Eye 1993;7: 350-70.

15. Donahue JG, Choo PW, Manson JE, et al. The incidence of herpes zoster. Arch Intern Med 1995;155: 1605-9.

16. Gnann JW, Whitley RJ. Herpes zoster. N Engl J Med 2002;347: 340-6.

17. Mitchell JD. Ocular emergencies. In: Tintinnalli JE,ed. Emergency medicine. A comprehensive study guide. 5th ed. New York:McGraw-Hill; 2000.

18. Helgason S, Petursson G, Gudmundsson S, et al. Prevalence of postherpetic neuralgia after a first episode of herpes zoster: prospective study with long term follow up. BMJ 2000;321: 794-6.

19. Goh CL, Khool L. A retrospective study on the clinical outcome of herpes zoster in patients treated with acyclovir or valaciclovir vs. patients not treated with antiviral. Int J Dermatol 1998;37: 544-6.

20. Whitley RJ, Weiss H, Gnann JW Jr, et al. Acyclovir with and without prednisone for the treatment of herpes zoster: a randomized, placebo-controlled trial. Ann Intern Med 1996;125: 376-83.

21. Wood MJ, Johnson RW, McKendrick MW, et al. A randomized trial of acyclovir for 7 days or 21 days with and without prednisolone for treatment of acute herpes zoster. N Engl J Med 1994;330:896-900.

22. Oxman MN, Levin MJ, Johnson GR, et al. A vaccine to prevent herpes zoster and postherpetic neuralgia in older adults. N Engl J Med 2005;352: 2271-84.

23. Gilbert DN, Moellering RC, Sande MA, et al. Sanford guide to antimicrobial therapy 2004, 34th ed. Hyde Park VT:Antimicrobial Therapy, Inc.; 2004:9. www.sanfordguide.com

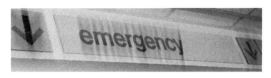

CASE 27

30 YEAR OLD PREGNANT FEMALE WITH ABDOMINAL PAIN

Commentary:
Gregory L. Henry, MD, FACEP

CEO, Medical Practice Risk Assessment, Inc., Ann Arbor, Michigan
Clinical Professor, Department of Emergency Medicine
    University of Michigan Medical School, Ann Arbor, Michigan
Past President, American College of Emergency Physicians (ACEP)

Discussion:
Robert Dart, MD, FACEP

Chief, Emergency Services, Quincy Medical Center, Quincy, Massachusetts
Associate Professor, Boston University
Vice-Chair, Department of Emergency Medicine
    Boston University School of Medicine, Boston, Massachusetts

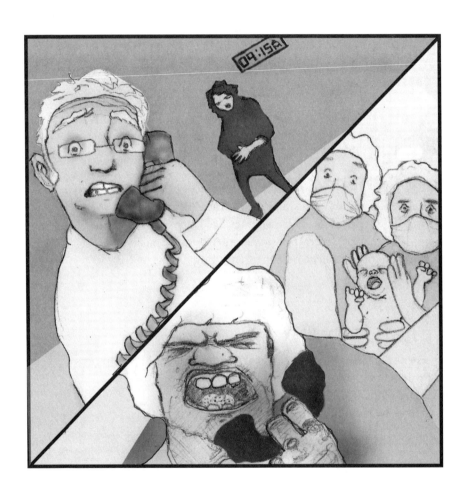

30 YEAR OLD PREGNANT FEMALE WITH ABDOMINAL PAIN

—Initial Visit*—

*Authors' Note: The history, exam and notes are the actual documentation of the physicians and providers, including abbreviations (and spelling errors)

CHIEF COMPLAINT (at 07:16): Twelve weeks pregnant having severe abdominal and back pain

```
VITAL SIGNS
Time     Temp(F)   Pulse   Resp   Syst   Diast   Pain Scale
07:19     98.6      112     18     114     72         7
08:28                       76
```

HISTORY OF PRESENT ILLNESS (at 08:01): Pt. is G1P0 with 12 week IUP with complaints of gradual onset of sharp, constant RLQ abdominal pain which radiates to the back and began yesterday. It has worsened in the last hour. She points just medial to the right ASIS as the location of the pain. She traces the radiation of the pain to the upper right inguinal ligament region. And she complains of some increased lumbosacral back pain. The pain has been constant. Increased movement causes increased pain. Yesterday she was very active including carrying a vacuum cleaner upstairs. The pain seemed to be worse after this. She took Tylenol for the pain. She states that the pain was greatly reduced for approximately 3½ hours and then the pain returned. Yesterday for breakfast she ate cereal. For lunch she ate Lasagna and for dinner she ate soup. She called her OB/GYN physician prior to coming to the Emergency department. She denies abdominal distension. She has had no fever, chills, anorexia. No nausea or vomiting, but did have diarrhea yesterday. No dysuria, hematuria, vaginal bleeding or discharge. No SOB, cough, lightheadedness or peripheral edema.

PAST MEDICAL HISTORY/TRIAGE:
Medications: None
Allergies: Sulfa
PMH: None
PSH: None

EXAM (at 08:04):
General: Well-appearing; well-nourished; in no acute respiratory distress
Head: Normocephalic; atraumatic
Eyes: PERRL; sclera anicteric, conjunctiva pink
Throat: Normal pharynx with no tonsillar hypertrophy
Neck: Supple; non-tender; no cervical lymphadenopathy; no masses or thyromegaly
Card: The heart has a regular rate and rhythm; there is no peripheral edema of the extremities.

Resp: Normal chest excursion with respiration; breath sounds clear and equal bilaterally; no wheezes, rhonchi, or rales

Abd: Normal appearance. Normal bowel sounds. Soft, non-distended; tender to palpation just lateral and inferior to McBurney's point in the RLQ and periumbilically, no rebound or guarding; no palpable organomegaly, no CVA tenderness. The uterus enlarged and nontender.

Skin: Normal for age and race; warm; dry; good turgor; no rash noted

Pelvic: No vaginal discharge or bleeding. Uterus just above pubis. Cervix closed. No CMT.

RESULTS (at 08:44):

Test	Flag	Value	Units	Ref. range
WBC	H	13.1	K/µL	4.6-10.2
HGB	L	13.2	G/DL	13.5-17.5
PLT		268	K/µL	142-424
NA		134	MMOL/L	135-144
K	L	3.4	MMOL/L	3.5-5.1
CL		103	MMOL/L	98-107
AGAP		12.4	MMOL/L	6.0-18.0
CO2		22	MMOL/L	22-29
GLU	H	129	MG/DL	70-119
BUN	H	22	MG/DL	7-18
CREAT		0.7	MG/DL	0.6-1.3

Serum hCG: 19,118
Urinalysis: WNL
FHT: 168

PROGRESS NOTES: Pt advised of round ligament pain. Pt also advised if pain increases, if N/V, if fever or other signs of worry to return to the ED for further evaluation and care. At 08:44, I called patient's OB office number, which was disconnected/changed. I then contacted the hospital where the office is located and was given both a beeper # and answering service # @ 08:55. At 09:15 I rec'd call from her OB, who said that he doesn't come to this hospital and wanted to know who was in charge of our policy to page doctors and re-page after 15 minutes. I tried to explain our policy but was hung up on. The OB's partner then also called back regarding pt at 09:20. I received another call from the patient's OB claiming that their new phone # is stated when calling old # - he took my name and re-stated "We don't go there!" and then hung up.

DIAGNOSIS (at 09:29):
1. Abdominal pain – RLQ
2. Pregnancy

DISPOSITION: Discharged to home ambulatory. Follow-up with OB/GYN if not improved in 1–2 days

Gregory L. Henry comments:

"The American public thinks 'if we can land men on the moon, we can easily diagnose appendicitis.' Nothing can be further from the truth"

Complaints during pregnancy always require analysis of 2 patients—the mother and the child. In this case it is the patient's first pregnancy; the general rule is that "primips" have no idea what abdominal sensations they are experiencing. A woman who has had several children is more experienced, and has a general feeling of what is normal and abnormal.

The chief complaint is nonspecific; this is a 30 year old woman with right lower quadrant pain and the fact that she was carrying a vacuum cleaner has very little to do with lower abdominal pathology. It is a mistake to attribute such symptoms to the activities of daily living. In addition, mild pain reduction with Tylenol should not lead to a presumptive diagnosis.

When a pregnant woman with lower abdominal pain comes to the emergency department, several problems must be considered. The first is the pregnancy itself; does this represent an ectopic? The presentation is certainly consistent with an ectopic pregnancy. Second, the urinary tract in pregnant women often is compromised. In addition, a woman with an expanding uterus can present with unusual symptomatology. The normal urinalysis in this case is reassuring. Lastly, pregnancy is not protective of any other disease process—the examination of the patient with abdominal pain should be carried out as if the pregnancy did not exist. The physician should ask the question, "If this patient was not pregnant, what might she have?"

The evaluation of this patient was reasonable, however, I would have liked to see documentation concerning whether an ultrasound had been performed—do we know that this is an intrauterine pregnancy? The physical examination revealed pain at McBurney's point. However, the vaginal examination does not comment on the adnexa or whether movement of the cervix and pelvic structures causes discomfort. A pregnant woman can be infected as often as a non-pregnant woman. No comment is made about rectal examination—literature would say that we have over-emphasized the rectal, and I find no specific criticism in omitting a rectal exam at this time.

Laboratory testing may be sensitive, but is very nonspecific. The white blood count of 13,100 is nonspecific, and could be associated with so many entities that it is impossible to ascribe a particular disease to this number. Patients with appendicitis, ruptured ectopic, viral gastroenteritis, and urinary tract infection could all have a 13,000 count. The normal urinalysis is helpful. Serum HCGs may be suggestive of problems in the pregnancy, but early on an ectopic may have perfectly normal hormone levels. A serum HCG of 19,000 does not tell you where the pregnancy is located, only that a pregnancy is progressing. A patient with an ectopic can certainly have an HCG of 19,000.

The documentation in this case is exemplary regarding the problems at time of discharge. The emergency physician was persistent in locating the patient's doctor, but if the doctor could not be located, the patient is still the ED physician's responsibility. For an OB physician to suggest that, because he/she does not come to a particular hospital, he/she should not be contacted about a patient, is ludicrous; the emergency physician needs to make proper contact. When telephone communication is going poorly, it is our job to find someone to take the patient. An appropriate alternative would have been to contact an obstetrician on the hospital staff who could take responsibility for follow up, if it could not be arranged in a civil manner by their own physician.

The laboratory evaluation obtained was perfectly adequate. However, it may have prompted me to obtain a vaginal ultrasound to confirm the presence of an intrauterine pregnancy. I would then be forced to ask serious questions about this right lower quadrant pain; the combination of appendicitis and pregnancy is certainly not unknown. The American public thinks "if we can land men on the moon, we can easily diagnose appendicitis." Nothing can be further from the truth. When there is guarding, rebound, and obvious tenderness at McBurney's point, anyone can make the diagnosis, but initially, with minimal discomfort and no peritoneal signs, the diagnosis can be difficult.

The use of CT scanning in this case merits further comment. In adults, CT scanning is unlikely to lead to enough radiation exposure to cause serious problems. This may not be the case for the fetus and we need to be careful about exposing early pregnancies to radiation without good cause. Intelligent re-evaluation and re-examination of the patient rather than immediate CT scanning is the most appropriate approach. A better follow up for this patient would be to see them back in 6 to 8 hours and evaluate how the pain is progressing. At that time, if the patient continues to have tenderness or guarding, surgical consultation can be obtained.

- **Thoroughness of Documentation:** 7 out of 10.
- **Thoroughness of Patient Evaluation:** 8 out of 10.
- **Risk of Serious Illness Being Missed:** Medium risk.
- **Risk Management Legal Rating:** Medium risk.

30 YEAR OLD PREGNANT WOMAN WITH ABDOMINAL PAIN

—Second Visit: 4 Days Later—

CHIEF COMPLAINT (at 22:27): Abdominal pain

```
VITAL SIGNS                                                    Pain
Time      Temp      Pulse     Resp      Syst      Diast     Scale
22:34     99.5      101       18        122       79        10
00:05               96        20        124       80        10
01:49               88        16        132       74
03:20     98.9      83        16        111       68        3
```

HISTORY OF PRESENT ILLNESS (at 23:01): Pt c/o generalized, severe, sharp abdominal pain and low back pain which has gotten worse, also has had night sweats but no body aches or fever. Was seen in ED 4 days ago for round ligament pain and has appointment with her OB tomorrow. Has been taking 2 Tylenol q4h without improvement. Pt denies fever, nausea, vomiting, diarrhea. No blood in stools, urinary frequency, hematuria, vaginal bleeding or discharge.

PAST MEDICAL HISTORY/TRIAGE:
 Medications: None
 Allergies: Sulfa
 PMH: None
 PSH: None

EXAM (at 23:19):
 General: Alert and oriented X3, well-nourished, well appearing, in no apparent distress
 Head: Normocephalic; atraumatic.
 Resp: Normal chest excursion with respiration; breath sounds clear and equal bilaterally; no wheezes, rhonchi, or rales
 Card: Regular rhythm, without murmurs, rub or gallop
 Abd: Non-distended; mildly tender general lower abdomen. No pain on palpation of low back or CVA tenderness. Abdomen is gravid and soft, without rigidity, rebound or guarding, negative heel tap, negative psoas; + McBurney's tenderness.
 Skin: Normal for age and race; warm and dry; no apparent lesions
 Pelvic: No lesions, masses, with thin yellow discharge in vaginal vault, cervical os is closed with no bleeding visible on exam. No cervical motion or adnexal tenderness to palpation.

ORDERS: Demerol 25 mg IVP, Phenergan 12.5 mg IVP, IV: .9NS-500cc bolus then to 125cc/hour

RESULTS (at 00:18)

Test	Flag	Value	Units	Ref. range
WBC	H	16.3	K/µL	4.6-10.2
HGB		11.9	G/DL	13.5-17.5
PLT		307	K/µL	142-424

Urinalysis

Test	Flag	Value	Ref. range
WBC	H	5-10	0-5/HPF
RBC	H	10-25	0-5/HPF
BACTERIA	H	RARE	NOT SEEN

PROGRESS NOTES: I spoke with the patient's OB/GYN (at 00:30) who agrees with surgical consultation. I also discussed with surgery (at 01:47), who came to evaluate the patient and will take her to the OR.

DIAGNOSIS (at 02:44):
Abdominal Pain – RLQ
Pregnancy

DISPOSITION: Admitted to surgical service

HOSPITAL COURSE:

********** **Operative Report** **********
POSTOPERATIVE DIAGNOSIS: Acute appendicitis with ruptured and walled-off pelvic abscess.
OPERATIONS: 1) Appendectomy. 2) Drainage of pelvic abscess. 3) Placement J-P drain

SUMMARY: The patient tolerated the operation well and left the hospital 4 days later without adverse effects to the fetus.

FINAL DIAGNOSIS: Ruptured appendix, secondary to appendicitis

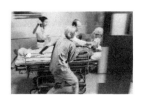

EVALUATION OF ABDOMINAL PAIN IN PREGNANCY AND APPENDICITIS IN PREGNANCY

Robert Dart, MD, FACEP

I. OVERVIEW OF ABDOMINAL PAIN IN PREGNANCY

Abdominal pain in pregnancy can present a number of unique challenges. The clinician needs to consider both pregnancy and non-pregnancy related causes of abdominal pain, as well as the effect of the gravid uterus on the intra-abdominal anatomy. In addition, the impact of pregnancy on the ordering of imaging studies as well as the interpretation of diagnostic tests needs to be incorporated into decision making. Finally, the treating physician needs to understand how pregnancy alters the approach to, and timing of, surgery, and how a delay in diagnosis might have a negative impact on fetal viability.

The differential diagnosis of abdominal pain in pregnant patients includes etiologies directly related to the pregnancy, etiologies unrelated to pregnancy, and etiologies which may occur in patients attempting to become pregnant. Examples of the first group would include ectopic pregnancy, nonviable pregnancy/spontaneous miscarriage, and placental abruption. Examples of the second group include appendicitis, ureteral colic, and cholecystitis. The third group includes the increased frequency of ovarian torsion, as well as ectopic pregnancy in patients who become pregnant as a result of in vitro fertilization, the use of ovulation induction agents, or both.[1,2]

II. ANATOMICAL CHANGES IN PREGNANCY

The gravid uterus increases in size and may displace intra-abdominal contents. Upward displacement of the appendix begins after the third month of pregnancy and reaches the level of the iliac crest by the end of 6 months. It returns to its normal position by day 10 postpartum.[3]

III. EVALUATION—CBC, CT, MRI, ULTRASOUND

A CBC is often obtained to in order to help differentiate surgical from nonsurgical causes of abdominal pain. While the presence of leukocytosis may be predictive of a surgical etiology in the nonpregnant patient, white blood counts up to 16,000 are normal findings in pregnancy. In fact, a number of recent studies have suggested that the WBC is not useful in confirming or excluding the diagnosis of appendicitis in the pregnant patient.[4,5] Our patient had a WBC count of 13,100 at her initial visit, which was not helpful in establishing a diagnosis. The WBC count, when she returned with a perforation, was 16,300, minimally above the normal range in pregnancy.

CT scan has become the imaging study of choice for the evaluation of patients with suspected appendicitis. However, while newer helical CT scans have decreased fetal radiation exposure to about 300 mrads, clinicians should avoid the use of this test in the first trimester when the fetus is most at risk.[6] Ultrasound is the best initial option and is an excellent test when complications of pregnancy are being considered.[7] In addition, ultrasound can confirm or exclude biliary tract disease. Unfortunately, as the pregnancy progresses into the third trimester, the increasing size of the gravid uterus can make visualization of the appendix more difficult.[8]

Recent studies suggest that MRI may be a useful imaging option when the ultrasound is nondiagnostic. MRI provides excellent visualization of pelvic and abdominal organs and soft tissue, without the need for radiation exposure.[9,10] The main draw back to MRI is its limited availability during off hours.

IV. LAPAROSCOPY

Laparoscopy has been performed with increasing frequency over the past decade. Most studies report excellent short-term fetal and maternal outcomes compared to laparotomy.[11] However, the long-term safety of this procedure in the pregnant patient has yet to be conclusively proven. The main concerns directly relate to carbon dioxide insufflation at the time of surgery—it has been postulated that the increased intra-abdominal pressure may lead to a decrease in uterine blood flow. Animal models suggest that CO_2 absorption may lead to the development of fetal acidosis.[12]

V. APPENDICITIS IN PREGNANCY

The classic clinical findings in patients with suspected appendicitis are RLQ abdominal pain, nausea, vomiting, anorexia, low-grade temperature and an elevated leukocyte count. However, in the well pregnant patient, nausea, vomiting, and anorexia are common findings, particularly in the first trimester. Neither an elevated leukocyte count nor the presence or absence of a fever discriminates between those with and without appendicitis at laparotomy.[4,5] Maintain a high index of suspicion and a low threshold for imaging studies and surgical consultation when appendicitis is considered during pregnancy.

Involvement of the patient's OB is always good practice, the timing of consultation and follow up are important when evaluating for appendicitis. The primary goal is to avoid appendiceal rupture, which can be minimized by obtaining a diagnosis and definitive therapy within 24 hours. An obstetric consult will be most useful if the patient is seen in the ED at the time of her initial visit. If discharge is being contemplated, a follow up exam should be arranged within 6–12 hours of discharge. In most cases, it is more practical to have the patient return to the ED, rather than go to the obstetrician's office. Despite the frustration of our ED physician in trying to arrange continuity of care for our patient, follow up in 24–48 hours was too long, since appendiceal rupture may occur before this time. In addition, the documentation of the conversation with the obstetrician does not suggest a reliable mechanism of follow up for this patient. If they speak like this to their peers, how do they treat their patients?

The greatest morbidity of appendicitis during pregnancy affects the fetus, as the maternal mortality rate is very low. Appendicitis often stimulates uterine contractions and can precipitate premature delivery.[4,5] The major risk to fetal viability relates to diagnostic delay. In pregnant patients with uncomplicated appendicitis, the fetal loss is only 1.5% when the appendix is unruptured at surgery.[13] However, when perforation occurs, the fetal loss rate may be as high as 36%.[13] In addition, appendiceal perforation occurs twice as often in the third trimester (69%), at a time where fetal viability is most likely an option,[14] compared to the first or second trimester (31%).

VI. SUMMARY

Pregnancy presents an expanded differential in patients presenting with abdominal pain, and can alter the diagnostic approach to the evaluation of these patients. Despite these challenges, clinicians should be aware of alternative diagnostic tests that are available and should make every effort to minimize diagnostic delay since this contributes to increased fetal mortality.

TEACHING POINTS ABOUT CASE 27:

- Pregnant patients with RLQ abdominal pain need to be evaluated for appendicitis.
- If follow up cannot be arranged with the patient's obstetrician, it is the responsibility of the ED physician to arrange alternative follow up; this is most easily accomplished in the ED.
- Delay in diagnosis of appendicitis is the major threat to fetal viability. If a diagnosis is not established during the initial encounter, follow up should be within 6–12 hours.
- Minimally elevated WBC counts are not helpful in diagnosing appendicitis in pregnancy; WBC counts up to 16,000 are normal in pregnancy.

REFERENCES

1. Fernandez H, Coste J, Job-Spira N. Controlled ovarian hyperstimulation as a risk factor for ectopic pregnancy. Obstet Gynecol 1991;78: 656-9.
2. Gorkemli H, Camus M, Clasen K. Adnexal torsion after gonadotropin induction for IVF or ICSI and its conservative treatment. Arch Gynecol Obstet 2002;267: 4-6.
3. Baer JL, Reis RA, Arens RA. Appendicitis in pregnancy with changes in position and axis of the normal appendix in pregnancy. JAMA 1932;52: 1359-64.
4. Andersen B, Nielsen TF. Appendicitis in pregnancy: diagnosis, management and complications. Acta Obstet Gynecol Scand 1999;78: 758-62.
5. Mourad J, Elliot JP, Erickson L, et al. Appendicitis in pregnancy: new information that contradicts long-held clinical beliefs. Am J Obstet Gynecol 2000;182: 1027-9.
6. Castro MA, Shipp TD, Castro EE, et al. The use of helical computed tomography in pregnancy for the diagnosis of appendicitis. Am J Obstet Gynecol 2001;184: 954-7.
7. Sharp HT. The acute abdomen during pregnancy. Clin Obstet Gynecol 2002;45: 405-13.
8. Lim HK, Bae, SH, Seo GS. Diagnosis of acute appendicitis in pregnant women: value of sonography. Am J Roentgenol 1992;159:539-42.
9. Birchard KR, Brown MA, Hyslop WB, et al. MRI of acute abdominal and pelvic pain in pregnant patients. Am J Roent 2005;184: 452-8.
10. Oto A, Ernst RD, Shah R, et. al. Right-lower-quadrant pain and suspected appendicitis in pregnant women: evaluation with MR imaging—initial experience. Radiology 2005;234:445-51.
11. Lackman E, Schienfeld A, Voss E, et al. Pregnancy and laparoscopic surgery. J Am Assoc Gynecol Laparosc 1999;6: 347-51.
12. Amos JD, Schorr SJ, Norman PF, et. al. Laparoscopic surgery during pregnancy. Am J Surg 1996;171:435-7 (Comment 1997; 174: 222).
13. Babaknia A, Parsa H, Woodruff JD. Appendicitis during pregnancy. Obstet Gynecol 1977;50: 40-44.
14. Weingold AB. Appendicitis in pregnancy. Clin Obstet Gynecol 1983;26:801-9.

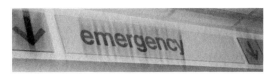

CASE 28

36 YEAR OLD MALE WITH
FEVER & MYALGIAS

Commentary:
Gregory L. Henry, MD, FACEP

CEO, Medical Practice Risk Assessment, Inc., Ann Arbor, Michigan
Clinical Professor, Department of Emergency Medicine
  University of Michigan Medical School, Ann Arbor, Michigan
Past President, American College of Emergency Physicians (ACEP)

Discussion:
David Hill, MD

Attending ED physician
  Mt. Carmel St. Ann's Emergency Department, Westerville, Ohio

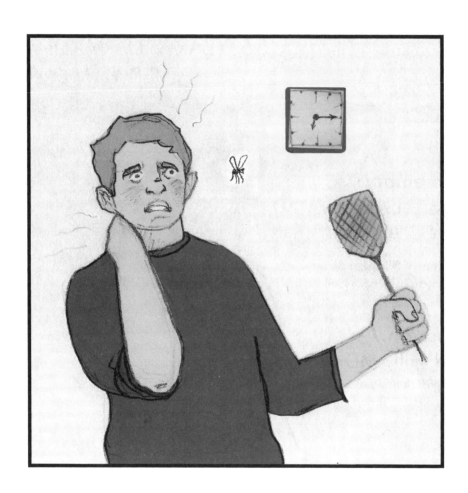

36 YEAR OLD MALE WITH FEVER & MYALGIAS

—Initial Visit—

*Authors' Note: The history, exam and notes are the actual documentation of the physicians and providers, including abbreviations (and spelling errors)

CHIEF COMPLAINT (at 12:37): Flu-like symptoms, having head and neck pain, dizziness

```
VITAL SIGNS
Time   Temp(F)  Rt. Pulse  Resp  Syst  Diast  Pos.  O2 Sat  O2%
12:48  100.2    Tym. 120   20    132   74     S     96      RA
```

HISTORY OF PRESENT ILLNESS (documented at 02:26, the next morning): The patient is a 36-year-old man who is presented by his wife to rule out West Nile Virus disease. The gentleman has had a low-grade fever, chills, and diffuse myalgia and fatigue for three days. He continues to drink excellent PO's and is making good urine. He is mildly anorexic and has had scant bowel movements but attributes this to his lack of food. His general overall decrease in energy, however denies any neurologic findings. He has no rash, or stiff neck, and only a moderate headache. He believes that he has the flu. Denies weight loss, n/v/d, chest pain, SOB, cough, rhinorrhea, dysuria, hematuria, dizziness, lymph node swelling or muscle cramps.

PAST MEDICAL HISTORY/TRIAGE
   Medication, common allergies: No known allergies.
   Current meds: Ibuprofen
   PMH: Heart murmur
   PSH: No significant surgical history.

EXAM (documented at 02:28, the next morning):
   General: Alert and oriented X3, well-nourished, ill but nontoxic appearing, in no apparent distress
   Head: Normocephalic; atraumatic.
   Eyes: PERRL, EOMI, nonicteric, noninjected.
   Nose: The nose is normal in appearance without rhinorrhea
   Neck: No jugular venous distention, no lymphadenopathy, supple without nucal rigidity.
   Throat: Normal without erythema, edema, exudate.
   Oral: Mucus membranes moist and intact
   Resp: Normal chest excursion with respiration; breath sounds clear and equal bilaterally; no wheezes, rhonchi, or rales
   Card: Regular tachycardic rhythm, without murmurs, rub or gallop
   Abd: Non-distended; non-tender, soft, without rigidity, rebound or guarding
   Skin: Normal for age and race; warm and dry; no apparent lesions

Neurological: Patient is alert and oriented times three. Cranial nerves III-XII are intact. Sensory and motor functions are intact. Strength is 5/5 for flexion and extension in all 4 extremities. Patellar DTRs are equal and intact. Finger to nose testing is equal and normal bilaterally.

DIAGNOSIS (at 13:45): Influenza

DISPOSITION (at 13:59): The patient was discharged to Home ambulatory, f/u PCP if not improved in 3 days, after care instructions viral syndrome.

Gregory L. Henry comments:

"When the chief complaint is vague and broad, a general review is essential"

Particularly during the winter months, there is no more common presentation than fever and myalgias, occasionally with some vomiting. The family often has a specific concern. In this case the wife inquired about West Nile Virus, which is not irrational thinking and needs to be addressed with the patient.

When the chief complaint is vague and broad, a general review is essential. Physical examination seems to be relatively complete and without specific findings.

The evaluation of these patients can vary from no testing to elaborate testing with about the same results. The conclusion of viral illness was perfectly reasonable, and the patient was sent home to be followed up with the family practice physician. This is also reasonable and acceptable in most cases.

Documentation of this visit seems adequate, as are the follow up instructions.

Risk management ratings follow the next visit…

36 YEAR OLD MALE WITH
FEVER AND MYALGIAS

—Second Visit: 1 Day Later—

CHIEF COMPLAINT (at 20:07): Fever

| VITAL SIGNS | | | | | | | | 02 | | Pain |
Time	Temp(F)	Rt.	Pulse	Resp	Syst	Diast	Pos.	Sat	O2%	Scale
20:25	100.6	Tym.	118	18	114	78	S	96	ra	4
22:06	98.8	Oral	80	18	120	68	S			
23:16			100	16	110	68	S			

HISTORY OF PRESENT ILLNESS (at 21:30): This is a 36 y/o male who presents with fever and generalized body aches. No weight change or malaise, visual changes, hearing changes, ear or throat pain, nasal discharge, neck stiffness, chest pain, SOB, cough, n/v/d, abd. pain, dysuria, hematuria, urinary frequency, muscle weakness, joint pain, back pain, HA, LOC, confusion, or rash.

EXAM (documented at 00:29):
  General: Well-appearing; well nourished; A&O X 3, in no apparent distress.
  Head: Normocephalic; atraumatic.
  Eyes: PERRL
  Ears: TM's normal
  Nose: Normal nose; no rhinorrhea;
  Throat: Normal pharynx with no tonsillar hypertrophy or exudate. Tongue and uvula midline. Buccal mucosa dry.
  Neck: Supple; non-tender; no cervical lymphadenopathy.
  Card: Regular rate and rhythm, no rubs or gallops. There is a LUSB systolic murmur II/VI.
  Resp: Normal chest excursion with respiration; breath sounds clear and equal bilaterally; no wheezes, rhonchi, or rales.
  Abd: Non-distended; +RLQ tenderness to palpation with guarding; BS + x 4, without rigidity, rebound. Neg Psoas, obtrurator, rovsing's, murphys.
  Skin: Normal for age and race; warm and dry; no apparent lesions
  Neurological: Patient is alert and oriented times three. Cranial nerves III-XII are intact. Sensory and motor functions are intact. Strength is 5/5 for flexion and extension in all 4 extremities. Patellar DTRs are equal and intact. No pronator drift.

ORDERS (at 21:23): .9NS – 1L bolus

RESULTS:

Test	Flag	Value	Units	Ref. Range
WBC	C	1.8	K/uL	4.6-10.2
HGB		14.3	G/DL	13.5-17.5
PLT	L	80	K/uL	142-424
Differential				
SEGS		39%		40-85
BANDS		23%		
LYMPHS		27%		5-46
MONOS		8%		0-12

Test	Flag	Value	Units	Ref. Range
NA	L	134	MMOL/L	135-144
K	L	3.1	MMOL/L	3.5-5.1
CL		98	MMOL/L	98-107
CO2		26	MMOL/L	22-29
BUN	H	19	MG/DL	7-18
CREAT		1.2	MG/DL	0.6-1.3

LFT's - WNL

Urine dip stick: WNL except: Protein; Results: 30 mg/dl

ORDERS (at 23:00): K-Lyte 50 meq PO

CONSULTATION (at 00:17): I spoke with the primary care doctor

DIAGNOSIS (at 00:30): 1. Fever, 2. Abnormal blood finding, 3. Abnormal blood chemistry, 4. Hypokalemia

DISPOSITION (at 00:38): Discharged home to f/u with PCP in 2-3 days as previously scheduled. After care instructions for viral infection. Prescription for KCl 10 mEq #10.

Additional comments by Gregory L. Henry:

The patient returned for a second visit one day later. More elaborate laboratory testing was done, which revealed a significant leukopenia. This, along with the systolic murmur and general malaise of the patient, is a tip off that further work up is necessary. In general, depressions of the white blood count are more a function of viral disease than bacterial. The emergency physician did speak with the primary care physician, but the patient was discharged home; with these abnormalities, admission, blood cultures, and prophylactic antibiotics might have been more reasonable.

- Thoroughness of Documentation: 8 out of 10.

- Thoroughness of Patient Evaluation: 8 out of 10.

- Risk of Serious Illness Being Missed: Medium risk.

- Risk Management Legal Rating: Medium risk.

36 YEAR OLD MALE WITH FEVER AND MYALGIAS

—Third Visit: 12 Days Later—

CHIEF COMPLAINT (at 22:55): Fever

```
VITAL SIGNS
Time    Temp(F)  Rt.   Pulse   Resp   Syst   Diast   Pos.
23:06   102.8    Tym.  122     18     111    77      S
00:56   100.1    Oral  87      18     102    62      S
03:24                  92      16     110    60      S
04:05   97.3     Oral
```

HISTORY OF PRESENT ILLNESS (at 23:26): 36 year old male c/o fever and low back pain x 2wks. States he was seen in this ER 2wks ago with similar sx's. Admits to abdominal bloating and bilateral lower back pain. States pain has increased and nothing makes it better or worse. Fever has been constant all week, tylenol has kept it low, but it rises after the tylenol wears off. Admits to generalized body myalgias and headache. He has had 6-8 pound weight loss and night sweats. No recent travel or TB exposure. No IVDA. Denies n/v/d, abdominal pain, dysuria, hematuria. Denies blood in stool, chest pain, SOB, cough, rhinorrhea, sore throat, ear pain, stiff neck, penile d/c, rash, lymph node swelling.

PAST MEDICAL HISTORY/TRIAGE
   Medication, common allergies: No known allergies.
   Current meds: Ibuprofen and tylenol
   PMH: Heart murmur

SOCIAL HISTORY: Patient is a smoker. Patient denies alcohol or drug use.

EXAM (documented at 02:57):
   General: Alert and oriented X3, well-nourished, ill appearing, in no apparent distress
   Head: Normocephalic; atraumatic.
   Eyes: PERRL sclera white and clear

Mouth: MMM post pharynx clear

Neck: Supple without LAN, Brudzinksi and Kernig's sign are negative.

Nose: The nose is normal in appearance without rhinorrhea

Resp: Normal chest excursion with respiration; breath sounds clear and equal bilaterally; no wheezes, rhonchi, or rales

Card: Regular rhythm, with a harsh holosystolic murmur, grade -5/6. No rubs or gallops .

Abd: Non-distended; diffusely tender, soft, without rigidity, rebound or guarding

Skin: Normal for age and race; warm and dry; no apparent lesions

Ext: No cyanosis or other deformity. nail beds are clear.

ORDERS (at 23:53): Ibuprofen 600mg PO, Acetaminophen 975 mg PO, IV: .9NS-125cc/ hour, 2DMMOD echo/colorflow

RESULTS:

Test	Value	Units	Ref. Range
WBC	5.3	K/uL	4.6-10.2
HGB	11.5	G/DL	13.5-17.5
PLT	247	K/uL	142-424
Differential:			
Auto seg	67.3%		40.0-85.0
Auto lymph	21.7%		5.0-46.0
Auto mono	10.1%		0-12.0

Test	Flag	Value	Units	Ref. Range
NA		135	MMOL/L	135-144
K		4.2	MMOL/L	3.5-5.1
CL		99	MMOL/L	98-107
CO2		25	MMOL/L	22-29
BUN	H	16	MG/DL	7-18
CREAT		1.2	MG/DL	0.6-1.3

LFT's, amylase/lipase - WNL

Test	Flag	Value	Units	Ref. Range
MONO		NEGATIVE		NEGATIVE
WSR	H	35	MM/HR	0-15

URINALYSIS - WNL

RADIOLOGY: CHEST: No acute cardiopulmonary disease is identified.

CT OF THE ABDOMEN/PELVIS WITH CONTRAST:

1. Mild cardiomegaly. 2. Mild splenomegaly measuring 15 cm. 3. Colonic diverticulosis. No acute pelvic findings.

CONSULTATION (at 03:10): I spoke with the infectious disease consultant for hospital admission and they recommended rocephin which was started.

DIAGNOSIS (at 03:20): 1. Febrile illness, 2. Splenomegaly

DISPOSITION (at 04:05): Was sent to medical surgical bed.

HOSPITAL COURSE

Initial note per infectious disease: Differential diagnosis includes bacterial endocarditis versus a viral infection. He has no epidemiologic history for an atypical bacterial infection such as Ehrlichia, or other unusual bacterial pathogens. Recent history of leukopenia and thrombocytopenia, along with mildly elevated liver function tests, which is compatible with a viral infection. This was unlikely to be a hematologic malignancy since his blood counts have normalized since then. Childhood history of heart murmur. Mild hepatitis, which has resolved. Plan is to await the three sets of blood cultures. Continue empiric Rocephin. Check 2D echocardiogram to rule out vegetation. We will check serology for epidermolysis bullosa dystrophica and CMB.

Results of blood culture: Streptococcus sanguis, viridans group isolated – Sensitive to all antibiotics except sulfa

Final diagnosis: Bacterial endocarditis

Additional comments by Gregory L. Henry:

It is interesting to note that the patient returned 12 days later. He is again febrile with new findings on cardiac ausculation of a 5/6 holosystolic murmur. This, and recurrent fever should cause one to consider an infective source. No petechiae, Roth spots, or Janeway lesions are noted; the lack of these findings certainly does not rule out bacterial endocarditis. The patient was then admitted, workup was undertaken, and blood cultures were positive for strep viridans. Parenthetically, this is a very difficult case. Early on, it is a bit much to expect that the emergency physician, without other findings, to make a correct diagnosis in this case.

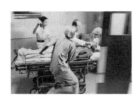

DIAGNOSIS AND MANAGEMENT OF INFLUENZA

David Hill, MD

I. SUMMARY OF CASE
Visit 1
Often, listening to a patient and the family will reveal the diagnosis; occasionally it will lead you astray. During the first visit, the physician was asked "Does my husband have West Nile Virus?" This question was correctly answered by the emergency physician, but the question which should have been focused on was: "Why does my husband have a fever."

The patient received a diagnosis of influenza. The chart records the time-of-day that entries are made, but we do not know the dates. Had this case occured in the middle of flu season, the diagnosis may have been supportable on the basis of clinical information and high pre-test probability. Since we don't know the season, the clinician may have gone too far out on a limb with the label of "influenza."

Limiting the formal diagnosis to what you can support from the chart is a more restrictive logical approach. In this case, "fever" would be accurate, and would tell subsequent clinicians that no causative etiology was identified. I think that this misstep played out in the next visit the following evening.

Visit 2
On this second visit, the HPI is quite abbreviated and really constitutes a review of symptoms (ROS) rather than a description of the current illness. Since this patient returned to the same ER, we hope that the second doctor would have read the first chart; in this case, I wonder if the same physician saw the patient on both the first and second visit. If this did occur, the abbreviated HPI makes more sense. The HPI isn't documenting an investigation into what the patient has— the doctor already "knows" what's wrong—he has the flu!

Lab work was ordered, but not well interpreted. The discovery of a very low WBC count should should raise some alarm and prompt further thinking about other etiologies of this finding. In this case, the manual differential shows 23% band forms, suggesting that the marrow isn't suppressing white cell formation but working hard to maintain an adequate number of cells in circulation.

Lastly, the new heart murmur heard on day #2 is ignored. The presence of a murmur in a febrile child may be regarded as a benign correlation to the hyperdynamic state induced by the fever. This may not be the case in adults. Furthermore, febrile murmurs are diastolic,[1] while an innocent flow murmur is systolic.[2] The physician may have assumed that it was an innocent febrile murmur.

The fever, neutropenic bandemia, and new cardiac murmur argue the case that the patient has something going on. The clinician may have recognized this; he changed the diagnosis from flu to a set of more descriptive diagnoses (implying that the etiology is unknown), but still provided the patient with the handout for viral illnesses.

Listening to the patient often gives you the diagnosis; on this second visit, the patient is saying (without words) "something is wrong."

Final Visit
This visit is an epilogue rather than another chapter. The patient had sufficient findings to trigger a quick evaluation and empiric treatment. I've never encountered a 5/6 murmur, but coupled with a fever and weight loss, admission is necessary. Fever and endocarditis are discussed at length in another chapter, the discussion below will focus on a discussion of West Nile Virus (briefly) and influenza.

II. WEST NILE VIRUS
West Nile Virus has been quite prominent in the media, despite only sporadic occurrences in the population. CDC data for the year 2003 shows just under 10,000 cases nationwide; of note, only 70% of these had fever on presentation. For Ohio, the state in question, a total of 108 cases in a population of 11.3 million were found,[3] equaling only 1 case per 100,000 persons per year, making this diagnosis unlikely. WNV infection ranges from asymptomatic to a full-blown meningitis or encephalitis presentation. The first clinician presumably dismissed the diagnosis of WNV and turned to a more statistically probable diagnosis.

We will now look at influenza in depth, which was diagnosed in error in this patient.

III. INFLUENZA—EPIDEMIOLOGY
For the vast majority of cases, influenza is an acute, non-specific illness characterized by fever, malaise, fatigue, and a host of other symptoms which leave the patient feeling miserable. In some at-risk patients, it progresses to pneumonia, hospitalization, and death.

Although influenza mortality is associated with extremes of age, the increase in morbidity (in the form of hospitalizations) is mostly in the < 65 year old age group. Influenza accounts for about 114,000 hospitalizations per year, but the number is quite variable, ranging from 16,000 during a mild flu season to 222,000 during an epidemic.[4]

The incubation period of influenza is relatively short, between 18 and 72 hours. The influenza virus may be shed as much as 1 day *prior* to the manifestation of symptoms by an infected individual.[5]

The great 1918 influenza pandemic caused 20 million deaths; its extreme virulence may have been due to a mutation which permitted very efficient transfer from human to human, rather than its traditional route of avian host to human. The estimated mortality was 2.5 – 3 %, far in excess of other "ordinary" influenza epidemics. Interestingly, the deaths of healthy adults between 15 and 35 years of age were responsible for much of the excess mortality.[6]

IV. INFLUENZA IMMUNIZATIONS

The CDC recommends yearly vaccination of patients over age 50, health care workers, residents of nursing homes or other high density living environments, and individuals with chronic medical conditions such as COPD, CRI, DM, cancer, HIV or any other immunosuppressive conditions. In addition, household contacts of individuals with chronic medical conditions should be vaccinated. Increasing emphasis is also being placed on the immunization of children aged 6–24 months (infants < 6 months old do not have an approved vaccine available). Lastly, women who will be pregnant during the flu season should be vaccinated.

The traditional vaccine is an intramuscular injection of inactivated influenza. The viral strains are different each year and are based on the predicted predominant strains for the next season. This vaccine is inactivated and safe for use in immunocompromised patients. A live attenuated vaccine is also available and is administered as an intranasal spray, mimicking the natural route of infection. Its use should be restricted to healthy patients, between the ages of 5 and 50.[7]

Inquire of the nursing home patient if the facility has had any outbreaks of influenza, and if they have routinely immunized their residents for that year or supplied prophylaxis during an outbreak.

V. DIAGNOSIS OF INFLUENZA

The diagnosis of a specific infectious etiology is an oft-sought, yet frequently elusive, goal of physicians. The typical symptoms of influenza—fever, myalgia, headache, malaise, dry cough, sore throat, and rhinitis—occur with most upper respiratory infections. Among adults, fever plus cough is reported to be 63% –78% sensitive and 55%–71% specific in diagnosing influenza. In children, one triad of symptoms—headache, sore throat, and cough—has a sensitivity of 80% and a likelihood ratio of positive viral culture of 3.7:1.[8] (Not a great sensitivity, but it approaches usefulness).

Like all evaluations, your pretest probability is paramount to interpreting your findings. In the middle of flu season, a kid with the triad of headache, sore throat, and cough will likely get an influenza diagnosis without much second guessing, but in the middle of summer you may wish to explore other possibilities. One pearl that I recall from my basic pathology was that the human body only has a few responses to any given pathologic process, thus the number of signs and symptoms of a given infection are going to be smaller than the number of causes. If different infections were to cause unique patterns of response (e.g., high fever and no myalgia and no rhinorrhea versus high fever and no myalgia and coryza) then we may be able to put together the patterns that I tried to learn as a resident, but even here we are not able to take advantage of the potential combinations of signs and symptoms. This stems from the fact that the immune response is mediated by an even smaller number of inflammatory hormones. Review the adverse effects of the interferon class of drugs and you will see "flu like symptoms" as a prominent item. If warranted, turn to laboratory analysis to assist with the identification of the offending agent.

Although many patients are often treated based on symptoms alone, it may be important to obtain a specific diagnosis. Influenza data is tracked; accurate data regarding its activity and location is invaluable to public health organizations to design and distribute vaccines for subsequent annual cycles. Furthermore, since the development of the neuraminidase inhibitors in 1999, we now can offer targeted interventions.

According to the CDC, a nasal swab for influenza has a sensitivity of 70% and specificity of 90%, although the manufacturers' specifications are somewhat better. The kit used at my hospital quotes sensitivities in the 70's but specificities in the high 90's.[9] A low sensitivity is not terribly surprising since it depends on proper sample collection, timely transportation, and correct processing. On the other hand, high specificity is expected since these tests are immunoassays based on monoclonal antibodies. The cost for these tests are in the range of $15–20 when purchased in case lots of 25 kits.

As with all tests, the sensitivity and specificity of these tests must be defined in terms of performance to a "gold standard" test. Monoclonal antibody screening tests are typically compared to cell cultures, but polymerase chain reaction studies have been cited as being the better test, and may become the new "gold standard."[10] With influenza, and RNA virus, reverse transcription needs to be performed prior to the standard PCR assay. Since both cell cultures and RT-PCR are not available in the typical ED laboratory, the speed and low cost of the CLIA-waived nasal swab screening tests make them acceptable compared to the gold or silver standards.

VI. MANAGEMENT OF INFLUENZA

A frequent frustration of emergency medicine is the evaluation of URI or other non-specific viral illness and explanation (again) that antibiotics will not cure the common cold. If we can diagnose influenza, we can now offer our patients a choice of antiviral therapies. A named diagnosis is sufficient for many patients ("I just want to know what's wrong"), and offering a specific treatment will provide reassurance that you are not just sending them home to "take two ibuprofen and call your doctor in the morning." The influenza drugs all share 2 significant Achilles heels: first, they must be started within the first 36–48 symptomatic hours to have any measurable effect; and second, their effect is minimal at best. They are advertised to reduce the symptom duration by 1–2 days, out of an expected 5–10 day duration without treatment.

Hemagglutin inhibitors—Amantadine and Rimantadine

Amantadine (Symmetrel) was initially approved by the FDA for the treatment of Asian Flu in 1966.[11] Since that time, its approved indications have been broadened to include any strain of type A influenza. The mechanism of action is competitive inhibition of the binding of viral hemagglutinin to cellular receptors; unfortunately, the rapid mutation rate of the RNA influenza virus leads to resistance.

In healthy adults, the dosage is 100 mg PO BID for 5 days—reductions are advised for elderly and debilitated patients (Table 1). Amantadine is cleared by the kidneys, and renal dosing is required based on the creatinine clearance of the patient. Because amantadine interferes with cellular infection, it can be used prophylactically; the FDA has approved it for this indication at 100 mg PO daily.

A similar drug, rimantadine (Flumadine), is less widely used but very similar in mechanism. Dosage is 100mg BID for 5 days. It is moderately more expensive than amantadine, but less than the newer agents discussed below.

Neuraminidase Inhibitors—Oseltamivir and Zanamivir

Neuraminidase is an enzyme used by type A and B influenza virus particles to cleave themselves from the infected cells. Zanamivir (Relenza) and oseltamivir (Tamiflu) are 2 new agents specifically designed to interfere with the active site of neuraminidase. Drug resistance is expected to be less than with the older drugs.

Oseltamivir is an absorbable pro-drug which crosses the GI tract before dissolving into a charged , active form of the drug.[12] Oseltamivir has won approval for prophylaxis. Zanamivir utilizes a positively charged guanidine moiety which prevents the drug from being efficiently absorbed across the GI tract; hence it is dispensed as a dry powder inhaler.[13] Doses are listed below.

The best choice depends on multiple factors such as the type of influenza present in the community, the ability of a patient to pay for the drug, and if a specific type of influenza is identified by nasal swab testing.

In summary, the antiviral drugs are limited in number, limited in window-of-opportunity, and limited in efficacy. Still, they are better than nothing and we should be familiar with all 4 of them. Mnemonic devices are one of my favorite techniques for learning, and this topic is no exception. I'll warn you that the last one is pretty weak—feel free to do better!

- *A*mantadine is only useful against influenza *A*
- Rimantadine *r*hymes with amantadine and is a "me-too" drug
- *T*amiflu comes in *T*ablets (capsules, actually) and
- *Z*anamivir uses one of those *z*any inhalers.

Table 1. Comparison of Influenza Antiviral Medications

Drug	Amantadine	Rimantadine	Oseltamivir	Zanamivir
Class	Hemagglutinin Inhibitors		Neuraminidase Inhibitors	
Target	A		A & B	
Cost	$	$$	$$$	
Window of opportunity	< 48 hours			
Treatment Dose	100 mg BID × 5 D or 100 mg Daily × 5 D if debilitated		75 mg BID × 5 D	10 mg (2 INH) BID × 5 D
Prophylaxis Dose	same		75 mg Daily × > 7 D	NA
Pediatric	>1 yr, 5 mg/kg/d PO divided BID × 5 d, 50 mg/5 mL		> 1 yr doses per insert, 60 mg/5 mL	> 7 yr

VII. OVERVIEW AND SUMMARY OF CASE

This patient initially presented with a fever, and the first physician was asked by the patient's wife to specifically evaluate for West Nile virus. His symptoms were nonspecific and he was diagnosed with influenza.

Though the review of symptoms at the second visit is extensive, the documentation of "the history of present illness" is only 5 words long: "…fever and generalized body aches." The physical exam is more complete, with documentation of a new heart murmur and right lower quadrant abdominal pain. Neither of these positive findings, nor his severe neutropenia, thrombocytopenia, or hypokalemia are commented on further. He receives K-lyte and is sent home for further follow up. These findings should have been addressed in more detail with further history and physical exam, an explanation as to the suspected etiology, and a definite plan for further evaluation. Return visits in the ED represent high risk encounters and the evaluation should be complete and detailed.

It is not possible to tell from the third visit if the patient had followed up with his primary care physician. We do have a history and physical exam which is no longer speaking, but screaming, to the ED doctor—this time, the message was heard and acted upon.

TEACHING POINTS ABOUT CASE 28:
- Positive findings from the history, physical exam, and other testing need to be specifically addressed. Unexpected findings during the exam or other testing may require further history to be taken. If a diagnosis is not possible, then a plan should be formed for further evaluation in the near future.
- Endocarditis is a difficult diagnosis to make definitively in the ED, but should remain in the differential diagnosis of patients with fever and heart murmur.

REFERENCES
1. Lilly LS. Pathophysiology of heart disease. Philadelphia:Lea & Febiger;1993: 27.
2. Tintinalli JE, ed. Emergency medicine. A comprehensive study guide. 5th ed. New York:McGraw-Hill; 2000: 382.
3. http://quickfacts.census.gov/qfd/states/39000.html
4. Harper SA, Fukuda K, Uyeki TM, et al. Prevention and control of influenza. MMWR, May 28, 2004;53 (RR06): 1-40.
5. Derlet R, Lawrence R. Influenza. http://www.emedicine.com/MED/topic1170.htm, reference date 5/15/05.
6. Taubenberger JK, Reid AH, Fanning TG. Capturing a killer flu virus. Scientific American, January 2005, 62-71.
7. Package insert. Influenza virus vaccine live, Intranasal FluMist® 2004-2005 Formula. MedImmune Vaccines, Inc. Gaithersburg, MD, March 2005.
8. Friedman MJ, Attia MW. Clinical predictors of influenza in children. Arch Pediatr Adolesc Med 2004;158: 391-4 (Comment 2004;158:1018).
9. Package insert. QuickVue® Influenza A+B Test, Quidel Corporation, San Diego, CA, April 2004.
10. Ruest A, Michaud S, Deslandes S, et al. Comparison of the Directigen Flu A+B Test, the QuickVue influenza test, and clinical case definition to viral culture and reverse transcription-PCR for rapid diagnosis of influenza virus infection. J Clin Microbiol 2003;41: 3487-93.
11. E.I. du Pont de Nemours and Company, web site: http://heritage.dupont.com/floater/fl_symmetrel/floater.shtml, as of May 2005
12. Lew W, Chen X, Kim CU, et al. Discovery and development of GS 4104 (oseltamivir): an orally active influenza neuraminidase inhibitor. Curr Med Chem 2000;7:663-7.
13. Laver WG, Bischofberger N, Webster RG. Disarming flu viruses. Scientific American , January 1999:78-87.

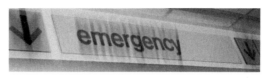

CASE29

29 YEAR OLD FEMALE WITH CHEST PAIN

Commentary:
Gregory L. Henry, MD, FACEP
CEO, Medical Practice Risk Assessment, Inc., Ann Arbor, Michigan
Clinical Professor, Department of Emergency Medicine
   University of Michigan Medical School, Ann Arbor, Michigan
Past President, American College of Emergency Physicians (ACEP)

Discussion:
Raymond Jackson MD, MS, FACEP
Research Director, William Beaumont Hospital, Royal Oak, Michigan
Clinical Professor, Wayne State University College of Medicine
   Detroit, Michigan

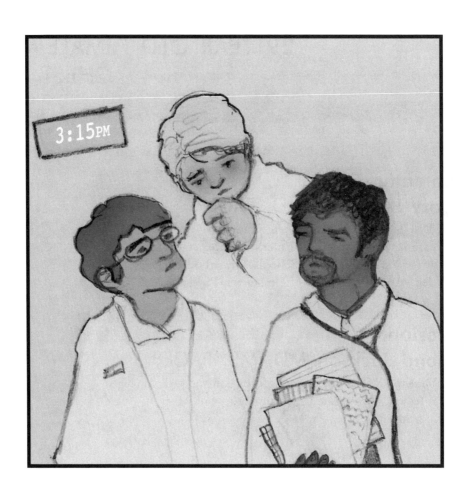

29 YEAR OLD FEMALE WITH CHEST PAIN

—Initial Visit*—

*Authors' Note: The history, exam and notes are the actual documentation of the physicians and providers, including abbreviations (and spelling errors)

CHIEF COMPLAINT (at 10:28): Chest pain, neck pain and hurts to breathe

```
VITAL SIGNS
Time      Temp     Pulse    Resp     Syst     Diast    O2 Sat   Pain
10:40     95.3     64       16       104      80       99%      6
15:07              68       16       84       60
16:10     97.4     64       16       90       58                2
```

HISTORY OF PRESENT ILLNESS (at 11:51): The patient with a past history of c-section term delivery 1 month ago arrives ambulatory and presents with complaints of moderate chest pain that began gradually 2 day(s) ago. The symptoms are constant. It is a heaviness pain located in the left chest area. The pain radiates to the left flank. The pain started while at rest. The patient complains of chest discomfort with deep breathing and twisting. The patient denies shortness of breath, diaphoresis, fever, nausea, vomiting, abdominal pain, cough. No history of ischemic disease.

PAST MEDICAL HISTORY/TRIAGE:
   Medications: None
   Allergies: No known allergies.
   PMH: None
   PSH: None
   SocHx: Tobacco use: (-), Drug use: (-)

EXAM (at 11:54):
   General: Well-appearing; thin; in no acute respiratory distress
   Head: Normocephalic; atraumatic
   Neck: Supple; non-tender; no cervical lymphadenopathy; no masses or thyromegaly, no JVD
   Card: The heart has a regular rate and rhythm; normal S1, S2; no S3 or S4; no murmurs, rubs, or gallops. The pulses are equal bilaterally and there is brisk capillary refill. There is no peripheral edema
   Resp: Breath sounds clear and equal bilaterally; no wheezes, rhonchi, or rales
   Chest: Symptoms easily reproduced with right thoracic rotation and palpation of the painful area.
   Ext: Normal ROM in all four extremities; calves non-tender to palpation
   Skin: Normal for age and race; warm; dry; good turgor; no rash noted

ORDERS (at 11:02): Torodol 30mg IM

PA AND LATERAL CHEST (ordered at 11:01): Normal PA and lateral chest.

RESULTS (results received at 12:36)

Test	Flag	Value	Units	Ref. Range
WBC		6.1	K/uL	4.6-10.2
HGB	L	11.4	G/DL	12.0-16.0
PLT		191	K/uL	142-424

Test	Flag	Value	Units	Ref. Range
D-Dimer	*	>1000	NG/ML	<500

Test	Flag	Value	Units	Ref. Range
CKMB		0.0	NG/ML	0.0-5.0
TROPI	H	.29	NG/ML	.00-.27
PROTIME		12.1	SEC	9.6-13.2
INR		1.0		

VENTILATION/PERFUSION LUNG SCAN (ordered at 12:28): Moderate sized pulmonary embolus to the posterior left lower lobe.

PROGRESS NOTES (at 14:53): Moderate probability for PE. Does have limited risk with BCP use. Will further evaluate through venous duplex scan of legs. (At 15:42) I ordered Lovenox 50 mg SQ and spoke with PCP for hospital admission.

DIAGNOSIS (at 15:31): Pulmonary – embolism

DISPOSITION (at 15:53): Patient assigned to Telemetry bed and released from the ED at 16:59.

INPATIENT COURSE

Per hospital physician: This is a 29-year-old female with a recent history of c-section with a two-day history of pleuritic chest pain on the left side. She had a VQ scan which per report from the emergency room was intermediate probability. I talked with the patient and according to the patient her chest discomfort had completely resolved and she was anxious to go home. The patient had Dopplers of the lower extremities, which were negative for any deep venous thromboses. A helical CT was performed to check for a pulmonary embolism. The Helical CT was negative for pulmonary embolism and the patient was discharged home. After the pain which brought her to the ED, she did not have any pain until the day of discharge, at which point she had a recurrent pain in her chest that she says she is unable to describe. The patient denied any fevers or chills.

DISPOSITION: Based on negative helical CT and negative venous Doppler exam, the anticoagulation was stopped and she was discharged from the hospital.

Gregory L. Henry comments:

"There is probably nothing less useful than an equivocal VQ scan"

Post-surgical patients have an increased risk of a pulmonary embolus (PE). It is the one disease entity where a statistical analysis of risk must predominate. Everything is based on probability theory—whether one uses the Wells criteria, Geneva criteria, or other criteria, the physician must have some logical base on which to make decisions. No one should be misled by the D-dimer. It is sensitive, but hardly specific. A patient with a major operation within the past month would have an elevated D-dimer, and it does not help with clinical decisions.

The patient with chest pain needs to have a careful history taken. Our patient's discomfort occurred with deep breathing and movement, which almost always signifies a musculoskeletal or pleural etiology. The lack of fever, diaphoresis, or cough argues against a post-operative infection. There is a discrepancy on the chart—the triage note indicates the patient is not taking medications, yet the progress note indicates that she is taking birth control pills. Inconsistencies on the chart need to be resolved and noted.

The evaluation of this patient is reasonable. The history notes an increase in pain with twisting and the physical exam documents that her pain is easily reproduced with thoracic rotation. Virtually no cardiac or mediastinal condition causes pain worsened with palpation. With the patient otherwise looking well, this is, to some extent, reassuring.

It is interesting that the patient's diagnosis was based on a ventilation and perfusion scan, which was considered mid-zone probability. Nothing is less useful than an equivocal V/Q scan. The reasonable workup of this patient, who had reproducible musculo-skeletal pain and a pulse ox of 99%, should include a Doppler of her lower extremity deep veins. The Doppler study in this case was negative, with an in-hospital negative helical CT scan. The helical CT is not perfect and may miss very small lesions, but, in combination with a negative Doppler study, puts the probability of PE at less than 1%. The decision to stop anticoagulation at this point is a reasonable one.

Risk management ratings follow…

29 YEAR OLD FEMALE WITH CHEST PAIN

—Second Visit: 2 Days Later—

CHIEF COMPLAINT (at 07:25): Chest pain

```
VITAL SIGNS
Time      Temp     Pulse    Resp     Syst     Diast    O2 Sat
07:36     98.2     84       16       114      77       99%
12:41              60       16       107      74
13:53              72       20       92       60
```

HISTORY OF PRESENT ILLNESS (at 08:56): The patient presents with complaints of severe, intermittent chest pain that began gradually 4 day(s) ago. She was here in the ED and had a V/Q scan which showed intermediate probability and was started on Lovenox and was admitted. A helical CT of the chest and venous Dopplers of the lower extremities were negative for PE, so the pt. was sent home yesterday. The discomfort is currently 5/10. The discomfort was previously 10/10. It is a pressure located in the left chest area, which radiates to the neck and began while she was sleeping. Patient denies chest discomfort with exertion. She does have associated SOB and nausea. Prior treatment includes Tylenol, which was not effective. She denies peripheral edema, fever, diaphoresis, vomiting, dizziness, calf muscle pain.

PAST MEDICAL HISTORY/TRIAGE:
  Medications: None
  Allergies: No known allergies.
  PMH: None
  PSH: None

EXAM (at 09:00):
  General: Alert and oriented X3, well-nourished, well appearing, in no apparent distress
  Head: Normocephalic; atraumatic.
  Eyes: PERRL
  Nose: The nose is normal in appearance without rhinorrhea
  Resp: Normal chest excursion with respiration; breath sounds clear and equal bilaterally; no wheezes, rhonchi, or rales
  Card: Regular rhythm, without murmurs, rubs or gallops
  Abd: Non-distended; non-tender, soft, without rigidity, rebound or guarding
  Skin: Normal for age and race; warm and dry; no apparent lesions
  Chest: Does have left chest and left neck pain with palpation
  Extremities: Pulses are 2 plus and equal times 4 extremities, no peripheral edema or calf muscle pain.

PROGRESS NOTES: I spoke with patient's primary care physician, the pulmonologist on call (10:30), and then the radiologist (10:30). I also spoke with interventional radiology (10:38) and they will come in to do a pulmonary angiogram.

ORDERS (at 10:52): Demerol 25 mg IV, Phenergan 12.5mg IV

RESULTS:
   PA and left lateral chest (at 08:22): Rather small left pleural effusion.
   Pulmonary angiogram (at 12:11) Angiographic finding is compatible with embolic disease to the left lower lobe.

PROGRESS NOTES (at 12:15): Will anticoagulate with lovenox 50mg SQ and coumadin 7.5mg PO. I spoke with the PCP for admission and they recommended a pulmonary consult. (At 12:55) I spoke with the pulmonologist.

DIAGNOSIS (at 12:19): Embolism - pulmonary w/ infarction

DISPOSITION (at 12:14): Admit to telemetry. Pt. discharged to the floor at 14:20.

INPATIENT COURSE

Per pulmonologist: This very pleasant 29-year-old Somalian female was status delivery of her first child via cesarean section 1 month ago. She is on Depo-Provera. She is a nonsmoker. She was admitted to the hospital via the Emergency Room earlier this weekend with chest pain and underwent ventilation/perfusion scanning. The primary physician and I discussed the case by telephone yesterday and, at that point, we were aware that the patient had what was read as an intermediate probability ventilation/perfusion scan. D-dimer was positive but lower extremity venous duplex were negative, and I advised that the patient get a CT scan with pulmonary embolus protocol. This was negative, and the patient was discharged. The patient returned to the Emergency Room today because her chest pain had recurred. It is in the left lower chest area, somewhat posterior and pleuritic in nature, worse with a deep breath in. She has not had any fevers, chills, sputum or hemoptysis. She has not noticed any lower extremity pain or edema. Venous duplex studies performed yesterday were negative. The patient has not had diaphoresis or rigor but did note a little bit of nausea without vomiting as well as some abdominal pain, which was transient in nature. The patient was evaluated, and I discussed the situation with the ED doctor. We agreed that it would be appropriate to check an angiogram, and this was positive, documenting a clot in the left lower lobe circulation. In retrospect, review of the ventilation/perfusion scan yesterday, as well as the dictation, lists it as not moderate probability but positive for a moderate size pulmonary embolus with a wedge-shaped perfusion defect, unmatched with ventilation deficit, in the left lower lobe extending out to the pleura.

IMPRESSION:
   1. Left lower lobe pulmonary embolus postpartum, with most likely source of embolus being the uterine veins status post cesarean section.
   2. Abnormal V/Q scan.
   3. Shortness of breath.
   4. Pleuritic chest pain.
   5. Left-sided pleural effusion with pleurisy.

PLANS: Treat the patient with bed rest and Lovenox anticoagulation. She is not breast-feeding, and we will go ahead and start Coumadin, and I will provide her with Coumadin literature. I will maintain pain control with nonsteroidal anti-inflammatory agents. I will maintain the patient on bed rest, despite the negative venous duplex, left. The venous duplex exams have missed a lower extremity clot. Forty-eight (48) hours from now, she can resume normal activity, however. I have told the patient her estimated length of stay is probably on the order of 4-5 days for therapeutic anticoagulation. I have encouraged her to remain off of her Depo-Provera birth control because of its association with thrombotic events and to use another form of birth control. We will probably be able to discontinue anticoagulation after 6-9 months. I would check her ventilation/perfusion scan at 4 months in order to determine resolution.

30 YEAR OLD FEMALE WITH CHEST PAIN

—Third Visit: 5 Months Later—

CHIEF COMPLAINT (AT 11:42): Chest pain

```
VITAL SIGNS
Time       Temp      Pulse    Resp     Syst     Diast    O2 Sat
11:43      98.0        71       16       96       65       99%
13:21                  59       16      138       82       99%
13:55                           16      143       85
14:47                  62       18      104       64
```

HISTORY OF PRESENT ILLNESS (at 13:08): 30 y/o Somali female, c/o intermittent gradual onset of intermittent left sided chest heaviness, radiating down left side of body to left knee, for last 2 weeks. She was sent over from her clinic due to her doctor thinking she had abnormal EKG today in office. She was admitted in November and December last year for possible PE, but sent home after no definitive labs for PE as well as neg Chest CT, neg Dopplers , although she did have a positive arteriogram later noted on the chart. . She was anticoagulated in hospital. She states this time she only has the CP at night and never during day. She is unable to sleep at night. She denies any dec. in activity, calf pain, no long car rides, or BCP's. She is on depo. She had a baby in Sept. 2002. She is a single mother taking care of 3 children under age 3. She doesn't eat very much or well at all. she states "no appetite". She missed her last Depo shot a few weeks ago, but has been on since her dx back in nov/dec. She states she went off Coumadin 1 month ago. She is in no pain currently on exam or thorough out her stay here. No chest discomfort with exertion, twisting, arm movement. She does have assoc. lightheadedness. Denies SOB, fever, cough, diaphoresis, abd. pain, n/v, calf muscle pain, syncope.

PAST MEDICAL HISTORY/TRIAGE (per RN): Sent in by doctor, have bad EKG
    Medications: None
    Allergies: No known allergies.

PMH: PE
PSH: None
SocHx: Nonsmoker

EXAM (at 13:12):

General: Very thin black female individual in no acute distress. af, nt, non tachycardic, VSS

Eyes: Pupils are equal, round and reactive to light.

Neck: The neck is supple and non-tender to palpation. There is no cervical lymphadenopathy.

Cardiovascular: The heart has a regular rate and rhythm. S1 and S2 are normal. There are no murmurs, rubs, or gallops. Pulses are equal bilaterally and there is brisk capillary refill. There is some mild left ant-lateral chest wall tenderness.

Respiratory: The respiratory rate and effort are normal. There is normal chest excursion with respiration. The lungs are clear to auscultation and percussion bilaterally.

GI: The abdomen is normal in appearance. There is no pain with palpation. No masses were palpated. No rigidity, rebound or guarding.

Musculoskeletal: There are no deformities noted in all four extremities.

Ext: No calf swelling, or tenderness bilat.

Skin: The skin appears normal for age and race. It is warm and dry. No diaphoresis.

RESULTS (AT14:34):

Test	Flag	Value	Units	Ref. Range
WBC		4.2	K/uL	4.6-10.2
HGB		12.0	G/DL	12.0-16.0
PLT		195	K/uL	142-424

Test	Flag	Value	Units	
D-dimer	H	793	NG/ML	<500

PA AND LATERAL CHEST (ordered at 12:48): Normal PA and lateral chest.

VENTILATION/PERFUSION LUNG SCAN (ordered at 14:45, results received by physician at 17:12): A fairly large area of at least one to two segments and perhaps two segmental perfusion/ventilation mismatch at the left lung base. This is intermediate to high probability for pulmonary embolus.

PROGRESS NOTES (at 17:19): Patient given Lovenox SQ. This patient states she feels like she can't stay and needs to go home tonight and "will return tomorrow—I have things to do tonight and can't stay." She feels as though she is not that sick because she doesn't have any pain right now. She is told not to leave as she needs to be admitted and she is still refusing. She has been informed of all risks, including death, by myself. She is still refusing to stay and will sign AMA form.

PROGRESS NOTES (per social work at 15:44):
Pt with 3 small children who are in daycare today and pt was to pick them up at 4:00 and stated she had no one to get them for her. However on the chart it was noted that pt has a spouse and a call

was placed to the home. Spoke with her husband and he states he can get the children. He asked for pt to give him a call. Talked to pt in room and helped her to a phone to place a call home. Will follow to see if additional needs arise.

DIAGNOSIS (at 17:13): PE (Pulmonary embolism)

DISPOSITION (at 18:13): RN notes: The patient states an intent to refuse admission. An AMA form was signed. She was instructed to return as soon as possible. Left the ED at 18:41.

30 YEAR OLD FEMALE WITH CHEST PAIN

—Fourth Visit: 1 Day Later—

CHIEF COMPLAINT (at 16:47): Chest pain – "I think I have a blood clot."

VITAL SIGNS						
Time	Temp	Pulse	Resp	Syst	Diast	O2 Sat
17:13	97.6	94	18	119	85	100%
19:05		76	16	96	60	100%

HISTORY OF PRESENT ILLNESS (at 18:52): The patient has returned with no change in her condition. I had seen her yesterday with a diagnosis of PE. She elected to sign out AMA yesterday. She was given a dose of Lovenox. She feels about the same. Complains of chest pain, SOB. Denies, fever, n/v, rhinorrhea, calf muscle pain.

PAST MEDICAL HISTORY/TRIAGE:
   Medications: None
   Allergies: No known allergies.
   PMH: PE
   PSH: None

EXAM (at 18:53):
   General: Alert and oriented X3, well-nourished, well appearing, in no apparent distress
   Head: Normocephalic; atraumatic.
   Eyes: PERRL
   Resp: Breath sounds clear and equal bilaterally; no wheezes, rhonchi, or rales
   Card: Regular rhythm, without murmurs, rubs or gallops
   Abd: Non-distended; non-tender, soft, without rigidity, rebound or guarding

ORDERS (at 18:50): CBC, PT, PTT, IV Heparin bolus and infusion

RESULTS:

Test	Flag	Value	Units	Ref. Range
WBC		5.3	K/uL	4.6-10.2
HGB		12.0	G/DL	12.0-16.0
PLT		200	K/uL	142-424
PROTIME		11.9	SEC	9.6-13.2
INR		1.0		

DIAGNOSIS (at 17:42): Pulmonary embolism

DISPOSITION (at 19:49): Patient assigned to telemetry

HOSPITAL COURSE

DISCUSSION PER PULMONOLOGIST: She has a probable recurrent left sided pulmonary embolus. We will rule out a hypercoagulable state. We will place the patient back on therapeutic anticoagulation. I will review the chart, but my expectation is to strongly recommend that the patient not be placed on Depo-Provera, and use an alternative form of birth control because of the likelihood it is producing a tendency toward thrombi. The patient may require life-long anticoagulation, because of her high-risk of recurrent pulmonary emboli and subsequent death from same.

Additional comments by Gregory L. Henry:

It just so happens that the patient did return, a PE was found, and therapy was required. However, the thought process involved during the initial ED visit and hospitalization was reasonable. Taking the patient off hormonal birth control, with a workup for a hypercoagulable state, is important and should be undertaken. The frustration of the patient is clear in this case.

Whenever a patient is noncompliant, the documentation needs to be excellent. On this patient's third visit, she left against medical advice; it is important to have incredibly careful documentation of the patient's capacity, family interaction, verbal communication, and subsequent referral/follow up.

Obviously, a patient who has had multiple PEs needs evaluation for more definitive therapy. The possibility that she may require a Greenfield filter needs to be entertained.

- Thoroughness of Documentation: 8 out of 10.

- Thoroughness of Patient Evaluation: 9 out of 10.

- Risk of Serious Illness Being Missed: Medium risk.

- Risk Management Legal Rating: Medium risk.

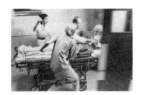

RISK AND EVALUATION OF VENOUS THROMBOEMBOLIC EVENTS IN THE ED, COMMUNICATION AND INTERPRETATION OF LAB RESULTS

Raymond Jackson MD, MS, FACEP

I. INTRODUCTION AND DIFFERENTIAL DIAGNOSIS OF CHEST PAIN

This instructive case addresses a number of important issues we encounter daily: 1) communication; 2) interpretation of test results; 3) how we resolve conflicting information; and 4) dealing with difficult patients.

I am impressed with the initial diagnostic evaluation by the emergency physician (EP) in this case. The primary symptom is left pleuritic chest pain that radiates to the back. Judging from the history, physical exam and pattern of ancillary test orders, the EP considered cardiac, respiratory, and thromboembolic etiologies. An initial differential diagnosis in a previously healthy young woman includes coronary artery disease, pulmonary embolism, pericarditis, pneumothorax, pneumonia, and musculoskeletal pain.

Her symptoms did not have characteristics of a gastrointestinal source. Aortic dissection is extremely unlikely given her age, no history of hypertension, and without mention of Marfanoid features. The onset was gradual, with no associated symptoms, including shortness of breath. The discomfort was worsened with twisting and deep breaths—this combination points to a musculoskeletal etiology, but does not exclude the other considerations. The vital signs and room air pulse oximetry were also normal, which does not exclude embolism, but also does not increase our suspicion. The initial history documented that she is not on any medications. Thiis is inconsistent with a progress note noting, "Does have limited risk with BCP use." In addition, the pulmonologist's inpatient note after the second ED visit stated that she is on Depo-Provera. This is communication failure #1. Finally, no family history is noted.

II. RISK FOR VENOUS THROMBOEMBOLIC EVENTS

Both the post-partum state and post-operative state increase the risk for venous thromboembolic (VTE) events. Our evaluation requires an increased level of suspicion for VTE, as patient presentations are rarely straightforward. Most emergency physicians use their experience to determine the pretest probability for pulmonary embolism; we typically look for classic "risk factors" such as advanced age, cancer, immobilization, recent surgery, personal or family history of VTE, pregnancy, and postpartum states. Typically this method works, but there is variation between individual physician assessments.

There are 2 validated methodologies to place patients into risk categories. The Canadian score[13] has 7 items, and requires the physician to determine if another diagnosis is more or less likely than PE, requiring a bit of circular logic. (Tables 1 and 2). In our case, the Canadian criteria would yield either a Low (3.6%) probability or Moderate (20.5%) probability, depending on whether the physician judged another diagnosis was less likely then PE.

Table 1. Canadian Score for Pretest Probability

Criteria	Points
Suspected DVT	3.0
Alternative Dx less likely then PE	3.0
Heart Rate > 100 /min	1.5
Immobilization or surgery in previous 4 weeks	1.5
Previous DVT/PE	1.5
Hemoptysis	1.5
Malignancy (on treatment, treated in past 6 mo., or palliative)	1.0

Table 2. Interpretation of Canadian Score

Score Range	Mean Probability of PE	Patients with Score	Interpretation
0-2	3.6%	40%	Low
3-6	20.5%	53%	Moderate
>6	66.7%	7%	High

The Charlotte score[5] has 6 items in the algorithm to determine if a patient requires immediate imaging, or can be safely ruled out with a negative D-dimer. (Figure 1) With the Charlotte score, our patient qualified to have a D-dimer rule-out. Regardless of which method was used, the emergency physician was obligated to obtain a D-dimer in this case.

Figure 1. Charlotte Score

The Probability for PE with a "safe" score is 13% which allows for a rule-out with a Turbidimetric or an ELISA D-dimer.

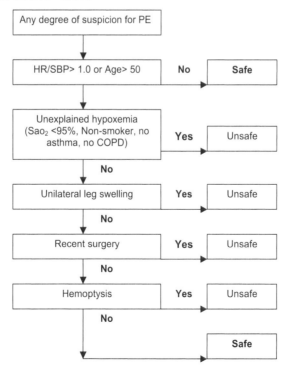

III. USE OF THE D-DIMER

The initial ED management of this case revealed a normal ECG, with an elevated D-Dimer and Troponin. The D-dimer was >1000. Though we are not certain which assay was used, with the commonly used VIDAS ELISA D-dimer, a level of >1000 has a positive Likelihood Ratio (LR+) of about 3.[4] This means that 3 out of every 4 such results are truly positive. Though this likelihood ratio does not make a D-dimer of >1000 diagnostic, defined as an LR+ of >10, it does increase the probability that this patient has a VTE. The exact timing of decreasing D-dimer levels after surgery or delivery has not been reliably established, but an elevated D-dimer level 4 weeks after surgery should definitely increase our suspicion.

The greatest utility for the D-dimer assay is in patients with a low pretest probability combined with a low D-Dimer. For the VIDAS ELISA D-dimer, a value < 500 reduces the VTE probability to < 1% for low-risk patients. In this case, we note an elevated Troponin level, indicating some myocardial damage. It is well known that a significant pulmonary embolism elevates the Troponin level, due to increased strain on the right ventricle; elevated troponin also signifies an increase in 30-day mortality.[8,9] Myocardial ischemia, coronary artery disease, renal disease, and myocarditis are unlikely causes for the elevated troponin, given our patient's sex, age, normal creatinine, and normal ECG. The only other explanations for an elevated Troponin are a pulmonary embolism or laboratory error.

IV. THE VENTILATION-PERFUSION (V/Q) SCAN

After the initial results are received, the EP correctly pursues a thromboembolic event by obtaining a Ventilatory-Perfusion (V/Q) scan, which is reported as showing a "moderately sized embolus in posterior left lower lobe." This report and location are consistent with the patient's history, symptoms, and elevated D-dimer and Troponin. What is inconsistent is the wording of the interpretation of the V/Q scan. We have become accustomed to the PIOPED definitions for interpretation of these tests. The PIOPED investigators clearly defined what constitutes high, intermediate, and low probability scans, as well as normal and indeterminate scans.[3]

Though the wording of the interpretation is in plain English, the confusion it wrought by straying from the exact PIOPED wording is instructive. This is communication error #2. The EP translated the wording "Moderate size" to "Moderate Probability" and eventually it became "Intermediate Probability." I may have done the same in the confusing, hectic environment of a busy ED. One of the biggest downfalls of the V/Q scan is the wording of the interpretation and its subsequent interpretation.

The PIOPED investigation revealed poor inter-rater reliability between Low and Intermediate Scan interpretations. Since neither interpretation significantly alters the probability of PE (LR for 'low' is 0.3 and LR for "intermediate" is 1.2), they both have been lumped into a "non-diagnostic" category. Despite all this, the EP correctly starts Lovenox, and admits the patient to a telemetry bed.

V. INPATIENT COURSE—MISCOMMUNICATION AND MISINTERPRETATION

The inpatient course revealed more miscommunication and misinterpretation. The inpatient physician relied on the EP report of the V/Q scan, noting it was an intermediate probability, not what appears on the radiology report to indicate a high probability scan with a moderately sized embolism. This leads the inpatient physician to doubt the diagnosis. Given this confusion, this physician ordered a Venous Doppler study and a helical CT. Does a normal Venous Doppler alter the probability of a pulmonary embolism? The answer is no.[2] Fully 50% of patients with a PE will have no evidence of a concurrent DVT, either because the source is the pelvic veins, or the clot has fully embolized.

However, a normal helical CT is problematic. Multi-row detector scanners are now considered the gold standard for pulmonary embolism.[10,11] Was this a 16 row multi-detector scanner? Was the patient able to breath-hold sufficiently? Was the radiologist aware of the V/Q result? Regardless, the inpatient physician now faces the following dilemma: Should I believe the CT or the V/Q? Most likely this physician interpreted the tests as an intermediate (read non-diagnostic) probability V/Q and a negative CT, with a negative venous Doppler. With the patient claiming to be asymptomatic and pushing to go home, who would not stop anticoagulation and discharge the patient?

VI. CONTINUATION OF CASE—HOSPITAL DISCHARGE AND ED RETURN

Two days after discharge the patient returns with continued pain. Vital signs and pulse oximetry are still normal. Is a normal room air pulse oximetry consistent with PE? The answer is yes. An unexplained low pulse oximetry (Less than 95% with no history of asthma, COPD, or smoking) increases the probability of PE, but a normal pulse oximetry does not alter the probabilities. If the patient has a PE, a low pulse oximtery increases the risk of mortality.[7] The emergency physician was faced with a symptomatic patient and conflicting test results. He needed a tie-breaker test and chose the Pulmonary Angiogram, which confirmed the V/Q results. Other options included reviewing and reinterpreting the prior scans if available, or echocardiography. If the ECHO revealed evidence of right heart dilatation, this would have supported the diagnosis of PE. The patient is again placed on anticoagulation and admitted. No testing for hypercoagulable states, such as Protein C and S deficiencies, was performed, since the inpatient physician assumed the VTE was due to the combination of surgery, post-partum state and Depo-Provera. This story should be over.

But the patient returns with left sided chest heaviness 5 months later, off Coumadin and on Depo-Provera! Her D-dimer is again elevated and her V/Q scan was interpreted as Intermediate to High probability for another PE. Again, this type of hedge interpretation does not help the treating physician. Is it Intermediate or High? During a 1-year period at our institution, we noted 10 different combinations of the PIOPED reporting definitions!

VII. LEAVING AGAINST MEDICAL ADVICE

Again, the patient talks the physician into letting her leave, this time against medical advice. She promises to return the next day, which she does. Though she signs the AMA form, does she understands the potential lethality of this condition? Should the physician have "protected her against her decision" by giving a dose of Lovenox? My philosophy is to let the patient go ahead and leave, but ask the patient to let me do my best to continue to treat you. Our responsibility does not end with the AMA form.

VIII. RISK OF MORTALITY AND FIBRINOLYTIC THERAPY IN ACUTE PE

What should we do when we confirm a diagnosis of a PE? We first must assess the risk for mortality. A patient's risk increases with an unexplained low room air pulse oximetry or a shock index (HR/ Systolic BP) of > 1. Evidence of right heart dilation on Echocardiography or helical CT scanning is also associated with increased mortality. Any rise in Troponin, CK-MB, or B-type Naturetic Peptide (BNP) may reflect right ventricular dysfunction. These are high-risk patients and we should consider the risks and benefits of fibrinolytic treatment. It is clear that in cases of hypotension from PE, we should strongly consider fibrinolytic therapy. Secondly, the inpatient physician needs to explore the underlying etiology for the VTE.

IX. LESSONS LEARNED FROM THIS CASE—COMMUNICATION, INTERPRETATION OF LAB RESULTS, AND CULTURAL BARRIERS

What can we learn from this complicated case? First, clear communication is a key component of medical care. It begins with communication between the physician and patient. It is not clear to me that this patient was able to clearly articulate her complaints and situation to the physicians, or maybe the physicians did not ask all the important questions. During one visit it was stated she was Somalian, and there may have been a language and/or cultural barrier that made this interaction more prone to error. Twice, on the first and third visits, she was able to convince the physicians to allow her to leave. We all fall into this trap of letting the patient make the decision for us; most of the time it is the right decision, this time it was not. There may have been cultural issues or home pressures that motivated her to push for leaving. The inconsistent documentation of her use of Depo-Provera could have altered the physician's perception of the probability of PE. The importance of communication continues with the importance of communication between physicians. We have already discussed the importance of precise wording in the interpretation of V/Q scans. Another failure is the lack of communication between the inpatient physician and her gynecologist—she continued to use depoprovera after her PE. Malpractice cases have an average of 9 teamwork failures, with communication being the greatest shortcoming.[12] This case had almost that many failures.

Proper interpretation of test results is key to good patient care, especially in the diagnosis of PE. We have discussed the importance of following the exact PIOPED definitions for interpretation of V/Q scans. With the advent of multi-row Helical Chest CT scanning, V/Q scans should only be ordered for patients with dye allergy, renal insufficiency or those too obese to fit in a CT scanner. If obtained, treating physicians should understand that the Low and Intermediate interpretations neither exclude nor confirm the diagnosis, and should be viewed as non-diagnostic results. I also see frequent misinterpretation of D-dimer results. First, we should only obtain this test in patients with a low (<15% probability) of a PE. A sufficiently low D-dimer value in this setting reduces the probability of PE to less than 1%. D-dimer rises with age, so its value for patients over age 70 is poor, though further research may determine a different cut-off value for the geriatric population. The confusion over D-dimer interpretation comes from higher values. Some D-dimer assays, such as the ELISA, report values in an interval scale up to 10,000 ng/mL. Our observations indicate increased likelihood of a VTE with increases in D-dimer values. Finally, I would like to reemphasize that a negative venous Doppler exam does not exclude the probability of PE, just the presence of a lower extremity DVT.

We frequently have conflicting data from the history, exam, laboratory and radiological tests. We weigh each factor using our experience and knowledge, but we often come to a point where we can neither exclude nor confirm the diagnosis. When this occurs, further testing, or re-evaluation of data, interpretations and assumptions, is required.

Certain patients' presentations represent high risk encounters for physicians. Problems with communication, either because of language barriers or dysphasia, rob physicians of the key to diagnosis: an accurate history. Cultural barriers can also lead to less than optimal physician-patient interactions. Personality conflicts are also high-risk encounters. In each of these situations, a more extensive diagnostic evaluation should be considered. As occurred during our patient's third visit, when a patient pushes to leave, we should consider alternate ways to treat the patient.

TEACHING POINTS ABOUT CASE 29:

- A normal heart rate and repiratory rate reading do not exclude the diagnosis of pulmonary embolism.
- An unexplained low pulse oximetry ($< 95\%$ with no history of Asthma, COPD, or smoking) increases the probability of PE, but a normal pulse oximetry does not alter the probabilities.
- The chart should be consistent and discrepancies between nursing and physician documentation addressed.
- A negative venous Doppler exam does not exclude the probability of PE, just the presence of a DVT.
- With the advent of multi-row Helical Chest CT scanning, V/Q scans should only be ordered for patients with dye allergy, renal insufficiency or those too obese to fit in a CT scanner.
- V/Q scans should be read per PIOPED definitions.

REFERENCES

1. Christiansen F, Anderson T, Rydman H, et al. Rater agreement in lung scintigraphy. Acta Radiologica 1996;37: 754-78.
2. Daniel KR, Jackson RE, Kline JA. Utility of lower extremity venous ultrasound scanning in the diagnosis and exclusion of pulmonary embolism in outpatients. Ann Emerg Med 2000;35: 547-54.
3. Gottschalk A, Sostman HD, Coleman RE, et al. Ventilation-perfusion scintigraphy in the PIOPED study. Part II. Evaluation of the scintigraphic criteria and interpretations. J Nucl Med 1993;34: 1119-26.
4. Jackson RE, Mattson J. Is the Current Diagnostic Cutoff for Enzyme-linked Immunosorbent Assay D-dimer Too Low? Acad Emerg Med (Abstract) 2005;12: 41.
5. Kline JA, Nelson RD, Jackson RE, et al. Criteria for the safe use of D-dimer testing in the emergency department with suspected pulmonary embolism: a multicenter United States study. Ann Emerg Med 2002;39:144-52.
6. Kline JA, Wells PS. Methodology for a rapid protocol to rule out pulmonary embolism in the emergency department. Ann Emerg Med 2003;42: 266-75.
7. Kline JA, Hernandez-Nino J, Newgard CD, et al. Use of pulse oximetry to predict in-hospital complications in normotensive patients with pulmonary embolism. Am J Med 2003;115: 203-8.
8. La Vecchia L, Ottani F, Favero L, et al. Increased cardiac troponin I on admission predicts in-hospital mortality in acute pulmonary embolism. Heart 2004;90: 633-7.
9. Pruszcyk P. Cardiac troponin T monitoring identifies high-risk group of normotensive patients with acute pulmonary embolism. Chest 2003;123: 1947-52.
10. Schoepf UJ, Costello P. CT angiography for diagnosis of pulmonary embolism: state of the art. Radiology 2004;230: 329
11. Schoepf UJ, Goldhaber SZ, Costello P. Spiral computed tomography for acute pulmonary embolism. Circulation 2004;109: 2160-7.

12. Schenkel S. Promoting patient safety and preventing medical error in emergency departments. Acad Emerg Med 2000;7: 1204-22.
13. Wells PS, Anderson DR, Rodger M, et al. Excluding pulmonary embolism at the bedside without diagnostic imaging: management of patients with suspected pulmonary embolism presenting to the emergency department by using a simple model. Ann Intern Med 2001;135: 98-107.

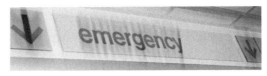

CASE 30

5 MONTH OLD MALE WITH A COUGH & EASY BRUISING

Commentary:
Gregory L. Henry, MD, FACEP

CEO, Medical Practice Risk Assessment, Inc., Ann Arbor, Michigan
Clinical Professor, Department of Emergency Medicine
   University of Michigan Medical School, Ann Arbor, Michigan
Past President, American College of Emergency Physicians (ACEP)

Discussion:
Sharon E. Mace, MD, FACEP, FAAP

Clinical Director, Observation Unit
Director, Pediatric Education/Quality Improvement
   Cleveland Clinic Foundation, Cleveland, Ohio
Author, *Pain Management and Sedation: Emergency Department Management*

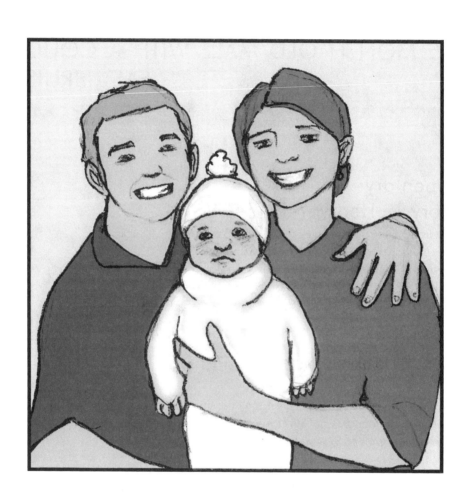

5 MONTH OLD MALE WITH A COUGH & EASY BRUISING

—Initial Visit*—

*Authors' Note: The history, exam and notes are the actual documentation of the physicians and providers, including abbreviations (and spelling errors)

CHIEF COMPLAINT (at 10:50): Cough

```
VITAL SIGNS
Time      Temp      Pulse      Resp  Pulse ox
10:53     100.1     140        24       92%
```

HISTORY OF PRESENT ILLNESS (at 11:21): 5 month old male with multiple visits for URI in the past with complaint of cough for 4 days associated with clear rhinorrhea and tugging at the ears. Taking fluids and bottle well. There have been 8 wet diapers. Does have diarrhea X 4. Mother complains of easy bruising and there is bruising at the external right ear and left wrist. Had been on an ATB 2-3 weeks ago – does not know name of ATB.

PAST MEDICAL HISTORY/TRIAGE (at 10:55):
  Past medical history: Chest colds.
  Immunization history: Immunizations are UTD

PHYSICAL EXAM (at 11:23):
  General: No acute distress
  Head: Ant. fontanelle is soft and concave
  Neck: Soft and supple without meningeal signs
  Oral: Mucous membranes are well hydrated
  Ears: TM's pink bilat
  Lungs: Coarse breath sounds without wheezing
  CV: RRR
  Abd: Soft, NT, positive bowel sounds
  Skin: Hyperkeratotic areas without petechiae/purpura to right temple area. Positive ecchymosis to superior helix right ear. No petechiae/purpura about torso or extremities or face

RADIOLOGY (read by ED doctor at 12:24): CXR: Possible right middle lobe infiltrate

ED COURSE (at 12:27): Rocephin 400mg IM

DIAGNOSIS: Acute early RML pneumonia

DISPOSITION: Pediazole, robitussin DM, aftercare instructions for fever, return to the ED tomorrow for recheck and with family doctor on Monday. Discharged from ED at 13:43.

Gregory L. Henry comments:

"The complaint of easy bruising is suspect"

The chief complaint in this case is fever and cough, but the complaint of easy bruising is suspect. This child does not have bruising everywhere on the body; it is localized to the external right ear and left wrist. Injuries such as this are usually from pressure of a striking hand or a slap.

The physical evaluation is, at the least, suspicious for child abuse. Bruises and petechiae in a disseminated fashion point to other diagnosis, but in a specific area (particularly on the head), these lesions are usually related to a direct blow.

Documentation in this case is reasonable, but again very little social information was obtained about the family.

- Thoroughness of Documentation: 7 out of 10.

- Thoroughness of Patient Evaluation: 7 out of 10.

- Risk of Serious Illness Being Missed: High risk.

- Risk Management Legal Rating: High risk.

5 MONTH OLD MALE WITH A COUGH & EASY BRUISING

—Second Visit: 3 Days Later—

CHIEF COMPLAINT (at 19:47) Full arrest

VITAL SIGNS				
Time	Temp	Pulse	Resp	Blood pressure
19:50	98.0	0	0	0

HISTORY OF PRESENT ILLNESS (at 19:47): 5 month old male, apparently was crying at home, as reported by mother and stopped crying. She stated the boyfriend went to check on the child and stated they called 911. Mother states that Fire dept. personnel arrived at the scene about 1 ½ minutes after the call went out. They found the child apneic with a pulse and then when the paramedics arrived the child was apneic without a pulse. They intubated the pt. and transported to the ED. Mother stated the child had been tugging at his ear, but was tolerating fluids well. A chest x-ray performed three days ago did show increased peri-hilar markings consistent with moderate bronchiolitis. The patient was treated with Pediazole and Robitussin and rocephin. During that exam a small amount of hyperkeratotic area was noted over the right temple and a slight amount of dark ecchymosis about the superior helix of the right ear. The mother did deny recent vomiting, but did admit to yellow and green stools which have occurred eight to 10 times per day over the last several days. The mother vehemently denies recent falls on the baby to the floor off of the bed or a couch. There is no history of trauma admitted to by the parents. No history of anything falling on the baby, per both parents who are interviewed.

PAST MEDICAL HISTORY/TRIAGE:

Past medical history: Chest colds and congestion
Social history: The parents are separated. The baby is exposed to secondary tobacco smoke.

PHYSICAL EXAM (at 19:49):

General: CPR is in progress. The patient is intubated and there is a left interosseous line present in the left anterior tibial region which did not seem to be functional during attempted fluid administration. There is no response to painful stimuli.
Head: There is no sign of head trauma noted
Eyes: The pupils are 5 to 6 mm and dilated, nonreactive bilaterally. The fundi were evaluated and retinal hemorrhages are noted about the fundus.
Neuro: There is no gag reflex, no corneal reflex.
Oral: There is blood in the oropharynx
Ears: There is no hemotympanum.
Lungs: There are no spontaneous breath sounds
CV: There are no spontaneous heart tones.
Abd: Unremarkable. Bowel sounds are absent.
Ext: There is deformity of about the right mid tibial region without evidence of laceration.

ED COURSE: The monitor initially showed asystole. The initial O2 saturation was 71%. The tube was noted to be in the esophagus and was pulled out and he was bagged.

At 19:58 the child was re-intubated on the first attempt with a 3.5 ET tube. Patient did receive epinephrine 0.7 cc in the endotracheal tube. Following intubation, the oxygen saturation was in the 92 to 93% range. ABG was drawn.

At 20:04 a second interosseous line was placed proximal to current interosseus line with good flow.

At 20:07 a right central line was attempted but was unsuccessful.

At 20:23 an elective chest tube was performed in the emergency Department.

At 20:27 results of arterial blood gas did show a pH of 7.19, PCO2 of 42, PO2 of 197 with an oxygen saturation of 99%.

At 20:33 the patient was given 700 mg of Rocephin IV.

At 21:12 the Sheriff's department and Child protective services were called for investigation of possible child abuse.

LAB TESTING: White blood cell count was 36,000, hemoglobin 7.2, platelet count 432. The liver function tests were normal except LDH 873. Stool culture and sensitivity, ova and parasite are pending.

RADIOLOGY TESTING: X-ray did show a right tibial fracture suggestive of a spiral fracture. Plain films of the skull showed possible skull fracture. A CAT scan of the head did not show skull fracture or intracerebral bleed or mass effect. A chest x-ray did show multiple rib fractures and suggestion of hemothorax on the right.

ED DIAGNOSIS: Acute right tibial fracture, multiple rib fractures, left hemothorax, status post cardiopulmonary arrest, hypoxic brain injury

DISPOSITION: Patient was admitted to the intensive care unit.

HOSPITAL COURSE AND SUBSEQUENT FOLLOW UP:

This patient did expire 1 day after admission to the intensive care unit. This became a Coroner's case.

FINAL DIAGNOSIS: (Per coroner report):
1. Acute traumatic encephalomalacia (hours) due to acute subdural hemorrhage (hours) due to blunt force trauma consistent with shaking (hours).
2. Other significant injuries include multiple rib fractures of varying age and fractures of the right tibia and fibula.

SUBSEQUENT FOLLOW UP: The police were not able to build a case against the boyfriend after this death. Four years later, though, the boyfriend was accused of beating to death a 4 year old child. The initial ED physician was then called to testify about the first death. The boyfriend was convicted, and sentenced to death, but one of the jurors did admit to watching the news on TV and a mistrial was called. A second trial was performed and the defendant was again sentenced to death. Newspaper reports stated that he showed no remorse, smirking and yawning throughout the hearing. Additional history revealed that the defendant had a long criminal record including juvenile conviction of cruelty to animals.

Additional comments by Gregory L. Henry:

Children deserve the aggressive protection of the state, and in your role as an emergency physician, you are an agent of the state. In most states, reporting suspected child abuse is required; failure to do so can result in criminal charges.

Signs of child abuse can be subtle. In this case, it is hard to blame the emergency physician for not picking up the problem. In many cases, the family dynamics cannot be understood; whenever there is a single male—usually the boyfriend of the mother—living in a house, the possibility of child abuse increases dramatically.

Unfortunately, when the child returned, everything became diagnostically clear. It is heart-wrenching for the emergency physician to know that this tragic outcome followed a delay in diagnosis. The outcome is due to the malignant boyfriend and not the emergency physician, but still the effect on the first physician will be felt for years. It is devastating to have been involved in such a case—I know.

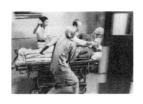

DIAGNOSIS AND MANAGEMENT OF CHILD ABUSE

Sharon E. Mace, MD, FACEP, FAAP

I. INTRODUCTION
Unfortunately, child abuse, more recently termed child maltreatment, is not uncommon.[1] Of the 3.2 million cases reported annually in the United States,[2] about one-third are substantiated,[2,3] which translates into one million abused children each year. Furthermore, the actual number of cases is estimated to be 3–5 times the number of reported cases. Each year, more than 140,000 children suffer serious injuries due to child abuse, of which 18,000 will have lifelong disabilities and 2,000 will die.[3] Every 10 seconds, a case of child maltreatment is reported,[5] and approximately one-third of all children are "seriously assaulted" by a caregiver.[6]

Child maltreatment is classified into 5 categories: neglect (54%), physical abuse (25%), sexual abuse (11%), emotional abuse (3%), and other (7%), (children may be in several categories).[6] Child maltreatment is found throughout the world in infants and children of all ages, in every culture, social/economic group, ethnic group, and religion. The emergency physician will encounter abused children whether he/she recognizes them or not. What then are the characteristics in the history and physical examination that will assist the physician in recognizing subtle, as well as obvious, child maltreatment? Concerns (red flags) during our patient's initial visit include the respiratory illness and easy bruising.

II. CHARACTERISTICS OF ABUSED CHILDREN AND ABUSERS
Characteristics occuring with increased frequency among abused children include parental expectations inconsistent with child's developmental capacity, accidental pregnancy or unwanted child, poor maternal child bonding, child born of a former relationship, hyperactivity, excessive crying or fussy behavior, and poor feeding.

Certain characteristics are associated with the "abuser." In this case the boyfriend had a criminal record with a history of animal abuse. Other characteristics reported frequently among child abusers include abuse as a child, substance abuse, domestic violence (spouse), antisocial personality disorder, single parent family, teenage parent, unrealistic expectations of the child, lack of a 'safety valve', and socioeconomically disadvantaged persons.

III. HISTORY
The lack of a "pediatric" history on the first visit is a problem—the history in any infant should include neonatal, developmental, family, and social history. Furthermore, it should be determined if the patient was a premature infant with respiratory distress at birth or the product of a complicated pregnancy, labor, and delivery. A 28-week premature infant would now have a 2-month-old "gestational" age (5 month old chronologic age) with pneumonia and a pulse oximetry of 92%. If this is the case,

admission should be considered since pneumonia or bronchiolitis at an early age can have significant morbidity and mortality.

Developmental history would indicate if this is a high-risk infant. Infants and children with delayed development, neurological disorders or "special healthcare needs" are often at higher risk for serious illnesses and child abuse. Previous medical problems may have led to poor maternal-infant bonding, a clue that the infant may be perceived by his caregivers as a "difficult" or "problem" infant.

The mother's report that this 5-month old has easy bruising is a major concern. A developmental history would corroborate your knowledge that this is a nonambulatory infant who should have little or no opportunity to fall and injure himself. A 5-month old's motor ability is limited. He may roll over in his crib, an activity that should incur no bruises. He is incapable of crawling out of his crib, standing, walking, falling or any other activity where he could injure or bruise himself. Therefore, bruises in a nonambulatory infant indicate either an underlying systemic disorder or inflicted trauma.

The infant has also had multiple chest colds, of which at least one was treated with antibiotics—this is a red flag. Recurrent respiratory illness in a 5 month old raises concerns for congenital problems, such as cardiac disease (congenital heart disease with failure), pulmonary disorders (tracheoesophageal fistula), or even an immunologic disorder. Neglected infants are often malnourished and at a greater risk for infection, including respiratory infections. A pulse oximetry of 92% is abnormal and should be, at least, repeated to see if it was a valid reading. If so, further evaluation and/or treatment are indicated, perhaps even admission. Family history may reveal congenital defects or bleeding diatheses in siblings, as many of these conditions have a genetic component.

Our patient's parents were separated and he was often left in the care of the mother's boyfriend (a frequent perpetrator in child abuse cases); this is important data. Social history may be relevant, especially if other siblings on previous visits had suspicious bruises, marks, or other findings suggestive of abuse. Sick contacts could explain acute communicable respiratory illness. It may also indicate predisposing factors for infections such as smoking in the home or daycare.

History of multiple emergency department (or clinic/office) visits should also be a red flag. Recurrent visits for apparently minor complaints, as documented in the first visit, often signify that the parent or caregiver is having trouble coping with the care of the infant.

Inquire in the family history about medical diseases (including those in the differential for child abuse), parental/caregiver history (spousal abuse, violence, substance abuse), sibling history (abuse or neglect), and any family crisis that might precipitate an abusive incident (such as job loss, marital strife, or financial problems). Document your observations in the ED, including how the parents are acting (aggressive or otherwise), the child's emotional/developmental state, the interactions (of parents, parent-child, etc.), and direct quotes of the child's story.

Thus, multiple concerns are found, as well as omissions, in the documentation on the first visit.

IV. PHYSICAL EXAMINATION

The location of the bruises on our patient suggest nonaccidental trauma. If this were from accidental trauma, such as a fall, then the bruises would not be limited to just the ear and wrist. Furthermore, the bruises would not be on opposite sides of the body (e.g., right ear and left wrist) but more likely on the same side of the body. Likewise, nonaccidental trauma would likely involve the entire exposed ear, not just the superior helix. The location on the superior helix suggests the infant was grabbed by the ear. Inspection of the ear should reveal bruising on both sides of the ear and a circular or oval shaped bruise from a fingerprint where the infant was grabbed. Similarly, if the bruises on the wrist are on both sides of the wrist, this may be from inflicted trauma where the infant was grabbed and held. If bruises are circumferential, they may be from the child being tied down. It is impossible for accidental trauma to cause a bruise on both sides of the wrist, without having bruises elsewhere on the arm. The wrist bruising is mentioned only in the history on visit 1, and not described in the physical exam.

The bruises on our patient have all the classic findings of inflicted bruises: regular uniform appearance, a distinct pattern, in a protected non-exposed area (pinnae of ear), and of various ages. The different colors of the bruise on the ear and the temple suggest bruises of different ages. Furthermore, they are present in a nonambulatory 5 month old with no possible way to injure himself.

On the physical examination, photograph any bruises/skin lesions/burns; use a ruler and color scale. Describe the shape, the location, associated findings (swelling, tenderness), color, and measure the size.

Finally, a weight is not documented on the first visit. If this infant's weight was < 10th percentile, he met the criteria for "failure to thrive" (FTT). FTT by itself is a reason for admission. More than half of all FTT is attributed to a "nonorganic" cause; if not from direct neglect, it is due to inadequate caloric intake secondary to feeding difficulties by the caregiver(s) in well over half of all FTT cases. Infections, especially respiratory infections in infants < 6 months old (particularly if undernourished) with low oxygen saturation, are a major concern and an indication for admission.

V. ACCIDENTAL AND NON-ACCIDENTAL BRUISING IN CHILDREN

Skin findings such as bruises or burns are the most frequent manifestation of physical abuse. The approximate incidence of the various presentations of physical abuse are: bruises/skin lesions (52%), central nervous system injuries (15%), burns (13%), skeletal injuries (8%), abdominal injuries (2%), and miscellaneous (10%) (e.g., toxic ingestions).

In the past, physicians attempted to "date" a bruise based on the color. However, we now know that the color of a bruise is affected by many variables, including: skin color, anatomic location, bruise depth, severity of impact, presence or absence of bleeding disorders, as well as timing of the injury. The recognition that the bruises are of varying ages is the important finding.

Non-accidental bruises often have a regular uniform appearance; have a distinct pattern, such as a circumferential linear appearance (from wrist being tied down); occur in non-exposed areas; and are of various ages. (Table 1)

Contrast this with the bruises found in a toddler learning to walk who has fallen several times. The toddler characteristically would have bruises on non-protected, exposed areas such as his shins, forearms, knees, chin, or elbow. They may have an irregular, non-uniform appearance and no recognizable shape. Bruises are usually of mild severity, limited in number, unilateral, asymmetric, and not circumferential.

Table 1. Characteristics Suggestive of Accidental vs. Non-accidental Bruises

CHARACTERISTIC	ACCIDENTAL	NON-ACCIDENTAL
General appearance	Irregular, non-uniform	Regular, uniform
Geometric shape or pattern	No recognizable shape (object) or pattern	Distinct pattern or shape (may be recognizable object)
Specific location	Non-protected "exposed" bony prominences (forehead, shins, knees, chin, elbows)	Protected non-exposed areas (chest, neck, axilla, ear pinnae, buttocks, genitalia, oral mucosa, inner aspects of arm, back of hands, inner thighs, small of back, back of knees)
General location	Peripheral distribution (lower extremity, arms, forehead)	More central (trunk)
Severity	Less severe	More severe, more extensive
Number/age	Few in numbers	Multiple, various ages
Unilateral/bilateral	Usually unilateral (e.g. a child who falls usually lands on one side, producing unilateral bruises)	Bilateral, symmetric (e.g. bilateral orbital contusions)
Suspicious location	--------------	Buttocks, thighs, genitalia, lower back, ear, gagging injuries (corners of mouth/lips): force-feeding injuries (inside mouth/palate); strangulation/restraining injuries (necks, ankles, wrists)
Symmetry/circumference	Asymmetric, unilateral, not circumferential	Circumferential, symmetric, bilateral
Typical patterns	Not recognizable pattern/object	Strangulation: circumferential linear marks on neck Tied down: circumferential linear marks on wrists/ankles Grabbed/shaker by ears or upper arms: circular bruises from adult fingers on pinna or upper arm Toilet-training punishment: bruises in genitalia, thighs, buttocks Tears of frenulum, mouth laceration: forced feeding To protect face: bruises on volar surface of forearms

VI. MANAGEMENT OF CHILD MALTREATMENT

First of all, any *suspected* child maltreatment must be reported. Mandated reporters, including physicians, are required to report suspected child maltreatment to the appropriate authorities. As long as the professional (physician, teacher, nurse, social worker, etc.) is reporting in good faith, they are immune from legal liability arising from the report. However, failure to report can result in both malpractice liability and criminal prosecution.

Typically, severely injured children have a history of prior "minor" injuries (as in this case) and/or a history of abuse in siblings; there may be an opportunity to prevent significant morbidity and mortality either to the "index" abused child or siblings.

In seriously injured children, resuscitation and stabilization is the first priority. Treatment of any specific illnesses or injuries should be prioritized. In children or infants whose medical condition allows for their discharge home, it should be determined if the home is safe for the patient, siblings, and spouse or significant others. If there is any question, admission or foster home placement is warranted. If the patient is discharged home, follow-up should occur with child protective services, the primary care physician, and appropriate specialist. Follow-up for the entire family (siblings, spouse, and any other household members, as well as the perpetrator) is necessary, since domestic violence can involve not only the children but also the domestic partner, elderly family members, and even the family pets.

Thorough documentation of the history and physical examination is essential. Use quotes, interview family/household members separately, including each parent, siblings (if old enough), grandparents, caregivers, and baby-sitters to detect discrepancies in the various histories. If any injury occurred, get specific details including how, when, where, and who was present. What is the mechanism of injury? Can it explain the injuries present?

Evaluate for other causes of bruising (Table 2 below). Laboratory testing may include a CBC and coagulation studies; negative laboratory tests can aid in ruling out systemic diseases. Child abusers will often claim that bruises are not due to abuse but to medications or an underlying disease. Such data makes it more difficult for a defense lawyer to plead the abuser's case in court. Involve social work and/or child protective services early. If this evaluation is not able to be thoroughly performed by the emergency physician, then transfer to a pediatric center is indicated.

Table 2. Differential Diagnosis of Possible Physical Abuse

A. Bruises
  Trauma
  • Accidental
  • Non-accidental (physical abuse)
  Hematologic Disorders
  • Platelet disorders or platelet dysfunction
        Platelet deficiencies (thrombocytopenia)
        Thrombotic thrombocytopenia purpura
        Idiopathic thrombocytopenia
        Drug or toxin induced
  • Factor deficiencies
        Hemophilia
        Hemorrhagic disease of the newborn
        Von Willebrand's disease
  Malignancies
  • Leukemia
  Infections
  • Viral infection/exanthems
  • Sepsis
  • Rickettsial infections
  • Streptococcal infections
  • Congenital syphilis
  Rheumatic/autoimmune/collagen vascular diseases
  • Systemic lupus erythematosis
  • Rheumatic fever
  • Acute glomerulonephritis
  • Henoch-Schonlein purpura
  Folk Remedies
  • Coining
  • Cupping
  • Spooning   (table continued on next page)

Skin lesions/dermatologic disorders
- Birthmarks/congenital lesions
- Mongolian spots
- Hemangiomas

Nutritional
- Vitamin C deficiency (scurvy)

Inborn errors of metabolism
- Letterer-Siwe disease
- Ehlers-Danlos syndrome
- Glutaric aciduria type 1

B. Burns

Vesiculobullous skin disorders
- Infectious (impetigo, toxic epidermal necrolysis, staphylococcal scalded skin syndrome, dermatitis herpetiformis, candidal diaper dermatitis, varicella, smallpox, scabies (vesicular presentation), herpes simplex, herpes zoster
- Noninfectious (phytodermatitis [contact dermatitis], sunburns, allergic diaper dermatitis, frostbite, dyshidrotic eczema, non-congenital dermatitis herpetiformis, bullous pemphigoid, bullous dermatitis)

Folk remedies (moxibustion)

Fixed drug eruptions

C. Skeletal Injuries
- Inherited disorders (osteogenesis imperfecta, inherited rickets, copper deficiency [menkos kinky hair syndrome])
- Acquired diseases (nutritional rickets, copper deficiency, scurvy)
- Drug-induced skeletal disorders
- Infections (congenital syphilis)
- Metabolic/endocrine diseases (osteoporosis)
- Miscellaneous (infantile cortical hyperplasia)

VII. SUMMARY

This patient presented like 10 others who are seen during every ED shift; a young patient with symptoms suggestive of a viral illness. Looking below the surface, though, some clues argued against a routine case of upper respiratory infection. He was high risk due to his frequent visits, and his oxygen saturation was low. The patient was nonambulatory, but had bruising in various locations and at various stages of healing, suggesting nonaccidental injury.

A thorough history and examination, with recheck of abnormal physical findings or vital signs, should be performed in all pediatric patients. If there is concern about maltreatment, transfer to a facility with resources and specialized expertise is indicated.

TEACHING POINTS ABOUT CASE 30:
- Bruises (or fractures) in a nonambulatory infant are child abuse until proven otherwise.
- Inflicted bruises typically have a regular uniform appearance, a distinct pattern, occur in protected, non-exposed areas, and are of different ages.
- Abnormal vital signs should be rechecked before ED discharge.
- Physicians are mandated to report any suspicion of child abuse. Failure to do so can lead to malpractice liability, as well as criminal penalties for the physician.

REFERENCES
1. Mace SE. Child physical abuse: a state of the art approach. Pediatric Emerg Med Prac 2004; 1(2): 1-20.
2. Peddle N, Wang CT. Current trends in child abuse reporting and fatalities. The results of the 1999 annual fifty-state survey. Chicago, IL: National Committee to Prevent Child Abuse; 2001.
3. Alexander RC. Statistics of child abuse. In Jones G, Levitt CJ, et al. American Academy of Pediatrics Section on Child Abuse and Neglect. A Guide to References and Resources in Child Abuse and Neglect. 2nd ed. Chicago, IL: American Academy of Pediatrics; 1998: 181-2.
4. Herman-Giddens ME, Brown G, Verbiest S, et al. Underascertainment of child abuse mortality in the United States. JAMA 1999 Aug 4; 282: 463-7.
5. Starr Commonwealth (Organization for Abused and Neglected Children). www.starr.org
6. Wang CT, Daro D. Current trends in child abuse reporting and fatalities: the results of the 1996 annual fifty-state survey. Chicago, IL: National Committee to Prevent Child Abuse; 1997.

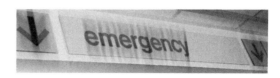

LEGAL CONSIDERATIONS

SO YOU WANT TO BE SUED FOR MALPRACTICE

Commentary:
Thomas R. Himmelspach, Esq.
Richard S. Milligan, Esq.
   Buckingham, Doolittle & Burroughs, LLP

Contributor:
Jeffrey D. Weinstock, Esq.
   Buckingham, Doolittle & Burroughs, LLP

SO YOU WANT TO BE SUED FOR MALPRACTICE

THE TOP-10 WAYS TO MAXIMIZE YOUR RISK

"Assume that you're the center of the universe, the only one who matters in any given situation. The truth is—and let me be the first to tell you—God went away on vacation and left you in charge!"

Ben Stein, *How to Ruin Your Life*[1]

While most doctors dread the prospect of defending a malpractice suit, some may have a different view. For those drawn to the drama and excitement of a courtroom experience, who yearn to see their names splashed across the daily paper, who are searching for ways to relieve themselves of needless sleep and extra cash, we offer these sure fire tips on how to land in court. Of course, if you found yourself agreeing with the above quote from Ben Stein, you're already halfway there. (In fact, it's likely that a malpractice suit would just be icing on the cake of your life.) Otherwise, sharpen your pencil and get ready to jot some notes as we run down the top ten list. Practice these and you'll be calling your malpractice carrier faster than you can say "ALL RISE"!

NUMBER **10**

Include unnecessary, inflammatory comments in the chart.

A derogatory comment or two in the chart about a patient never hurt anyone. Now is the time to get even with that obnoxious patient. No doubt the patient deserves whatever you write. As an added benefit, everyone will clearly then know your thoughts about the value of the patient.

Some examples from actual cases might be helpful to you:

- "Patient is 55 years old and obese, smelly and unpleasant female in no need of emergency department services."

- For the patient who needs to exit the ER ASAP—put in the record "get them out of here via ambulance, train, plane, whatever." So what if the patient becomes a quadriplegic in the ensuing hours. You *do* want to be sued, right?

NUMBER 9
Use tunnel vision in evaluating patients.

Assume the best. I mean, what are the chances that your patient has a life-threatening illness? Why waste time and health care resources disproving the unlikely outcome?

One great suggestion is to use, freely and often, the word "just" in describing your patient's condition. This is particularly useful in describing the elderly, where dismissive assumptions can shortcut an otherwise complicated workup. For example, never hesitate to say "it's *just* old age"; "it's *just* a fall"; "it's *just* heartburn"; "it's *just* dizziness"; "he's *just* depressed." Such terminology makes it far more likely that you'll miss a serious condition.[2] And that's what you're after, right?

NUMBER 8
Go it alone: don't get a consult.

Just because EMTALA requires the availability of on call consultants doesn't mean you actually have to take advantage of them. You're smart enough and skilled enough to handle most patient problems. Why call a consultant? Show a little spine.

As Dr. Henry points out in his analysis, Case 21 is an example of a situation where a consult should have been obtained.

NUMBER 7
Assume that frequent fliers are not acutely ill.

Nothing's a bigger hassle for you than the frequent flier.[3] Never really sick. Taking time away from the *real* patients. Not paying for care.

Here's a great tip. Keep a *list* of your frequent fliers and when they come in, pass them through a quick exam and GET THEM OUT! That way you can bill for your services and move on to a real patient. As a bonus, a malpractice suit may follow! And if that happens, your frequent flier list can be used to prove that the patient got the care he deserved!

Case 12 is an example of a frequent flier which was evaluated appropriately with each visit.

NUMBER 6
Never document that you've reviewed lab results and have acted on them.

Sure, you ordered the lab tests. So what? Why should you bother looking at the results or documenting that you did? It should be obvious to everyone that you must have looked at them since you ordered them, right? Why waste time documenting the fact? What could it possibly matter?

Case 5 is an example of this. In that case, the blood pressure reading of 72 was abnormally low. Although it was documented in the chart, the physician did not address the condition which contributed to the undesirable outcome.

NUMBER 5

Don't order a timely follow-up visit with a physician.

When you've seen a patient, made your diagnosis, and provided the care, you need to assume the case is *closed.* You're that good. Why order a follow-up visit? No use wasting your time ordering something the patient won't do anyway. Remember, your goal is to help the plaintiff's lawyer, and nothing's more discouraging to a lawyer than finding out his client didn't do what the ER doc ordered. Why not just avoid that risk by not ordering the follow up? And guess what? Since you didn't pass off care to another physician there's no one else to blame for the bad outcome! A malpractice suit is sure to follow and it's all yours!

For a contrary view, see Dr. Henry's comments to case 18. Cases 2, 6 and 27 are both cases where Dr. Henry feels the follow up time was too long.

NUMBER 4

On discharge, don't record that patient is stable.

While EMTALA requires a patient to be stabilized prior to discharge or transfer, you really don't need to address the discharge condition in your documentation. After all, the maximum EMTALA fine is only $50,000, and everybody knows fines are rarely imposed. Right?

See Case 10 in which the patient was transferred in an unstable condition, but the benefits of transfer were deemed to be greater than the risks associated with transfer. The patient did die in transfer, but both Dr. Henry and Dr. Hollander agree that transfer was the right thing to do.

NUMBER 3

Make sure you blame someone else for what happened —if someone is to be held responsible for the outcome, why should it be you?

This is a big one. Why should you take the fall? Blame somebody else. While this might increase the chances a malpractice case will be filed, it probably won't be against you! If you're sued anyway, you now have documentation that another physician or the hospital or nurses are at fault.

Here are some examples to get you started:

- Following an unsuccessful resuscitation effort: "All attending the code made a valiant effort to save the patient, but the defibrillator failed."

- "Hospital failed to timely obtain prior record for me."

- "Radiology failed to STAT scan the patient."

- "Neurologist on call was golfing."

NUMBER 2
After disaster strikes, freely alter the chart to CYA.

Cardinal Rule #1: When disaster strikes, find the medical records as soon as possible and change them to exonerate yourself.

You know what needs to be in there to CYA. Add it. If something is in the chart that "didn't happen," use the white-out you keep in your pocket to change it. That's what it's for!

If you need to add something to your handwritten notes, just squeeze it in. No one will ever know, especially if you use the same pen. You're much too clever to get caught at this.

Your dictated note may not be helpful. What do you do? That's right—*destroy* it and recreate it! Even if it's months later. You can always claim that you were behind in your chart review.

NUMBER 1
Treat your patients badly; they are wasting your time!

We can't stress this one enough. Rule number one is treat your patients *badly*; they probably deserve it and they're wasting *your* valuable time. Treated badly, patients are much more likely to do exactly what you want—like go see a lawyer.

Let's face it. You're the *doctor*. Doesn't that make you more important than the patient? Time is money. How can you be expected to earn your fair share if you have to waste time on undeserving patients who don't pay their bills!

SO YOU'VE BEEN SUED. WHAT SHOULD YOU DO?

The frequency of malpractice lawsuits makes it unlikely that you will go through your career without being a defendant. Being sued can be a profoundly unsettling event. For the first time, someone will be challenging your professional judgment. You will be called upon to spend substantial uncompensated time in your own defense.

Here are some tips on what to do when you are sued.

- **Do not discuss the case with others**
  The temptation to discuss a newly filed case with your friends and colleagues will be enormous. Don't do it.

  You will be deposed by the lawyer for the patient. One of the first questions that will be asked is who you have spoken with about the case. You will be forced to reveal you conversations, whether they help you or not.

  Your discussions with your lawyer are confidential and privileged. Conversations with anyone else are not. Do not unwittingly make your colleagues and friends witnesses in your case. It may hurt both of you.

- **Secure the chart**
  The chart needs to be locked up so that its contents may not be altered. There is no more certain way to an adverse result than a patient being able to prove a physician altered the chart to protect him or herself. A lost chart can also become a source of an additional claim against you.

- **Get to know your lawyer**
  The lawsuit is about you, not the insurance company. You need to play a central role in the defense of your case. Meet with your lawyer. He or she will want to fully understand the medical issues involved and your assessment of the care that was provided.

- **Tell your lawyer everything**
  You have a confidential relationship with your lawyer. The lawyer will rely on you being candid about what took place. If there are bad facts, tell your lawyer so he can plan on how best to deal with them. Nothing can be more devastating to your case than the sudden disclosure of adverse facts. Do not let it happen.

- **Let your lawyer investigate the case and obtain expert witnesses**
  As tempting as it will be, do not engage in your own independent investigation of the medical or factual issues in your case.

Nothing is more helpful to the opposing lawyer than you doing medical research and providing him with the results. Any material in the research you find that is adverse will be used against you.

If investigation is needed, let your lawyer do it. It will remain confidential. Your investigation will not.

- **Control your emotions**
  Your natural anger at being sued needs to be focused on your defense and not directed at the court, the jury, or the plaintiff. It is counter-productive to do so. You need to be in control so that your emotions do not adversely influence the outcome.

  Juries and judges generally hold physicians in very high esteem. This is one reason why physicians win most medical malpractice trials. Do not forfeit that tremendous advantage by being disrespectful to the court, lawyers, or other parties.

- **Be patient**
  Even in the best of jurisdictions, the judicial process moves slowly. Steel yourself for the long haul.

A SHORT OVERVIEW ON EMTALA

- **What is it?**
  EMTALA is a federal law that poses unique liability risks in the area of emergency medicine. In 1986, Congress enacted the Emergency Medical Treatment and Active Labor Act ("EMTALA"),[4] commonly known as the "Patient Anti-Dumping Act." As that name implies, EMTALA was enacted to prevent facilities from refusing emergency medical treatment to patients who are unable to pay or transferring them before emergency conditions are stabilized."[5]

  EMTALA applies to hospitals that accept Medicare reimbursement and to all their patients, not just those covered by Medicare.[6]

  Hospital emergency departments have two duties under EMTALA: (1) to provide an "appropriate medical screening examination" to determine whether an emergency condition exists and, if so; (2) to stabilize the condition before discharging or transferring the patient to another medical facility.[7]

  From a liability standpoint, the key features of EMTALA are (1) that conduct is judged under a statutory framework and the tort law standard-of-care analysis doesn't apply; (2) the claims qualify for federal court jurisdiction; (3) state law damage caps on medical negligence claims might not apply; and (4) violators are subject to fines.

- **What's "appropriate screening"?**
  EMTALA requires that hospitals provide "an *appropriate* medical screening examination within the capability of the hospital's emergency department…." A screening is "appropriate" if it (1) conforms to the hospital's screening procedures, and (2) is reasonably calculated to identify critical medical conditions that may be afflicting the patient. It isn't a guarantee of a proper diagnosis, and the question of whether a provider met the screening requirement isn't decided under a negligence standard. Rather, an appropriate screening is one that is applied uniformly to all emergency room patients.

  When a hospital fails to give an emergency room patient the same screening it regularly gives to others under similar circumstances, and the variation is significant, it can be liable for damages under EMTALA. For example, in *Correa v. Hospital of San Francisco*,[8] a woman who entered a hospital with complaints of chest pain was given a number (forty-seven) and told to wait. She left the hospital after waiting over 2 hours and went to another facility where she died from hypovolemic shock. The court held that the hospital violated the EMTALA screening requirement.

  The requirements for an "appropriate" screening are necessarily vague and courts apply a rule of reason in enforcing them; minor deviations between customary screening practice and the screening given to a particular patient aren't violations.

  For example, in *Johnson v. Nacogdoches County Hospital*,[10] an R.N. met a patient, Betty Johnson, in the hallway leading to the ER, asked about her complaints, and wheeled her to the triage nurse. The nurse started an assessment 22 minutes later and completed it within 15 minutes, classifying Mrs. Johnson's condition as non-urgent. Johnson then sat, moaning in the ER waiting room for 25 minutes before her family took her to another facility. There, she was diagnosed with meningitis from which she later died. Her estate sued the first hospital, alleging EMTALA liability for failing to provide an appropriate screening. Noting that the hospital's utilization policy required that patients "will be spoken with within 10 minutes of arrival," plaintiff argued that the hospital had failed to provide an appropriate screening, since 22 minutes had passed before the triage nurse began her assessment. The court held, however, that the 12-minute delay wasn't a material deviation from the standard procedure, particularly in light of the RN's evaluation before Johnson reached the ER.

- **What are the stabilization requirements?**
If the screening discloses that the patient has an emergency medical condition, the provider must stabilize the patient before discharge or transfer. Most courts have held the requirement applies only when the provider has actually identified an emergency condition. In other words, if the provider did an appropriate screening and discharged the patient without identifying an emergency medical condition, it isn't liable under EMTALA, even though it may have been negligent in failing to diagnose the condition.

Once the provider determines that the patient has an emergency medical condition, it must use measures appropriate under the circumstances to stabilize the patient. The duty applies only where the patient is discharged or transferred; most courts have held it doesn't continue after the patient is admitted.

What does a provider have to do to "stabilize" a patient? Like the screening requirement, EMTALA doesn't give the patient any guarantees. In the trial of an EMTALA claim, the jury will consider whether the treatment and subsequent release or transfer were "reasonable in view of the circumstances that existed at the time the hospital discharged or transferred the individual." EMTALA requires the provider "assure, within reasonable medical probability, that no material deterioration of the condition is likely to result from or occur during the transfer" or discharge.

Whether or not the patient is stabilized at the time of discharge or transfer is typically a judgment call, and courts will review the record for signs of acute distress. Hospitals transferring or discharging patients from emergency rooms face liability risks where the patient's stabilization is tenuous. The risks underscore the importance of thorough documentation of patient care, monitoring, and assessment.

- **What happens if I violate EMTALA?**
As noted earlier, a patient who is injured or suffers damages as a result of an EMTALA violation is entitled to recover damages for the loss. While the statute provides for a cause of action only against the hospital and not against an individual physician for violating EMTALA, it does provide for fines that can be imposed against both hospitals and individual physicians.

The physician penalties include fines of up to $50,000 for each violation. In cases of gross and flagrant violations, the physician can be excluded from Medicare and Medicaid programs.

The government is increasingly aggressive in enforcing EMTALA. The Office of the Inspector General reported that in 2000, $1.17 million in fines were assessed for EMTALA violations. That's as much as were assessed in the first 10 years of the Act.

A FEW WORDS ON RAPPORT AND SYMPATHY

Lawsuits happen for many reasons. The more you know about the dynamics of the process, the better your chances of avoiding litigation. One major factor leading to medical lawsuits—maybe *the* major factor—is that the doctor didn't connect with the patient on a human level.

A critical time to make that connection is when the patient has suffered a bad outcome. At that point, the patient is searching for emotional support. The expectation is that it will first be found among those connected with the loss, and a doctor who is involved in a bad result has that connection.

At a recent symposium in Ohio, a trial court judge observed that the overwhelming majority of medical negligence cases in his court are there because, at the time of a bad outcome, the doctor didn't connect with the patient or his or her family. He's talking about sympathy.

In our culture, there's a notion that apologies and expressions of sympathy only increase the risk of liability. Look at the insurer's brochure in your glove box on what to do in the event of an accident. Chances are it warns you against saying anything apologetic. Some insurers won't cover liability when a driver says the word "Sorry."

In fact, there's evidence that offering an apology or expressing sympathy doesn't increase the risk of liability. For example, in Vermont, the state supreme court held that that a physician's apology for an "inadequate" operation wasn't an admission of liability.[11] In another case, the Vermont court held that a plaintiff hadn't established negligence based only on the apology of a surgeon for a serious mistake during surgery.[11] (Plaintiff presented evidence that the surgeon said she'd "made a mistake, that she was sorry, and that [the perforation of the uterus] had never happened before.") One Utah lawyer who has represented plaintiffs and defendants in medical negligence cases wrote recently that in 20 years of practice he's never seen a case where someone was sued because he or she apologized.

With skyrocketing costs of malpractice insurance and the resulting pressures on medical care providers, state legislatures have sought solutions to the liability problems facing physicians. One approach that has spread quickly over the past couple years is aimed at encouraging apologies or words of sympathy from doctors for bad results. Several states now provide by statute or evidence rules that apologies or statements of sympathy are not admissible as evidence in a case of medical negligence. Laws that promote apologies or expressions of sympathy give legislators the rare opportunity to provide meaningful improvements to the system at minimal cost.

In 2005, Ohio enacted an apology statute typical of the broad provisions now being adopted nationally, saying "All statements, affirmations, gestures, or conduct expressing apology, sympathy, commiseration, condolence, compassion or a general sense of benevolence" are inadmissible. A medical professional practicing in Ohio should make full use of the statutory protection. In that regard, we suggest that you (1) make your contact with the patient or family early and preempt any perception that you're uncaring; (2) be forthright in explaining what happened and in answering questions; (3) and, most importantly, be empathetic, and offer your sympathy.

Whether or not a doctor's apology or statement of sympathy avoids litigation altogether, there is evidence that it can make any litigation less adversarial and, accordingly, easier to settle. The apology can address the intangible injury a patient may feel from the sense of being wronged, whether willfully or negligently. While it won't compensate the physical injury or address recovery expenses, an apology can remove the emotional sting.

One account of a doctor's poor treatment of a patient recently made national news. In 1994, a doctor in New York City telephoned a woman late at night with a report that she had a rare form of cancer (mesothelioma) for which there was no available treatment. Then he hung up. The woman, living alone, had no one to comfort her after receiving the news.

She decided to leave a bequest to a medical college in her hometown, not for the treatment of cancer, but for another use she found more urgent. With a $1.9 million gift, the College of Medicine of Ohio has developed the Ruth Hillebrand Clinical Skills Center, where health-care professionals learn interpersonal skills. Director, Judy Riggle, says "Qualities such as listening carefully, noticing body language, and showing empathy to patients have proven to be a very effective method of developing rapport with patients."[12]

Recent studies have shown that doctors who develop a rapport with their patients are far less likely to be sued. What are the signs of good communication? The appropriate use of humor; soliciting patient opinions; checking for patient understanding; and generally, encouraging patients to talk.[13] And, in the event of a bad result, it is most important that the patient or family hear some expression of concern, condolence, or sympathy.

Thomas R. Himmelspach is a Partner in the Health & Medicine Practice Group of Buckingham, Doolittle & Burroughs, LLP. He has extensive experience in insurance coverage disputes, railroad litigation, conflicts of law disputes, workers' compensation subrogation, and state and federal appellate practice. He can be reached at thimmelspach@bdblaw.com or 330.491.5284.

Richard S. Milligan is a shareholder in the Health and Medicine Practice Group of Buckingham, Doolittle & Burroughs, LLP. He is a trial lawyer who defends hospitals, physicians and nurses in medical malpractice lawsuits. Mr. Milligan speaks regularly on risk management for health care providers. He can be reached at rmilligan@bdblaw.com or 330. 491.5280.

Jeffrey D. Weinstock is an attorney in the Boca Raton, Florida office of Buckingham, Doolittle & Burroughs, LLP. He represents physicians, physician practice groups and other health care companies in business and operational issues, including formation, structuring, contracting, employment agreements, buy-ins, buy-outs and shareholder issues. He can be reached at jweinstock@bdblaw.com or 561.241.0414.

REFERENCES

1. Ben Stein, How to Ruin Your Life, Copyright 2002, Hay House, Inc., Carlsbad, CA.
2. See "Geriatric Patients in the Emergency Department Aren't 'Just Another…,'" by W.S. Ernoehazy, Jr., M.D., F.A.C.E.P., Geriatric Times, May/June 2001, Vol. II, Issue 3
3. Also sometimes known as "GOMERs,", i.e., Get Out of My Emergency Room. The liberal use of these funny terms is highly recommended.
4. 42 U.S.C. 1282.
5. Power v. Arlington Hosp. Assn. (C.A. 4, 1994), 42 F.3d 851, 856. See also H.R. Rep. No. 241, 99th Cong. 1st Sess. 27 (1986), U.S.C.C.A.N. 42, 605, 726-27. One study, from 1986, reported that 87% of hospitals transferring patients cited the lack of insurance as the sole reason for the transfer. Schiff RL, Ansell DA, Schlosser JE, et al. Transfers to a public hospital. A prospective study of 467 patients. N Engl J Med 1986; 314(9):552-7.
6. See, e.g., Brooker v. Desert Hosp. Corp. (C.A. 9, 1991), 947 F.2d 412, 414. Recent regulations, however, clarify that a "hospital's obligations under EMTALA end once an individual is admitted for in-patient care." 42 CFR. 489.24(d)(2). The rules further prohibit a hospital from admitting a patient in bad faith only as a way of avoiding EMTALA liability for a later inappropriate transfer.
7. 42 U.S.C. 1395dd(c)(1).
8. (C.A. 1, 2002), 69 F.3d 1184.
9. 2003 Tex. App. LEXIS 7230.
10. Phinney v. Vinson (Vt. 1992), 605 A.2d 849.
11. Senesac v. Associates in Obstetrics and Gynecology (1982), 449 A.2d 900.
12. MCO News, Feb. 28– March 11, 2005.
13. Levinson W., Roter DL, Mullooly JP, et al. Physician-patient communication; the relationship with malpractice claims among primary care physicians and surgeons.; Hickson GB. Federspiel CF, Pichert JW, et al. Patient complaints and malpractice risk. JAMA 2002; 287: 2951-7.

APPENDIX

ANSWERS TO CASES & TITLES OF DISCUSSION SECTIONS

LIST OF CHIEF COMPLAINTS BY SYSTEM, INCLUDING
1. Chapter titles
2. Final diagnoses
3. Titles and authors of discussion sections

A. CARDIOVASCULAR
   1. Evaluation of chest pain (main discussion of diagnosis of chest pain)
      a. Case 7–38 year old male with chest pain
      b. Final diagnosis–Acute myocardial infarction
      c. Discussion (Amal Mattu)–Evaluation of chest pain and diagnosis of acute coronary syndrome
   2. Diagnosis and management of arrhythmias and acute MI
      a. Case 10–50 year old male with "gallbladder inflammation"
      b. Final diagnosis–Acute anterolateral myocardial infarction with wide complex tachycardia and hypotension
      c. Discussion (Jud Hollander and Esther Chen)–Evaluation of acute coronary syndrome and management of cardiac arrhythmias
   3. Diagnosis and management of atrial fibrillation and anxiety
      a. Case 19–57 year old male with heart fluttering and lightheadedness
      b. Final diagnosis–New onset atrial fibrillation/flutter
      c. Discussion (Sandy Craig)–Evaluation and management of tachycardias and atrial flutter
   4. Evaluation of and admission criteria for syncope
      a. Case 20–76 year old female with syncope
      b. Final diagnosis: Ruptured abdominal aortic aneurysm
      c. Discussion (Wyatt Decker)–Evaluation and management of syncope (Note: See case 3 for discussion of diagnosis of ruptured AAA)
   5. Evaluation and diagnosis of chest pain and pulmonary embolism
      a. Case 29–29 year old female with chest pain
      b. Final diagnosis: Pulmonary embolism
      c. Discussion (Raymond Jackson)–Risk and evaluation of venous thromboembolic events in the ED, communication (including issues surrounding leaving AMA), and interpretation of lab results

B. **SHORTNESS OF BREATH**
1. **Diagnosis and evaluation of pulmonary embolism**
   a. Case 9–34 year old male with leg pain
   b. Final diagnosis–Pulmonary embolism
   c. Discussion (Jeff Kline)–Diagnosis and management of pulmonary embolism
2. **Evaluation of shortness of breath (main discussion of SOB) and diagnosis and management of cardiomyopathy**
   a. Case 15–45 year old man with cough and sore throat
   b. Final diagnosis–Cardiomyopathy, acute renal failure, shock liver
   c. Discussion (Michael Weinstock)–Evaluation of shortness of breath, diagnosis and management of heart failure
3. Also see Chapter 22 (28 year old pregnant female with shortness of breath) for discussion of evaluation of shortness of breath and cardiomyopathy in pregnancy

C. **HEADACHE**
1. **Evaluation of HA in adults**
   a. Case 4–37 year old female with headache and flu-like symptoms
   b. Final diagnosis–Carotid artery dissection
   c. Discussion (Andy Jagoda and John Bruns)–Evaluation of headaches in adults and discussion of carotid artery dissection
2. **Evaluation of HA in patients with HIV/AIDS**
   a. Case 11–37 year old male with headaches
   b. Final diagnosis–Cryptococcal meningitis, AIDS
   c. Discussion (Michael Para)–Diagnosis of HIV, evaluation of headaches in patients with HIV/AIDS, and cryptococcal meningitis
3. **Evaluation of HA in patients with eye pain**
   a. Case 26–53 year old female with headache and eye pain
   b. Final diagnosis–Herpes zoster ophthalmicus
   c. Discussion (Frank and Michael Weinstock)–Evaluation of nontraumatic eye pain, discussion of varicella zoster virus and zoster ophthalmicus
4. Also see Case 5 for evaluation of headache in children (17 year old male with fever and headache) and Case 12 for evaluation of headache in drug seeking patients (42 year old female with headache)

D. **ABDOMINAL PAIN**
1. **Evaluation of abdominal pain in adults (focus on testing/imaging)**
   a. Case 2–33 year old male with abdominal pain
   b. Final diagnosis–Ruptured appendicitis and postoperative ileus
   c. Discussion (Scott Melanson)–Diagnosis and management of abdominal pain
2. **Evaluation of abdominal pain in adults (main discussion)**
   a. Case 6–24 year old male with abdominal pain
   b. Final diagnosis (by autopsy)–Infarction of small bowel, mesenteric vein thrombosis, multiple other sites of thrombi
   c. Discussion (Steve Colucciello)–Evaluation and diagnosis of abdominal pain in adults

3. **Evaluation of abdominal pain in children**
   a. Case 25–6 year old male with abdominal pain
   b. Final diagnosis–Ruptured appendix
   c. Discussion (Ann Dietrich)–Evaluation of abdominal pain in children and diagnosis of appendicitis in children
4. Also see chapter 8 (38 year old female with abdominal pain) for discussion of abdominal pain and ruptured ectopic and chapter 27 (30 year-old pregnant female with abdominal pain) for discussion of abdominal pain and appendicitis in pregnancy, and chapter 14 (55 year old male with LUQ abdominal pain s/p MVA) for discussion of blunt abdominal trauma

E. **MUSCULOSKELETAL COMPLAINTS *AND* ED ULTRASOUND**
   1. **Diagnosis and management of AAA, bedside ED ultrasound**
      a. Case 3–71 year old male with back pain
      b. Final diagnosis–Ruptured abdominal aortic aneurysm (AAA)
      c. Discussion (Jake Ott)–Evaluation for abdominal aortic aneurysm and bedside ED ultrasound
   2. **Evaluation of neck pain (main discussion of non-traumatic neck pain)**
      a. Case 16–46 year old male with neck and upper back pain
      b. Final diagnosis–Cervical epidural abscess with spinal cord compression
      c. Discussion (Ed Boudreau)–Atraumatic neck pain and diagnosis/management of spinal epidural abscess
   3. **Evaluation of back pain (main discussion of back pain) and red flags for cancer**
      a. Case 23–51 year old male with back pain
      b. Final diagnosis–Renal cell cancer with metastasis
      c. Discussion (Michael Weinstock)–Diagnosis and management of non-traumatic low back pain and renal cell cancer

F. **INFECTIOUS DISEASE**
   1. **Evaluation of fever in children (main discussion of fever without source in children)**
      a. Case 5–17 year old male with fever and headache
      b. Final diagnosis–bacterial meningitis
      c. Discussion (Ann Dietrich)–Discussion of fever without source and meningitis in children
   2. **Evaluation of fever in adults (main discussion of adult fevers)**
      a. Case 24–48 year old male with back pain and fevers
      b. Final diagnosis–Culture negative endocarditis
      c. Discussion (Frank Orth)–Evaluation of fever in adults and infectious endocarditis
   3. **Diagnosis and management of influenza**
      a. Case 28–36 year old male with fevers and myalgias
      b. Final diagnosis–Bacterial endocarditis
      c. Discussion (Dave Hill)–Diagnosis and management of influenza

G PREGNANCY
1. **Evaluation of shortness of breath in pregnancy and issues about leaving AMA**
    a. Case 22–28 year old pregnant female with shortness of breath
    b. Final diagnosis–Cardiomyopathy secondary to severe mitral regurgitation and pregnancy
    c. Discussion (Ryan Longstreth)–Evaluation of shortness of breath, hypertensive disorders, and cardiomyopathy in pregnancy
2. **Evaluation of abdominal pain in pregnant women**
    a. Case 27–30 year old pregnant female with abdominal pain
    b. Final diagnosis–Ruptured appendix
    c. Discussion (Robert Dart)–Evaluation of abdominal pain in pregnancy and appendicitis in pregnancy
3. **Diagnosis and management of ectopic pregnancy**
    a. Case 8–38 year old female with abdominal pain
    b. Final diagnosis–Ruptured tubal pregnancy
    c. Discussion (William Mallon)–Discussion of ectopic pregnancy with a risk management focus

H. TRAUMA
1. **Evaluation of ocular trauma**
    a. Case 18–10 year old male with eye pain
    b. Final diagnosis–Globe rupture
    c. Discussion (Grace Kim, Lance Brown)–Evaluation and management of eye injuries in children
2. **Evaluation of trauma and MVC's in community hospitals**
    a. Case 14–55 year old male with LUQ abdominal pain s/p MVA
    b. Final diagnosis–Acute traumatic splenic rupture
    c. Discussion (Tom Lukens)–Evaluation of patients with blunt abdominal trauma
3. **Child abuse: Diagnosis and management of child abuse**
    a. Case 30–5 month old male with a cough and easy bruising
    b. Final diagnosis (per coroner report)–Acute subdural hemorrhage due to shaking, multiple rib fractures, right tibia and fibula fractures
    c. Discussion (Sharon Mace)–Diagnosis and management of child abuse
4. **Hand injuries: Evaluation and management of hand injuries**
    a. Case 1–18 year old male with hand pain
    b. Final diagnosis–Hand laceration secondary to human bite wound
    c. Discussion (Wes Eilbert)–Discussion of clench fist injuries, animal bite wounds, and adherence to therapy

I. PSYCHIATRIC ISSUES
1. **Evaluation of patients with mental health issues and diagnosis of cancer**
    a. Case 13–71 year old female with bipolar disorder and shoulder pain
    b. Final diagnosis–Adenocarcinoma of the GI tract with metastases to the brain, bone, lungs, liver, and pelvis

c. Discussion (Stephen Pariser, Doug Rund)–Evaluation of patients with known psychiatric illness, discussion of bipolar mood disorder and lithium treatment

2. **Evaluation of HA in frequent ED visitors**
   a. Case 12–42 year old female with headache
   b. Final diagnosis–Headache, probable drug-seeking behavior
   c. Discussion (Stephen Karas)–Evaluation and management of frequent-headache patients and potential drug-seeking behavior

J. **FLANK PAIN/UTI/URETERAL OBSTRUCTION**
   Evaluation of flank pain and UTI's
   a. Case 21–47 year old female with flank pain
   b. Final diagnosis–Acute pyelonephritis
   c. Discussion (Patrick Pettengill)–Evaluation of flank pain, diagnosis and management of ureterolithiasis

K. **TOXICOLOGY**
   Diagnosis and management of common overdoses (main discussion of toxicology)
   a. Case 17–82 year old female with generalized weakness
   b. Final diagnosis–Delerium secondary to chronic salicylate toxicity
   c. Discussion (Ryan Longstreth)–Evaluation of the poisoned patient, management of acetaminophen and salicylate toxicities

During the last 10 years, I have changed my approach to emergency medicine from a textbook oriented new grad, to a "wizened" physician trying to practice of art of medicine. Lectures from the "greats" in emergency medicine have inspired me to not only practice state of the art medicine, but to make sure the patients and their families *know* that I am practicing good medicine. Sometimes this job really is, as Greg Henry has said many times; "Show business for ugly people!"

Several years ago I had the "pleasure" of being the subject of a deposition; a sobering experience. I was the physician on the second visit of Case 24—the 48 year old man with back pain and fevers that turned out to have endocarditis. Fortunately, the physician assistant who dictated the chart did an excellent job, and the case was eventually dropped, but during the two years when it was pending, I had plenty of time to think about the evaluation and documentation of that patient's visit. Since then, I have moved endocarditis higher in my differential diagnosis for prolonged fevers. I have also become more cognizant of how a chart looks, as any of our patients could "bounce back."

This point rang out loud and clear in the discussion sections in this book; emergency medicine is more about proving what a patient *doesn't* have, than it is about proving what a patient does have! When that cannot be accomplished in the ED, the thought process needs to be put down in a progress note, and a plan made for follow up. Patients with possible appendicitis should not be asked to follow up in 1–2 days, a time frame when rupture is likely to occur. This was the situation in Case 27, a 30 year old pregnant woman with RLQ pain, and Case 2, a 33 year old man with abdominal pain. Patients with abdominal pain should be re-examined before leaving the ED and seen again in 8–12 hours if their pain persists.

If the diagnosis is not consistent with the history and physical, as in Case 3, a 71 year old man with back pain who turned out to have a ruptured AAA, this discrepancy needs to be explained, addressing why the physician *doesn't* think the more serious diagnosis is occurring. When a test is ordered and comes back positive, as in Case 21, the 47 year old diabetic woman with flank pain who was diagnosed with an infected ureteral stone, the result needs to be acted upon. These tenets are basic principles that everyone would normally follow, but in a busy ED with patients who stand up, shake your hand, look great, and ask to leave, abnormalities can be overlooked.

Infants with bruising, as in Case 30, should be evaluated for possible child abuse, and elderly patients with a laceration secondary to a syncopal episode, as in Case 20, the 76 year old woman with syncope, should have the laceration, as well as the syncope, adequately evaluated. I have listened for more bruits on patients with headache and neck pain, inspired by the 37 year old woman in Case 4, but have not yet diagnosed a carotid artery dissection. I have also been more acutely aware of the accuracy as well as timeliness of management, a technique which will hopefully avoid the disastrous consequences which could have occurred in Case 8, the 38 year old woman with abdominal pain who turned out to have a ruptured tubal pregnancy, (despite the WBC count that was "too high," quant. HCG "too low," and Hb "not low enough")— I swear this is a true case—the OB/GYN's didn't just say that to make this a better chapter!

How did we pick the cases for this book? We tried to create a comprehensive arrangement of cases. Symptoms with potential for bad outcomes, such as chest pain and abdominal pain, are repeated several times. We have not concentrated on the "zebras," but on common presentations and diagnoses— judging from the discussions, there is plenty of thought and controversy surrounding these!

For those who would like to participate in future versions of this book, either with true "bounce back" cases, or by writing a discussion of a case, I would love to hear from you at: mweinstock@ihainc.org.

I would first like to thank Ryan—level-headed, enthusiastic, supportive, and knowledgeable—I have enjoyed working on this project with you almost as much as I have enjoyed drinking a cold one after a long shift. I would like to thank Greg Henry, whose words echo every time I see a patient with a knuckle laceration or a patient with "heart fluttering" that seems to be due to anxiety. May his colorful comments and wisdom enter your brain, as it has mine, and refuse to leave like a bad song which keeps going round and round, and round and round…. Thank you to our panel of experts—they have brought a collective wisdom and contemporary thought on management, as if one were still in training and precepted on each patient by a renowned expert in each field. I hope this collection has exceeded your expectations, making you proud to have participated. To the physicians, physician assistants, and staff at Mt. Carmel St. Ann's Emergency Department—it has been a pleasure working together for the last 10 years—many more to come! And to my brother Jeffrey Weinstock, Thomas Himmelspach, and Richard Milligan—thanks for rounding things out so beautifully (and humorously) from a legal perspective!

I'm not sure how Hudson (Margaret B Meredith), was able to so successfully capture the essence of each case with her brilliant illustrations, without giving away the final diagnosis. Her work has enlightened the book, making the reading easier and more memorable!

Special and heartfelt thanks to my wife, Beth Weinstock, a family physician who somehow always knows the diagnosis when I tell her about my "interesting" ED cases. She went through a whole package of pens (*after* I had presented her with my final, edited version of the chapters) correcting grammar and improving clarity, while still working and taking care of three young kids. She was just the right amount removed from these experts to comfortably change their words while focusing their message. The book is so much better for your wisdom. My children Olivia (7), Eli (5), and Theo (1), have kept me focused on the important things; playing, reading, scavenger hunts, and lots of hugs….

My great grandfather was a barber-surgeon in Russia (he may have had a few cases for this book) and both of my grandfathers were general surgeons. How I would have loved for them to be able to read this book… I'm sure some cases would have sounded familiar. My father is an ophthalmologist, husband, grandfather, passionate exerciser, traveler, and prolific writer—I was proud to have been able to co-author with him on Case 23, the 53 year old woman with headache. May we have many more years of collaborating on projects!

Thanks to Anadem Publishing, Will, Mike, Helen, Kate and Tony, and for all of your help and support. Your professionalism, attention to detail, and enthusiasm seem unmatched in the publishing industry. It's been pure pleasure to work with you. Thanks for the reviews of select chapters by Brad McGwire, MD (ID), Rajiv Hede, MD (cardiology), and Johnny Joon Huh, MD (ID); your expertise has rounded out these chapters beautifully. And thanks to my great friend Rob Crane, MD, for the title "Bouncebacks!"

Finally, thanks to the patients who place their trust in us. Hopefully, we treat you with respect, good clinical acumen, and compassion. And when we fail, as is occasionally bound to happen, may appropriate follow up been arranged in a timely fashion!

Thanks again to the contributors to this book… because of you, I am a better physician.

Michael Weinstock
June 17, 2006

I can't imagine doing anything else. Emergency medicine has been the most rewarding career choice I could have made and I feel fortunate that I enjoy my job as much as I do. I hope those of you reading this feel as fulfilled by your careers as I.

None of this would mean anything without Amy, my wife. You have been so flexible. You have put your career on hold numerous times as I moved around the Midwest in pursuit of my dream. You have also brought two wonderful children into our lives. If I were $\frac{1}{10}$ as selfless as you, I would be a much better person. For all of this, I thank you and I love you.

To Max and Drew, my two young children, you have given me so much joy in the short time you have been here. I know you wish I weren't stuck at work all hours of the day. I truly enjoy my career, but it doesn't compare with being a father!

To my parents and the rest of my family and friends who have given me lots of support and encouragement along the way—I wouldn't be in a position to write this book without you.

To those educators who helped me become the physician I am today (there are too many to name), I must also say thank you. Keith Wilkinson—you are truly a great role model in the field of medicine and I feel privileged to have learned from you. Ray Jackson—thanks for everything and good luck with your golf game!

Greg—thank you for lending your insight on each of these cases. You have a unique perspective and have added so much to the book.

And of course, thank you Mike for having included me in this one-of-a-kind project. This was so much fun to work on. It has been truly satisfying to see this come together. We can still share a cold one after this is done!

I hope you find this book fun and educational, and I think your patients will be glad you read this.

Happy reading!

Ryan Longstreth

Index

Ventricular fibrillation 145–146
Ventricular tachycardia 145–146
  vs. SVT with aberrancy 146
Visual fields 387
Volvulus 372
VZV 160

W

Waddell's signs 342
WBC
  pregnancy 401
West nile virus 415

X

Xanthochromia 57

Z

Zanamivir 417, 418
Zoster ophthalmicus 389–390

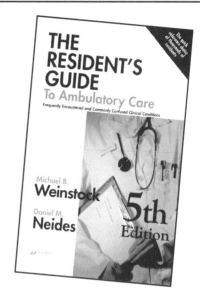

"A helpful review of common problems and errors in emergency medicine. Use this book ... you will see most of these troublesome cases during your career and you want to do them right the first time!"

Stephen V. Cantrill, MD/FACEP
Associate Director, Emergency Medicine
Assistant Professor, University of Colorado Health Sciences Center
Department of Surgery, Division of Emergency Medicine

REVIEWS FROM SPECIALISTS IN FAMILY MEDICINE:

"This book is fascinating reading for the reflective physician. It has a compelling message about listening carefully and acting deliberately. Exposing the evolution of cases allows everyone the opportunity to find quality improvement targets. Students will benefit by realizing that healthcare is a continuum that doesn't end after each visit or hospitalization."

Edward T. Bope, MD , FAAFP
Director of the Family Practice Residency Program, Riverside Methodist Hospitals
Clinical Professor of Family Medicine, The Ohio State University, Columbus, Ohio
Editor, *Conn's Current Therapy, 2006*, *Saunder's Review of Family Practice*, and *Family Practice Desk Reference*
Past president, American Board of Family Practice

"This book is a good review of difficult cases that are seen by emergency medicine physicians. It helps to remind us that we must know our differential diagnosis in order to focus our history, our physical exam, our diagnostic studies and our treatment plan appropriately for the undifferentiated patient."

Mary Jo Welker, MD
Chair and Professor of Clinical Family Medicine
Associate Dean for Primary Care, The Ohio State University College of Medicine
Board of Directors of the American Academy of Family Physicians (AAFP), 2002–2005

REVIEWS FROM MEMBERS OF THE BOARD OF THE SOCIETY OF EMERGENCY MEDICINE PHYSICIAN ASSISTANTS (SEMPA):

"The first of its kind EM project, which highlights those cases that cause EM providers the most angst. The case review format was easy to interpret, and will help guide my EM practice for years to come. Your expert panel discusses the realm of issues surrounding each case, from the medical to the legal. Looking forward to future editions."

Brian McCambley, MS, PA-C
Board of directors, Society of Emergency Medicine Physician Assistants (SEMPA)

"*Bouncebacks* is an excellent book for reviewing cases. The format keeps it interesting. Dr. Henry's comments as always are insightful and candid. The discussion is a complete review of each issue. The legal chapter is a great review for general risk management. An excellent resource for Emergency Physicians and PA's. Also great review for discussions with students and residents."

Jeff Callard, PA-C
Vice president and member Executive Board of directors, Society of Emergency Medicine Physician Assistants (SEMPA)

Advance Praise for Bouncebacks!
(More comments in front)

"The unique format and real-life presentations in Bouncebacks! Emergency Department Cases: ED Returns make it a pleasure to read, and outstandingly educational. Readers learn best when they can identify with a specific case or set of facts, and picture themselves 'on the line.' The format of including discussion along the way, and after the fact keeps your interest, and the more academic discussion that follows has the perfect setting- the actual case at hand. The academic discussions are concise and up to date. A great read for all Emergency and primary care physicians!"

Neal Little, MD, FACEP
Clinical instructor, University of Michigan Medical School
Co-author, *Neurologic Emergencies: A Symptom-Oriented Approach, 2nd ed.*
Co-presentor, Medical practice risk assessment: Continuing medical education for Emergency Physicians

"The format of exploring all the management options including diagnostic studies and therapies is educational, current and comprehensive. Dr. Henry's comments provide expert insight, valuable lessons and a bit of humor.

Weinstock and Longstreth have covered all of the diagnostics pitfalls and risks associated with Emergency Medicine. This is a valuable read for both the resident and the seasoned attending."

Michael Cetta, MD FACEP
Chief of Emergency Medicine, St. Mary's Hospital, Leonardtown MD
Member, ACEP Task Force on Health Care and the Uninsured

"While an edited Dr. Henry is not quite so mind jarring and entertaining as Dr. Henry live and on stage, his erudition and immense closed case experience make this book a must read for every emergency and primary care physician. Drs. Weinstock and Longstreth and their co-authors have done a superb job of presenting the spectrum of all those "obvious" diagnoses that can sometimes lead us astray.

An emergency physician can practice a lifetime and still be drawing stick figures when it comes to the art of medicine. Two of the skills of a master are an ever present sense of what can go wrong and a high index of suspicion for things being not as they first appear. Reading Drs. Weinstock, Longstreth and Henry's *Bouncebacks* and incorporating its lessons into your practice should take you a long way toward one day making your masterpiece diagnosis.

One of the problems with the lifetime practice of EM and primary care is that so much of what's wrong coming through the door is obvious. The trouble with the narcotizing effect of obvious is that it is only accurate 99% of the time. Drs. Weinstock, Longstreth and Henry's *Bouncebacks* provides the two things we need to outwit 'obvious' - an ever present sense of what can go wrong and a high index of suspicion for things being not as they first appear. This book is a must read for every emergency and primary care physician."

Ronald A. Hellstern, M.D.
Board Examiner for the American Board of Emergency Medicine
ACEP James D. Mills Award for Outstanding Contribution to the Field of Emergency Medicine, 1992
Member, ACEP Emergency Medicine Practice Committee
Past president, Texas ACEP

NOTES

NOTES